CW01676780

NATN Standards and Recommendations

for Safe Perioperative Practice

Chairman's Foreword

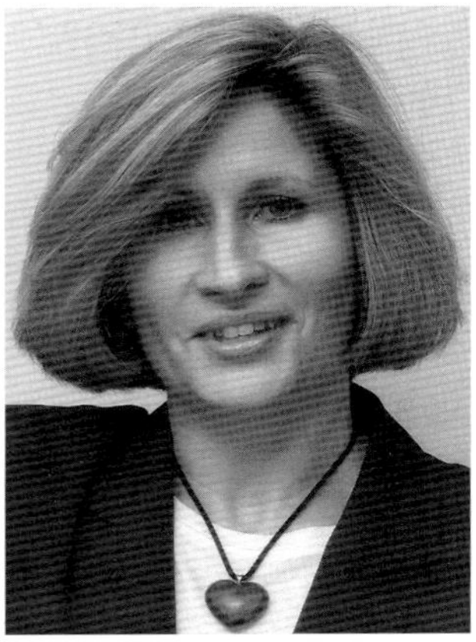

This publication introduces the National Association of Theatre Nurses' (NATN) standards and recommendations for perioperative patient care. It replaces the NATN publication *Principles of Safe Practice in the Perioperative Environment* (1998). These generic standards were developed by the Professional Officers in conjunction with the NATN Education Committee, Practitioners Panel and Anaesthetic and Recovery Forum. The standards and recommendations were developed in consultation with other professional associations and external agencies relevant to perioperative practice.

Standards are a key component of the quality assurance process and are integral to clinical governance within any hospital organisation. NATN standards and recommendations are often cited as the benchmark for the standard of care expected in the perioperative setting by the legal profession, risk agencies and other organisations investigating adverse incidents.

This publication will enable perioperative managers and practitioners to ensure that the care administered to their patients is up to date and meets national recommendations and standards. The referencing of the publication is comprehensive, and practitioners and managers are recommended to use the references and further reading to broaden their understanding of risk management and clinical effectiveness in the perioperative setting.

Evidence-based practice occurs through the integration of clinical expertise with the best available evidence from systematic research. This publication should ensure that perioperative practitioners are confident that their clinical and managerial interventions are informed by a current knowledge base. Practices, policies and guidelines can then be audited against agreed national standards at a local level and can be updated to comply with these recommendations where applicable. It is recommended that this publication is used in conjunction with the NATN publication *Risk and Quality Management System* (2002).

These guidelines promote the delivery of safe and effective patient care within the perioperative setting. I highly recommended this document to you.

Melanie van Limborgh

Melanie van Limborgh
NATN Chairman

Acknowledgements

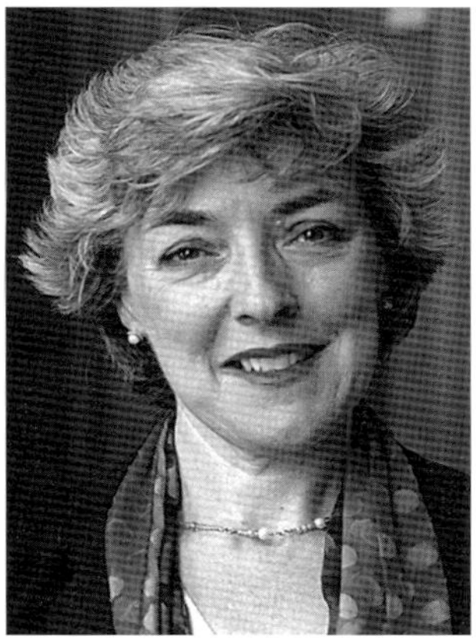

Safe perioperative practice is what every patient expects and deserves. The tremendous team effort that has been put into developing these standards and recommendations for perioperative care will help to ensure that not only patients but also staff will benefit. I would like to thank all the individuals and organisations that have contributed to this edition which should be widely used wherever perioperative patient care occurs.

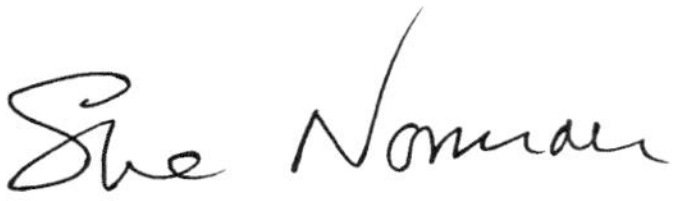

Sue Norman
NATN President (2002–2004)

NATN gratefully acknowledges the participation and contributions of the following people in the revision of the 1998 *Principles of Safe Practice in the Perioperative Environment*. Their involvement in this project supported the achievement of this 2004 edition of *NATN Standards and Recommendations for Safe Perioperative Practice*.

Christine Allan
Wendy Christie
Cynthia Clark
Tracy Coates
Joanna Connor
Sally Couzens
Felicia Cox
Chris Earl
Jill Ferbrache
Caroline Figueiredo
Helen Ford
Eleanor Freeman
Diane Gilmour
Tuija Hirva
Kathryn Kitson
Sue Lord
Mary McGeough
Amanda Parker
Anton Philpott
Rosanne Robinson
Grace Rogers
Fiona Wakely
Sarah Wilde
Edwina Williams

The Editors are grateful to the following people for their involvement and consultation on this publication:

Angela Haken Marketing Co-ordinator, Central Medical Supplies

Sue Shelley Professional Officer in Radiology, The College of Radiographers

Elizabeth Qua Principal Nurse, Department of Health and Social Services Public Health and Safety

Beverly McNeil Theatre Sister, East Kent Hospitals NHS Trust

Carole Coombs Theatre Skills Training, Golden Jubilee National Hospital, Clydebank

Diane Irvine Theatre Skills Training, Golden Jubilee National Hospital, Clydebank

Jean White Theatre Manager, Golden Jubilee National Hospital, Clydebank

Alan Nixon Head of Medical Physics, Golden Jubilee National Hospital, Clydebank

Jane Curle Business Development Manager, Health Edge Solutions

Lynn Graham Professional Advisor, Health Professions Wales

Jean White Professional Advisor, Health Professions Wales

Kate Woodhead Independent Nurse Consultant, President of the International Federation of Perioperative Nurses

Gill Hawkins Clinical Product Specialist, Kimberley-Clark

Jonathan Plumb Nursing Advisor, Medicines Healthcare products Regulatory Agency

Val O'Brien Project Co-ordinator (Decontamination), NHS Estates

Ron Eunson Authorised Person (Sterilizers), NHS Scotland

Peter Furness Clinical Speciality Advisor for Pathology, National Patient Safety Agency

Maggie O'Donovan Assistant Director, National Patient Safety Agency

Clive Tomsett Assistant Director, National Patient Safety Agency

Christine Morrow Infection Control Nurse, North Staffordshire NHS Trust

Linda Coultrop Training Co-ordinator, Peterborough DGH

Christine Elding Donor Liaison Sister, Royal Sussex County Hospital

Hazel Parkinson Lecturer Practitioner, St James University Hospital, Leeds

Fiona Morrison UK Marketing Manager, Tyco Healthcare

Pat Hutchinson Infection Control Nurse, Walsall DGH

Contents

3 MANAGEMENT/HUMAN RESOURCES

4 INFECTION CONTROL

5 DECONTAMINATION

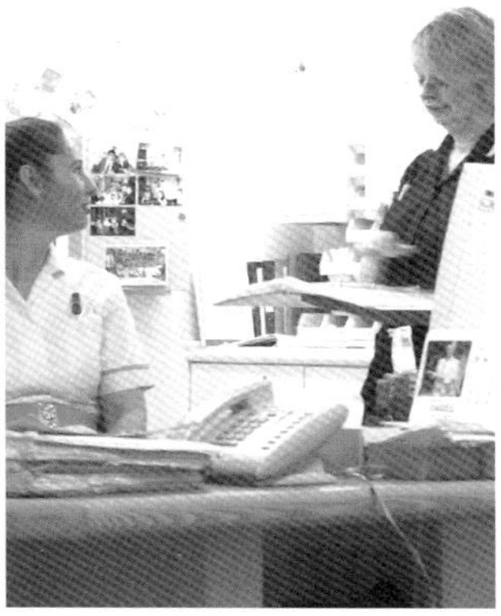

LEGAL AND ETHICAL ISSUES

1.1 MEDICAL LAW

STANDARD Personnel working in the perioperative setting understand their personal professional accountability and the standard of care expected of them.

Legal issues are fast becoming one of the main areas of concern to all health professionals. The NHS *Complaints Procedure* and *The Patients' Charter* have helped to raise the expectations of patients and their relatives and made them more aware of their civil legal rights. The NHS faces an annual legal bill of around £200 million in the area of clinical negligence alone. The current estimate for ongoing total healthcare litigation is nearly £5.6 billion. Bearing in mind this enormous financial pressure, all health professionals should become more aware of their personal responsibilities and accountability, especially with regard to areas in which problems can arise which can lead to legal actions and subsequent payment of damages.

There is always a risk in the day-to-day work carried out by any healthcare professional. Critical care has specific concerns which involve both ethical and moral dilemmas and also legal problems. This is further compounded by constraints of financial resources and manpower availability.

As medicine advances, the role of staff working within the perioperative setting continues to develop, and with this comes the inevitable increase of workload and responsibility. Working within theatres is a highly specialised and technical role and the boundaries between the medical and nursing professions are becoming less clear. Issues of law which impact professional accountability and personal responsibility therefore remain high on the agenda.

Reduction in junior doctors' hours and the expansion of the role of the nurse has generated the need for an increased understanding of the accountability and legal implications of day-to-day practice in all areas of healthcare.

Every day moral and ethical dilemmas are an important part of every healthcare professional's agenda. However, the law often remains 'two steps behind' current medical thinking. This does not give the health professional the excuse of pleading ignorance of the law, and it is not a defence in court.

Law as it exists today is based on a set of rules which are derived from common law and statutes. 'Common law' is the term used for the laws and customs which were applied by the Royal Courts following the Norman Conquest. As decisions of these courts were recorded and published, a practice developed by which past decisions would be cited as argument before the court and these were regarded as being 'persuasive' or 'binding authority'. Common law is 'judge-made' law and is a benchmark which is applied in all courts. Common law is changed frequently and can be modified by senior courts depending upon current social and judicial attitudes.

'Statutory law' is law which is set by Parliament. Governments are elected every four to five years and they are given a mandate to enact on our behalf and to introduce any laws which they think appropriate. Parliament can overrule common law and can abolish previous statutes in order to bring in fresh legislation if it is necessary.

Common law decisions are referred to as 'case law', for example 'The Bolam Test', Bolam v Friern Hospital Management Committee (1957). Statutory law is referred to as an 'Act', for example The Data Protection Act (HMSO 1998a) and The Mental Health Act (HMSO 1983).

Law has many functions: it seeks to encourage good conduct and to reduce or prevent bad conduct. It is used as a method of settling disputes and as an 'avenue' to pursue legal redress and claims for compensation. Law is used to punish those who are found guilty of criminal charges.

'Medical law' is seen as being a 'duty' based law. Healthcare professionals are part of a 'public authority' and are empowered with the duty of providing healthcare. The effect of failing to meet the terms of this duty (whether deliberate or accidental) can result in either civil or criminal liability.

Civil liability has the following characteristics:

- The wrong is between individuals.
- One individual takes action against another (A v B).
- The action is taken to remedy the wrong, often with compensation.
- Judgement is taken in the civil courts.
- The standard of proof is the 'balance of probabilities'.
- The person is sued and is found 'liable' or 'not liable'.

Criminal liability has the following characteristics:

- The wrong is regarded as being against society.
- The action is taken in the name of the ruling monarch (R v XYZ).
- The aim is to punish the offender.
- The standard of proof is 'beyond all reasonable doubt'.
- The person is prosecuted and found 'guilty' or 'not guilty'.

'Civil law' is the area which should mostly concern health professionals. When patients or their relatives sue hospitals, GP practices, NHS trusts, health authorities and private practices, it is through the process of civil law. However, criminal law and civil law can overlap – the most recent case being that of Harold Shipman, where claims were lodged both in the criminal and civil courts against his actions with patients.

1.2 TYPES OF COURT (ENGLAND AND WALES)*

MAGISTRATES' COURT

These are the inferior criminal courts. They also hear some family law, administrative law and minor civil disputes. They are involved in some way in nearly all criminal prosecutions and refer cases to the Crown Court.

The court is normally comprised of three Justices of the Peace (JPs) or 'lay' magistrates. Stipendiary magistrates, who are generally barristers, normally sit on their own. In cases where a juvenile court needs to be set up it must comprise no more than three justices and must normally include a man and a woman. Since the Children Act (HMSO 1989a) most care proceedings are transferred from juvenile court to the family proceedings courts.

NB Criminal proceedings cannot be instituted against children under the age of ten. Where children aged 10–14 are prosecuted it must be proved that they were children of a 'mischievous discretion' and that they knew that they were committing a legal or moral wrong. Those over 14 years are regarded as being fully responsible for their actions.

COUNTY COURT

Established by the County Courts Act of 1846, the County Courts deal with almost the whole range of civil proceedings. They are presided over by a circuit judge who must be a barrister of at least seven years standing. An action of clinical negligence would commence in the County Court as a summons up to the value of £50,000.

CROWN COURT

The Crown Courts are used for both criminal and civil cases and are visited by High Court judges, circuit judges and recorders. They deal with criminal cases, which have been referred by the Magistrates' Court, as well as those cases which may be tried by a jury. Crown Courts also deal with appeals against conviction from the Magistrates' Court.

HIGH COURT

This court has jurisdiction over criminal and civil matters and is presided over by a High Court judge. The High Court deals with child and civil matters relating to clinical negligence over £50,000. Actions are commenced as a writ.

* NATN acknowledges that the legal system and court structure are different in Scotland and Northern Ireland. This will be addressed in the next edition of this publication.

COURT OF APPEAL

This court hears appeals against decisions made in the County Court, Crown Court, and the High Court. The Court of Appeal can be presided over by High Court judges, Law Lords, Lord Justices and the Master of the Rolls (currently Lord Woolf).

HOUSE OF LORDS

The House of Lords hears appeals from the High Court and the Court of Appeal on issues such as points of law which are of importance to the general public. An appeal cannot be heard unless at least three of the following are present:

- The Lord Chancellor
- The Lords of Appeal in the Ordinary
- Any peer who has held one of the high judicial offices of Lord Chancellor:
  - Judicial Committee of the Privy Council
  - Lord of Appeal in the Ordinary
  - Judge of the Supreme Court
  - Judge of the Court of Session.

EUROPEAN COURT OF JUSTICE

Created by the treaties which established the European Communities, the European Court of Justice consists of 15 judges assisted by nine advocates general, chosen by agreement of the 15 member states. They are appointed for a term of six years. Only one judgement is delivered and it is not revealed whether it was unanimous or reached by a majority. All judgements are binding to all member states.

1.3 THE LAW OF TORT

The term 'tort' comes from the Latin 'tortus' which means 'twisted'. The word has developed over the years to mean 'wrong'. In law, a civil 'wrong' is known as a 'tort'. The law of tort is concerned with the allocation or prevention of losses to one person by another. This is known as 'tortuous liability'. There have been numerous attempts to define tort, the most widely accepted being that of Winfield and Jolowicz: *'Tortuous liability arises from the breach of duty primarily fixed by law; this duty is towards persons generally and its breach is redressible by an action for unliquidated damages'* (Rogers 1998).

Therefore in law there is an imposition of duty on persons to respect the legal rights of others. If this duty is breached it allows the injured party to sue in common law for damages. This is the prime existence of the law of tort. It is developed by judges, usually in reaction to the social circumstances and economic conditions in force at the time of judgement. Hence many decisions appear to be in conflict and often there appears to be no logical reasoning for some decisions.

Crimes are deemed as being against the state and prosecution will be dealt with by the criminal courts. If found guilty the 'accused' will be punished by a prison sentence, community service, fine etc. A tort is against the person and is not therefore punitive (punishable). The injured party sues for negligence and, if successful, damages in the form of money are awarded. In most cases there is no jury involvement.

Crimes and torts can however overlap, that is there may be dual liability. For example a person may be convicted of a crime against a patient (a criminal offence) and they may also be sued in the civil courts for damages.

In the realm of healthcare, the law of tort is the most likely basis of a claim for compensation for the following:

- **Negligence** Injuries sustained as a result of a medical error during the course of an operation
- **Assault and/or battery** Treating a competent person without their consent
- **False imprisonment** Deprivation of a person's freedom of movement by locking room and ward doors
- **Defamation** Loss sustained to a person's reputation through unthinking spoken word (slander) or through written comments (libel) such as patient records.

As with all law there are rules which govern the bringing of an action in tort. Anyone of full age can sue or be sued and the law divides the parties as follows:

- **The claimant** – generally the person who suffers loss or injury or damage to their person or property as a result of a negligent act or omission by another
- **The defendant** – generally the person who causes the loss or injury or damage to another or their property as a result of their negligent act or omission
- **The next friend (or litigation friend)** – usually someone who acts as a support and help for certain groups, for example minors or patients with a mental health disability.

The Limitations Act (HMSO 1980) sets out the limitation period in which claims can be brought. As a general rule a claim in tort cannot be brought more than six years from the date on which the claimant's cause of action began. The date from which the time begins will either be when it happened, or in tort (where damage is caused) it will be the date of the damage. However there are exceptions to this general rule and these are of particular importance to clinical negligence claims:

- **Personal injury claims** There is a limitation period of three years from the date on which the cause of action occurred. Or alternatively, this time begins from the date when the claimant had knowledge of the damage. Children can commence an action when they become of full age. For example, if the injury occurred at birth, applying the three-year rule, an action could begin 21 years after the child was born.
- **Death occurring as a result of the defendant's action** In these cases where the death occurs within the three years of the cause of the action, a fresh three-year period commences in the favour of the dependants or personal representative. This period runs from the date of death or the date of knowledge of death.

It is widely accepted that the law of tort is not concerned with motives. It is not normally necessary to prove that the defendant intended the consequences of their act or omission. In general they are liable only for failing to act where there was a positive duty of care.

1.4 NEGLIGENCE

The majority of law on negligence is based on common law decisions. Negligence establishes that in certain circumstances everyone will have a duty of care to others and, if someone breaches that duty of care and causes damage, they must compensate the injured party. To prove liability in negligence, the claimant must establish three essential elements:

- The existence of a duty to care which is owed by the defendant to the claimant
- The failure to attain the standard of care thereby committing a breach of such duty
- That the resultant damage or harm was caused by the defendant's breach of duty.

All three elements must be present to establish the tort of negligence.

A duty of care is not difficult to establish. Once a GP or consultant has accepted a patient for treatment, a duty of care is automatically acknowledged. The law does not require 'Good Samaritans', therefore there is no duty of care when the individual is not at work. However, professional codes of conduct often advocate the opposite principle.

Breach of duty is harder to establish simply because many professionals have different types of practice concerning the same type of patient. One of the best examples is a patient with breast cancer: she may be offered a lumpectomy, a mastectomy – partial or full, and either of these treatments with a combination of chemotherapy and/or radiotherapy. A surgeon would not be in breach for offering one therapy over any of the others, because there is still no conclusive evidence that one is better than the others. It is simply a matter of choice – both for the woman and the surgeon.

Breach of duty is easier to establish when it is likely that there has been an error, for example, a patient receiving a burn from electrosurgery. If used correctly electrosurgery devices should not cause skin burns, so the resultant burn would suggest that a breach has occurred.

'Res ipsa loquiter' cases

There are other cases that are so obvious that a defence seems unlikely: for example, surgical instruments and swabs left in body cavities. In cases of this nature the term 'Res ipsa loquiter' is used – 'the facts speak for themselves'. In cases of this nature the claimant does not have to know the facts, or to prove causation. The fact that the object has been left inside the claimant advertises the fact that a mistake has been made. Should a defence be made it would be up to the defendant to show how these objects were left inside without there being negligence. In reality, these cases are very embarrassing and the majority are settled out of court, thus avoiding any damage to public confidence.

To prove causation, the claimant has to be able to show that the defendant's action actually caused the resulting damage. This can be difficult when an injury has occurred in a medical/surgical circumstance. Mistakes can be one explanation for the patient's injury, but there is also the progression of natural disease.

In order for a successful claim in negligence to be brought, the judge has to satisfy himself that no reasonable doctor or nurse would have behaved in that manner. The test used is the one established in the case of Bolam v Frien HMC (1957). Mr Bolam had agreed to electro-convulsive therapy (ECT) in order to help relieve his depression. He suffered fractures as a result of the treatment and sued for negligence – citing that the doctor was aware of the risks but had failed to inform him, and that no restraints or muscle relaxants had been used. The case was lost because the judge was satisfied that any ordinary reasonable doctor would not inform the patient of these risks, and that restraints, whether chemical or mechanical, were by no means uniform practice.

There is no allowance in negligence for inexperience. Juniors must be competent to practice, or they should refuse to do so. This also applies to nurses and operating department practitioners (ODPs) who extend their roles. From the moment they practise their new role, they are expected to do so at the level of the person who normally does the role. This has implications for perioperative practitioners working in the advanced scrub practitioner and surgical care practitioner role. A good example of this is someone trained to take the leg vein of a patient undergoing bypass surgery. Before undergoing such work, they need to be absolutely certain that their practice is as good and safe as a surgical registrar and that the hospital indemnity insurance has been altered to cover their practice.

It can be said that the law is seeking to protect the patient from the defence of staff learning curves.

Bolitho v City and Hackney HA (1997) challenged the Bolam standard. Before the ruling, if the doctor could show that he/she had acted in accordance with a body of medical opinion, this was admitted in defence of an action. The ruling in Bolitho stated that showing a doctor had acted according to medical opinion was not enough, medical opinion also had to be found by the court to be reasonable.

It must be said that if negligence were always automatically proven by any difference between one professional and the rest of their colleagues, then the art of medicine would never progress. There is always someone willing to take risks when performing new surgical techniques. However, two things are required before undertaking such risks. Firstly, it is good practice to inform the patient that they are being used as a guinea pig. This affords them the chance to refuse the treatment and may prevent a case being brought at a later date. Secondly, if a case is brought, the defendant must prove that they were not negligent in departing from the accepted practice. In other words – there must be a good reason for doing things differently.

A good example of this is the case of Clarke v MacLennan (1983) where the claimant suffered stress incontinence following the birth of her baby. After 1 month and 11 days of conservative treatment, Mr MacLennan operated to repair the weakness in her bladder and muscles. The claimant haemorrhaged and the repair broke down. Following two further unsuccessful operations to repair the surgical damage, she was left with permanent stress incontinence. A case of negligence was brought on the grounds that the surgeon had departed from the conventional practice of waiting three months post delivery to repair, which is established practice because of the known risks of haemorrhage and breakdown. The case was successful.

Any harm has to be reasonably foreseeable. Once again the Bolam standard is used. Would the ordinary reasonable practitioner foresee the harm and act to avoid it? For example, if during the course of an operation the patient has spillage of their bowel contents into the peritoneal cavity, it is reasonably foreseeable that the patient will develop peritonitis. Antibiotics should therefore be prescribed immediately. If this is not done, the patient can sue and may indeed succeed in a negligence case. However, if the patient develops peritonitis one year after an appendectomy, the defence of remoteness would apply. That is assuming that no surgical instruments or swabs were the cause!

1.5 RESPONSIBILITY AND ACCOUNTABILITY

A patient claiming against a doctor or a hospital usually has little difficulty in establishing that the defendant owes them a duty of care.

The duty of care that health professionals owe to patients can be found as a deep-seated core within their professional codes of conduct. The Nursing and Midwifery Council *Code of Professional Conduct* (NMC 2002a) Section 6.2 states: *'To practice competently, you must possess the knowledge, skills and abilities required for lawful, safe and effective practice without direct supervision, you must acknowledge the limits of your professional competence and only undertake practice and accept responsibilities for those activities in which you are competent.'*

We can assess whether liability would be found by the courts by taking a look at a situation in hand (eg: poor equipment, low staffing levels, lack of qualified staff) and then assess what would be 'reasonably foreseeable' and what would be the 'logical and natural outcome'. For example, a sharps bin left on the floor of an unlocked room – what would be a reasonable foreseeable consequence of an unsupervised child entering that room?

When care is given privately (ie: outside the NHS), the doctor-patient relationship is governed by a contract for services. One result of this is that in addition to the duty of care, the doctor also owes a contemporaneous contractual duty. This is almost identical in terms of care – the doctor is obliged to exercise reasonable care and skill while discharging his contractual obligations (the Supply of Goods and Services Act 1982, Section 13).

1.6 VICARIOUS LIABILITY

In employment terms vicarious liability signifies the liability which the employer may incur for the damage caused to the patient by the negligence of one of its employees. Patients in hospital are treated by the employees of the hospital or trust. The patient has no choice in the selection of the doctor, nurse or health professional. The employer is liable because they select the employees and allocate their duties and responsibilities.

In the case of a negligent drug administration it is clear that the giving of drugs would be in the continuance of the interests of the 'master' (employer) while caring for the patient. However, giving the wrong drug because of carelessness would be negligent as it would constitute a breach of duty of care. It is possible that as well as suing the 'master', the patient could sue the health professional directly. This is unlikely because of the probable inability of the health professional to pay any damages awarded.

PROTECTION FROM LIABILITY

What can be done to protect nurses and doctors and other healthcare professionals from negligent liability? Healthcare professionals can:

- be sure of their personal competence and limitations
- document all patient care clearly and carefully
- take immediate action following patient disputes or allegations
- take all complaints seriously and follow hospital policies/procedures
- check that professional indemnity insurance is adequate and suitable for work undertaken
- check contract of employment and terms and conditions
- know and follow all hospital policies and guidelines
- ensure that their employer knows about and authorises all healthcare activities that are undertaken
- check that the job description is robust
- document with the manager and employer any additional responsibilities which become part of the workload
- if working for agencies or a 'bank', ensure that they have adequate professional indemnity insurance.

1.7 CLINICAL RESPONSIBILITIES

All doctors, nurses and health professionals have a duty of professional accountability, which makes them responsible for the outcome of their professional actions. Health professionals are not only accountable through general law but also through their contract of employment. They are also subject to regulation through the governing body of their profession. Health professionals are required to be placed upon a regulatory register and are bound by professional codes of conduct and practice. In the case of nurses it is the Nursing and Midwifery Council (NMC) and for operating department practitioners the Health Professions Council (HPC). Failure to comply with these could result in disciplinary action and/or removal from such registers and losing of the licence to practice.

It is important that all professions should be sufficiently competent and qualified to carry out a task. The case of Wilsher v Essex AHA (1988) clearly demonstrates this. In this example a three-month premature baby could not breathe properly and was fitted with an umbilical catheter to allow for administration of extra oxygen. A senior house officer (SHO) fitted the catheter to a vein instead of an artery resulting in false oxygen level readings. These readings were questioned and an x-ray was performed. This showed the catheter to be in the wrong place and was replaced by a registrar – who mistakenly replaced it into the vein. Despite further x-rays this mistake was not noticed. The baby received excessive levels of oxygen and contracted retrolental fibroplasias.

At trial and appeal there was no dispute of the negligence. The duty of care is related to the post that the healthcare professional holds – the registrar was negligent, but the SHO was not as he was entitled to rely on his work being checked by a more experienced doctor. This case has implications on the level of competence expected for particular tasks.

In theatre, the surgeon bears overall responsibility for the safety and efficacy of the operation. However, a scrub practitioner who fails to manage the count properly may cause real problems for the patient at a later stage of healing. This could result in a case of negligence which will nearly always be successful. The practitioner could avoid direct legal consequences but will almost certainly be dealt with by the trust and/or the regulatory body.

There will be many occasions when the nurse/ODP will be requested by the surgeon to act as advanced scrub practitioner, also known as first assistant, and thus take an active part in the operation. From a legal perspective this is potentially risky, as there is a clear demarcation between the role of the surgeon and any other professional. Often first assistants take very active and crucial roles in the operation – especially at night. An SHO will not have the degree of expertise of the consultant surgeon. This can lead to surgery becoming dangerous and, if placed in this situation, a practitioner has to consider at what point their legal duty of care should lead them to do something which is preventative. If the practitioner admits to having extra skills and practices, they will be judged as being the competent professional in that position. The Perioperative Care Collaborative (2003) published a position statement on this issue *'The Provision of the Non-medical Perioperative Practitioner Working as First Assistant to the Surgeon'*. The guidance recommends that the role of the advanced scrub practitioner must be undertaken by a competent practitioner who has received recognised training in this role.

ARE CODES OF PRACTICE LAW?

It is sometimes said that people will be breaking the law if they do or don't do certain procedures. There is some confusion regarding these issues: Parliament granted the power to professional bodies to draft detailed rules and regulations connected with healthcare that have already been considered in general terms within a statute. For example, the United Kingdom Central Council (UKCC – the predecessor to the NMC) *Code of Professional Conduct* (UKCC 1992) is seen as 'nursing law' or quasi law which is put together to allow nurses to meet certain professional standards. The same will apply for operating department practitioners and the Health Professions Council as their regulator.

If a clause of that code is breached it is likely that the person will be in breach of the common law, with the consequence that someone will be hurt and a claim for damages will follow. Although codes talk of personal responsibility, in 99% of cases it will be the trust that will be sued through the process of vicarious liability.

There are those who feel that hospital policies, although not law in themselves, should be written to reflect current law. It is not uncommon for hospital policies to be scrutinised in a court of law. Therefore it is essential that policies are regularly reviewed and are updated to promote the delivery of care which is based on current evidence, best practice and the recommendations of professional bodies such as NATN.

1.8 CONSCIENTIOUS OBJECTION

Conscientious objection is an ever-present ethical dilemma in the provision of perioperative care within the UK and is present when members of nursing staff refuse to be involved in some or all aspects of a patient's care. This objection may be based on personal, moral or religious beliefs, which can make participation in the patient's care difficult for the individual practitioner. However, it is pertinent to note that the right to conscientious objection does not exist if the practitioner is involved in an emergency situation where a life is at risk (Clarke & Jones 1998).

The NMC *Code of Professional Conduct* (2002a) states in Section 2.5 that *'you must report to a relevant person or authority, at the earliest possible time, any conscientious objection that may be relevant to your practice. You must continue to provide care to the best of your ability until alternative arrangements are implemented.'* However, in an emergency situation the nurse would be expected to provide care – they do not have the right to refuse in emergency treatment: *'In an emergency, in or outside the work setting, you have a professional duty to provide care. The care provided would be judged against what could reasonably be expected from someone with your knowledge, skills and abilities when placed in those particular circumstances.'*

At present, a perioperative practitioner has the right to conscientiously object to participate in patient care in two distinct areas. One of these is participation in abortion as detailed in the Abortion Act of 1967 (Scotland, England and Wales). The Human Fertilisation and Embryology Act of 1990 allows an individual the right to refuse to be involved in technological procedures to achieve conception and pregnancy.

However, it is important to be aware that conscientious objection does not just focus on abortion and assisted fertility procedures. There are many other procedures in which practitioners may not wish to participate. One such example would be patients undergoing gender reassignment surgery. The NMC *Code of Professional Conduct* (Section 2.2) states: *'You are personally accountable for ensuring that you promote and protect the interests and dignity of patients and clients, irrespective of gender, age, race, ability, sexuality, economic status, lifestyle, culture and religious or political beliefs.'*

Regardless of this requirement, many individuals are uncomfortable with issues surrounding this type of surgery, and as such, should be given the opportunity to discuss their concerns with their line manager.

Managing conscientious objection

Having established that conscientious objection exists, how can it be effectively managed in the workplace and in particular, in the perioperative setting? It is good practice to inform potential applicants for vacancies of the types of surgery that are carried out and for the applicant to be open and honest in response. It is clearly unacceptable to take a job in a department that regularly undertakes terminations of pregnancy if the individual has conscientious objections to the procedure. However, if as a result of service reorganisation, this type of surgery is introduced to a department, then it is necessary to be aware of, and to respect, any objections that staff may have to the procedure.

Confusion can occur about exactly where in the patient's journey that conscientious objection allows a practitioner to withdraw from participating in patient care. In the first instance, the individual has to be clear themselves on their interpretation of conscientious objection and where this fits in relation to the patient's journey. Some people feel so strongly that they do not wish to participate at all whereas others do not wish to be present or participate in the intraoperative phase. It is important that they have discussed and agreed with their manager exactly what aspects of care they are prepared to be involved in. It is also imperative that a manager is informed of these issues with sufficient time to manage them. In this way, the manager is able to allocate staff accordingly, and ensure that the patient still receives optimum care without prejudice. By achieving compromise in this way, the duty of care that is incumbent on all practitioners is fulfilled.

It is important that those who do exercise their legal right of non-participation are not discriminated against in any way as this in turn could be interpreted as a breach of the NMC *Code of Professional Conduct* Section 4.2 which states: *'You are expected to work co-operatively within teams and to respect the skills, expertise and contributions of your colleagues. You must treat them fairly and without discrimination.'*

If there is discord in the perioperative team that is not resolved quickly, then there is potential for another breach of the NMC *Code of Professional Conduct*. Section 8.1 states: *'You must work with other members of the team to promote healthcare environments that are conducive to safe, therapeutic and ethical practice.'*

RECOMMENDATIONS FOR LOCAL POLICY

RECOMMENDATION **1.8.1** Identify the operative procedures that have the potential for staff to action their right to conscientious objection.

RECOMMENDATION **1.8.2** Inform staff at interview that these procedures are undertaken in the operating department and indicate the frequency of these procedures.

RECOMMENDATION **1.8.3** In the event that these procedures are incorporated into an existing operating department as a result of service organisation, existing staff must be supported in the transitional stage if they have concerns relating to conscientious objection.

RECOMMENDATION **1.8.4** Identify, if appropriate, the stages at which a practitioner may withdraw from patient care during the perioperative journey of a patient undergoing a procedure identified in 1.8.1 above.

RECOMMENDATION **1.8.5** Outline the procedure by which staff should notify the appropriate person of authority, or their designated deputy, of their intention or stated conscientious objection in relation to their practice in the operating department.

RECOMMENDATION **1.8.6** Outline the process for ensuring that alternative staff are available to care for the patient at the stages of their perioperative journey where a practitioner has withdrawn care through conscientious objection.

RECOMMENDATION **1.8.7** It is important that staff members who action their right to conscientious objection do not suffer any discrimination from the perioperative team.

The issue of conscientious objection is complex, both for the practitioner who has the objection and also for other members of the perioperative team involved in the patient's care. Nevertheless, the overriding concern of all involved has to be the patient's right to non-judgmental optimum care.

1.9 CONSENT AND REFUSAL OF CONSENT

Many aspects of healthcare involve close and often intimate contact with the patient. Indeed many procedures are accompanied by discomfort and sometimes pain. Health professionals must understand that the potential for an accusation of trespass to a patient is very real if any of the following occur:

- The application of any intentional or negligent physical force.
- Treatment and contact is threatened, implied, or takes place without the consent of the patient.
- The patient is kept in hospital without their expressed consent.

Trespass to the person is a wrong that requires intention and is expressed in one of three forms:

- Assault
- Battery
- False imprisonment.

You will often hear the terms assault and battery together, however in law these terms are totally different.

Assault is the fear or threat of impending harm. The fear or threat can be physical, verbal or both. For example, giving a patient an injection could be termed an assault if the patient has not expressly given permission to receive the injection. The patient interprets the action as a threat to their person.

Battery is the unlawful application of force or any unwanted touching. The nurse may face a charge of battery if they proceed with the injection against the will of the patient.

False imprisonment is the infliction of bodily restraint which is not expressly authorised or implied by the law. For example, a doctor who authorises a ward to be locked to stop a patient wandering for his own safety may be accused of false imprisonment on behalf of the other patients in the ward.

There are several rules to follow when obtaining consent from a patient:

- In order to gain a valid consent the patient must be competent to understand the information given to them. Consent can be expressed – that is, on a legal document (consent form), or it can be implied – such as rolling up a sleeve in order to give a blood sample.

- The patient must be conscious. No adult can consent for another. In the case of a patient who is not able to consent it is the responsibility of the doctor to give consent, although family members may be consulted as to the known wishes of the patient. But the final responsibility lies with the doctor.
- The patient must have mental capacity. This means that they must be able to understand the information given to them. Basic law takes this to mean anyone over the age of 18, but there are special rules governing those with known mental disorders.
- The patient must have the relevant information in order to give a true consent. This includes knowing the risks of the proposed treatment, and the risk of not having the treatment.
- The patient must have understood the information given. This means that all risks are discussed and understood, but there are no hard or fast rules as to what constitutes understanding.
- The patient must have given consent voluntarily, that is without the coercion of the medical staff or family. It has to be the decision of the patient alone.

There is no agreed standard of competence as this is dependent on the treatment to be given. A lesser degree of competence will be required for the taking of a blood sample compared with that for major surgery where the nature of the surgery can have an impact on body image and carries with it inherent risks.

Any information should be given in a form which the patient can readily understand. The onus of this rests with the person gaining consent. The legal standard is again that of Bolam (1957). What information would a reasonable person give in order to secure consent? However, this edict could be challenged by the Human Rights Act (HMSO 1998b) article 10, which requires that a patient *'receives and imparts information without interference'*. This could be seen as a move towards the patient deciding his or her own standard of information-giving in order to consent with full knowledge.

The most common cases of negligence with regard to consent are those concerning non-disclosure of risks. Sidaway v Bethlem Royal Hospital Governors (1985) is still seen as a leading case in informed consent issues. Mrs Sidaway was informed of the risk of nerve damage during spinal surgery, but not of the risk to the spinal cord. She suffered spinal cord damage and was left severely disabled. She sued, claiming that had she known of the potential damage, she would have refused to consent and thus the consent she gave was invalid. The claim was lost in the High Court, with the Bolam test cited as the standard.

However the Bolam test has been challenged in court in the case of Chester v Afshar (2002). In this case the neurosurgeon did not give any warnings about the risk involved in surgery to remove three discs. Following surgery the claimant's left leg was left disabled due to nerve damage. The court established that, although the surgeon was not negligent in conducting the operation, he was negligent in failing to warn the patient of any possible risk involved. At appeal the surgeon was told that a patient has the right to make a choice as to what should or should not be done to their body. The doctor owed a duty to take the care expected of a reasonable doctor in the circumstances. In this case the patient had not been told of the risk of paralysis before consent was given and the doctor was in breach of duty. There was no negligence on the part of the surgeon during surgery but the claimant could claim compensation – the justification being that, had she been told of the risks involved, she would have sought a second or third opinion before consenting to surgery.

REFUSING TO CONSENT

It would seem logical to assume that if patients have the right to consent to treatment then they have the right to refuse consent. In most cases this is true, but there are still some areas where the 'paternalistic' view comes into play. In the past this view was used to validate the overruling of a refusal, stating that it was in 'the best interests of the patient'. These cases would be brought in battery and were often overturned because a good case could be made as to why it was the appropriate responsibility of the doctor to act in this way.

An exception to this has been Jehovah's Witnesses who have refused to accept blood transfusions. Over the years many patients have found it difficult to get their refusal to consent accepted. This may change with the introduction of the Human Rights Act, Article 3 (inhumane and degrading treatment) which will put the onus on medical staff to justify why any refusal should be overruled. One of the most bizarre but successful cases is that of Allen v New Mount Sinai Hospital (1980). This involved a patient about to undergo an anaesthetic who insisted that the cannulae be placed in her right arm and not her left. The anaesthetist ignored her request, the cannula was placed in her left as she drifted off to sleep, and during the operation her left arm began to swell. The resulting case of battery was successful, as she had clearly refused to consent to having the cannula placed in her left arm. Cases of this type are beginning to appear more regularly and all medical staff should take note and listen to patient refusals and act upon them accordingly.

There are some refusals where it is necessary for legal intervention to play a major part, for example where an enforced caesarean section is necessary in order to save the life of the baby and in some cases the mother. Here the consultant must seek a court order, which will rule that surgery is lawful and not battery.

Prisoners can be recipients of enforced treatment if their medical condition warrants intervention. They are allowed to consent but not to refuse. Most prisoners do not want to die in custody so refusal is rarely a problem – however cases like that of Ian Brady have highlighted the issue of refusal, as has the introduction of the Human Rights Act, Article 3.

A medical and legal loophole is that of competence, as in order to obtain a valid consent competence has to be established. For patients who are not competent the 'paternalistic best interests' of medicine will provide the legal justification for operating if the patient has not consented – without the threat of being sued in battery.

MENTAL HEALTH

The Mental Health Act (HMSO 1983) provides for treatment without consent, but only that which relates to mental illness. There is no proviso for enforced surgery of any other kind. There is still the 'best interests' where the surgeon must be able to justify not seeking or gaining consent, or overruling refusal – usually connected with life-saving or emergency treatment. For those patients who are incompetent through organic brain disease or who are congenitally mentally handicapped, there is no provision for obtaining consent. As with other adults no one may consent on his or her behalf. The medical staff must justify that they are acting in the patient's best interests.

1.10 CHILDREN AND CONSENT

Children are a unique group for whom the law makes specific rules. The definition of adulthood for the purpose of consent is variable in the UK: it is 16 in England and Wales, 12 in Scotland and 17 in Northern Ireland. The legal age for consent is generally accepted as 18, however there is a special allowance for those aged 16 plus, governed by Section 8 of the Family Law Reforms Act 1969. Basically it allows doctors to take consent from those who are aged 16 plus and deemed competent, without the threat of legal attacks from parents.

The law provides for parental consent for those under this age because it assumes that the parents will act in the best interests of the child. If there is a dispute between the medical staff and parents, the child can be made a ward of court and a judge will decide on the disputed medical treatment. Consent is signed on behalf of the judge by a social worker who is acting for the judge. In an emergency the case notes should be signed by two doctors to show that verbal permission has been granted through the court.

For those aged 12–14 it is common practice for parental consent to be sought. This is not a legal practice but is seen as a common sense one. Parents will be required to sign the consent form. A child currently has no legal right to refuse surgery and the decision is that of the parents or medical staff. In the case of non-life-threatening minor surgery which could wait a few years, it would be prudent to wait until the child is of an age to decide for itself. However in most cases where the surgery is of a life-saving nature, a refusal will be overruled. In a recent case a child refused to have a heart transplant; the child's decision was overruled and surgery was allowed to take place. The courts are unwilling to allow children to die, even if the child considers it to be preferable to what lies ahead.

There is a different ruling for those aged 14–16. This is known as 'Gillick Competence' named after the case which sought to change the way competency for this group of children was seen. It was a test case involving a daughter of Mrs Gillick – a 15 year old who sought a prescription from her GP for the oral contraceptive. Mrs Gillick objected to the GP prescribing and sought an action in court. It was ruled that if it could be shown that any child (within this age group) was indeed competent it would be lawful for them to consent to treatment without their parent's permission. The ruling went further to state that healthcare professionals owed a duty of care with regard to the confidentiality of those deemed Gillick Competent.

Establishing Gillick Competency

In ruling, the House of Lords set out a test which is used today to establish Gillick Competency. A child under the age of 16 can give consent if they can understand all of the following:

- The medical advice
- Details of the medical treatment proposed
- Any ethical questions related to the treatment
- Any family problems
- Any long-term emotional effects.

However this test cannot be used to test competency when treatment is refused.

1.11 CONSENT TO PHOTOGRAPHY AND RECORDING

STANDARD A system is in place for managing clinical photography and video recordings. Patient consent is always obtained and documented before clinical photography and video recordings are authorised.

Audio or video recordings and clinical photography are often used by medical staff in the provision of care. They can be used as case records, teaching tools, or for audit or research. The incidence of misuse of medical images taken without patient consent has challenged existing hospital standards and policies.

RECOMMENDATIONS FOR LOCAL POLICY

RECOMMENDATION **1.11.1** Although certain recordings such as x-rays are implicit to the patient's consent to treatment, perioperative staff should ensure that patients know in advance if any photographic or video recording will result from that procedure (DH 2001a).

RECOMMENDATION **1.11.2** Medical staff must give patients the opportunity to give their consent for medical photography.

RECOMMENDATION **1.11.3** This must be documented in order to comply with the Caldicott recommendations on data protection and patient confidentiality. If consent is not obtained and confidentiality is breached, the legal charge would be trespass to the patient.

RECOMMENDATION **1.11.4** Patients must be aware that they can refuse consent without their care being compromised and that, if required, the video or photograph can be anonymised.

RECOMMENDATION **1.11.5** The availability and ease of use of small digital cameras has brought about a change in practice. It is a popular misconception that if a patient cannot be identified in a photograph, then consent to take or indeed publish the image is not required. Consent is a legal requirement for all photographic work whether video, digital or conventional photographic images.

RECOMMENDATION **1.11.6** Photographic and video recordings which are made for treating or assessing a patient must not be used for any purpose other than the patient's care or the audit of that care, without the consent of the patient.

RECOMMENDATION **1.11.7** Patients must know that they are free to stop the recording at any time and that they are entitled to view the video or photographs if they wish. If the patient does not want the video or photographs to be used then they must be destroyed. If a recording or photographs are taken for education purposes and the patient is unconscious, consent for their use must be received as soon as the patient regains capacity. If the patient does not consent to any form of use, the recording must be destroyed.

RECOMMENDATION 1.11.8 Informed written consent is a prerequisite for the release of photographs. If the image is to be used for a purpose which differs from that to which the patient consented, then further consent is required, for instance if the clinician wishes to publish the photographs. The *Good Practice in Consent Implementation Guide* (DH 2001b) makes it clear that all clinical photography, including conventional or digital video recordings, form part of the patient's records and require written informed consent. The guide also states that the patient should be made fully aware of the possible uses of the material obtained.

1.12 RECORD KEEPING AND DOCUMENTATION

STANDARD The patient's surgical care pathway is documented, including: preoperative assessment, identification of problems, planning and evaluation of care. Perioperative personnel understand the legal status of record keeping as a means of providing proof that care has been administered. Accurate records relating to the production, procurement, modification, maintenance and use of medical devices are kept as proof of non-liability.

All records are potentially legal documents. Patient records may be used as evidence in many different circumstances such as a court of law, during an investigation of a complaint locally or by the NMC/HPC Professional Conduct Committee. The need for concise documentation has been compounded by the increase in litigation in recent years. Documentation is often required many years after the event. The approach to record keeping which courts of law tend to adopt is: if it is not recorded, it has not been done. Record keeping must therefore be seen as a key clinical skill to protect healthcare staff from potential litigation.

Accurate record keeping is essential for the delivery of care of the individual patient in the operating theatre. The quality of record keeping is a reflection of the standard of professional practice expected of professional practitioners.

The NMC *Code of Professional Conduct* (2002a) states: *'Healthcare records are a tool of communication within the team. You must ensure that the healthcare record for the patient or client is an accurate account of treatment, care planning and delivery. It should be consecutive, written with the involvement of the patient or client wherever practicable and completed as soon as possible after an event has occurred. It should provide clear evidence of the care planned, the decisions made, the care delivered and the information shared.'*

The NMC (2002b) recommends: *'Record keeping is an integral part of nursing, midwifery and health visiting practice. It is a tool of professional practice and one which should help the care process. It is not separate from this process and it is not an optional extra to be fitted in if circumstances allow.'*

Operating departments should avoid using a variety of records and documents as this may increase the risk of errors. Documentation should be consistent and used hospital-wide where applicable.

INTEGRATED CARE PATHWAYS

An integrated care pathway is a structured multidisciplinary care plan that identifies key steps and anticipates outcomes in patients with specific clinical problems or who are undergoing a specific surgical procedure (Chilcott & Hunt 2001). They may also be referred to as critical care pathways, clinical care pathways or integrated care management using multidisciplinary care pathways.

An integrated care pathway will be used by all healthcare professionals involved in the care of that patient and will provide a single document relating to that particular patient admission. Integrated care pathways utilised in this way will replace separate documentation such as case note entries by medical staff and nursing care plans including perioperative documents. These care plans will also facilitate collaboration between members of the multidisciplinary team in the assessment, planning implementation and evaluation of patient care.

One important feature of an integrated care pathway is the facility to record details of everyone involved in the patient's care. Most integrated care pathways achieve this by having a specific sheet at the beginning of the care plan which enables individual staff members to enter their full name, position, discipline, full signature and initials. This is a major improvement on traditional documentation as every entry made in the integrated care pathway is initialled by the professional recording the entry. This has obvious benefits for improving documentation, particularly in the event of an adverse incident or potential litigation actions.

An integrated care pathway is based on the principle of exception reporting. This means that any event that has or has not occurred as expected in the pathway is recorded as a variance. It is possible to predict much of a patient's care when admitted for a specific procedure, thus facilitating the development of a care pathway that will chart their progress but remains flexible to respond to individual patient need and preference. Consequently each integrated care pathway requires space for the variance to be recorded and the actions taken to resolve the variance. A variance can be either a positive or negative event that is either avoidable or non-avoidable. Variance analysis can be utilised as an evaluation tool that can be incorporated into a clinical audit programme.

RECOMMENDATIONS FOR LOCAL POLICY

General considerations

RECOMMENDATION **1.12.1** Patient records in the perioperative setting should be (NMC 2002b):

- factual, consistent and accurate
- written as soon as possible after the event has occurred, providing current information on the care and condition of the patient or client
- written clearly and in such a manner that the text cannot be erased
- written in a manner that any alterations or additions are dated, timed and signed in such a way that the original entry can still be read clearly
- accurately dated, timed and signed, with the signature printed alongside the first entry
- free from abbreviations, jargon, meaningless phrases, and irrelevant speculation
- written in black ink to make photocopies readable.

Swab counts

RECOMMENDATION **1.12.2** The completed intraoperative record of all accountable items should be signed legibly and placed in the patient's record in compliance with local guidelines.

Recording of implant/prosthesis

RECOMMENDATION **1.12.3** Documentation of implant/prosthesis should comply with the Consumer Protection Act (HMSO 1987). The minimum information recorded should include:

- manufacturer
- product source
- type of implant/prosthesis
- code number
- batch/lot number
- size
- sterilisation date/date of manufacturer
- expiry date
- any amendments or adaptation made.

Tracking and traceability

RECOMMENDATION **1.12.4** The Consumer Protection Act 1987, in particular regarding product liability, has implications for the reprocessing of devices used for patient care. In particular it is essential to maintain adequate records that demonstrate how a particular device was processed, a description of the methods employed and details of available trained personnel with the copies of training records. These records must be linked to the patient's notes. Further guidance is given in the NHS Executive publications HSC 1999/178 and HSC 2000/032 (NHS Executive 1999, 2000).

PROCESSING ENDOSCOPES

RECOMMENDATION **1.12.5** Health Technical Memoranda *HTM 2010 Sterilisation* and *SHTM 2010* (Scotland) (NHS Estates 1997) requires the documentation of:

- date and time the solution was activated
- solution lot number
- expiry date of the solution
- name of the person who activated the solution
- age of the activated solution
- scopes processed
- duration of processing
- persons responsible for processing
- identity of the patient that the scope was being used on.

THEATRE REGISTER

RECOMMENDATION **1.12.6** A theatre register should be kept in every theatre to record the essential details of all surgical procedures. It may be recorded either on paper, in a book format or as part of a computer-held information system.

Computer-held records have the advantage of being easier to read. But any computerised system should have a local policy based on the requirements of the Data Protection Act (HMSO 1984) and the Consumer Protection Act (HMSO 1987).

RECOMMENDATION **1.12.7** The Bevan Report (NHS Executive 1989) outlined that the theatre register should include:

- procedures which were undertaken (both surgical and the type of anaesthetic)
- the names (and signatures) of surgeon, anaesthetist and a list of support staff
- the time each patient entered and left theatre
- the patient's name, date of birth, sex, hospital number
- the name of the scrub and circulating practitioner
- details of any implanted materials
- any untoward incidents.

The theatre record is not a patient record. It is the theatre's own record of procedures, but it could still be used for evidence in a litigation case and should therefore be retained.

RECOMMENDATION **1.12.8** There are specific legal requirements for the keeping of a patient's records (Audit Commission 1995):

- Obstetric records can be kept for 25 years.
- Records for children and young people are kept until the patient's 25th birthday.
- Other records are kept for a minimum of eight years after completion of treatment or death.

ADMISSION AND LABELLING PROCEDURE

RECOMMENDATION **1.12.9** All patients admitted for invasive inpatient or day surgery procedures should have an identity bracelet. This should be of a reliable, tamper-proof design and should bear the patient's full name, hospital number and date of birth in indelible ink.

RECOMMENDATION **1.12.10** If the identity bracelet is removed from a patient for any reason, special care must be taken to ensure that no mistake is made about future identification. The patient should have the identity label replaced as soon as possible. According to the Association of Anaesthetists of Great Britain and Ireland guidelines (AAGBI 1995), where an identity bracelet cannot be used or is removed, the patient's identity should be marked on the skin with an indelible marker.

RECOMMENDATION **1.12.11** It is recommended that patients undergoing general anaesthesia and those who are not competent should wear two identity bracelets.

THE PROCEDURE LIST

RECOMMENDATION **1.12.12** Responsibility for the completion of the procedure list in a recognised printed format must be taken by the clinician undertaking the procedure or a designated member of the team.

RECOMMENDATION **1.12.13** The list should include: surname, forename, hospital number, date of birth of the patient, ward, procedure, type of anaesthetic, surgeon, anaesthetist, theatre name (number), and start time.

RECOMMENDATION **1.12.14** Abbreviations must not be used when describing side or site of the procedure. To avoid ambiguity about the digit on which the operation is to be performed, fingers should be described as thumb, index, middle, ring and little. Toes should be described as hallux or big toe, second, third, fourth and fifth or little.

CANCELLATION/CHANGES TO THE OPERATING LIST

RECOMMENDATION **1.12.15** Operating lists should arrive in theatre 16–24 hours in advance of a scheduled session in order to ensure patient safety and effective utilisation of resources.

RECOMMENDATION **1.12.16** Alterations or cancellations to the operating list must be relayed to the person in charge of the operating list immediately.

RECOMMENDATION **1.12.17** All copies of the operating list or send-for slips must be amended as appropriate by the person making the changes to ensure that all appropriate members of staff are notified of them (AAGBI 1995).

RECOMMENDATION **1.12.18** The persons making the amendments must sign and add a note to the side of the list 'Note Change to Order'. The appropriate untoward incident form should be completed detailing the reasons why the change in order was required/indicated.

RECOMMENDATION **1.12.19** All relevant staff should be informed, including the wards and radiological departments and support services as appropriate.

RECOMMENDATION **1.12.20** It must be acknowledged by all staff that to change the order of an operating list creates the potential for error/oversight and that changes to a published schedule should only occur in extreme circumstances and only where absolutely necessary. The importance of documenting the circumstances of any change via the appropriate untoward incident form should be viewed as essential and fundamental to securing improvements in future scheduling practice.

ELECTIVE SURGERY VERIFICATION CHECKLIST

RECOMMENDATION **1.12.21** It is the responsibility of the surgical practitioner performing the operative procedure to ensure that where side or site could be confused, the operation site is marked with an indelible marker.

RECOMMENDATION **1.12.22** This should be confirmed with the patient's clinical records, radiographs and the procedure list and with the patient wherever possible.

RECOMMENDATION **1.12.23** A registered practitioner at the reception area of theatre should identify the patient and the procedure by checking the full name, date of birth, consent form and hospital unit number on the patient's identity bracelet with the patient's notes. Checks should also be made with the accompanying nurse (NATN 1998).

RECOMMENDATION **1.12.24** For procedures where the patient is undergoing general anaesthesia or sedation, the person performing the procedure has a duty to see the patient or if unavailable, delegate a member of the operative team, before induction of anaesthesia or sedation commences. This person should check the consent form and examine the patient's records to ensure that they relate to the patient, and that the correct procedure and operative site is identified.

RECOMMENDATION **1.12.25** The scrub practitioner should verify that the correct side is to be operated on by checking the patient's records and confirming correct details with the operating surgeon (NMC 2002a).

Ensuring the correct patient undergoes the correct procedure is part of a team effort for minimising the risk of an adverse incident occurring that could be detrimental to patient outcome. The clinician undertaking the procedure is ultimately responsible for managing the risk.

Equipment-related records

RECOMMENDATION **1.12.26** The following equipment-related records should be maintained by the operating department staff in conjunction with estates and medical physics departments, medical devices companies and sterile supplies units:

- Record of purchase
- Any product trials information which may be held by the company
- Identification number for individual items for the purpose of tracking and locating
- Working history/maintenance records
- Capital assets register
- Maintenance contract
- Manufacturer's warranties
- Planned preventative maintenance
- Record of defective instruments sent for repair
- Calibration
- Lending of equipment
- Documentation and tracking of instruments used.

Personal staff-related records

RECOMMENDATION **1.12.27** Making and keeping records is an essential part of human resource management and an individual's file should be kept in a secure location.

It should contain:

- their application for employment
- records of policies issued

- occupational health records
- education and training records
- absence records
- appraisal records.

Accident/incident reporting and statement writing

RECOMMENDATION **1.12.28** All accidents, whether they concern staff or patients, must be reported and documented as soon as possible. When writing a statement/report it is important to concentrate on the facts: what happened, what was said or written at the time and any observations that were made.

RECOMMENDATION **1.12.29** The report should be a clear and comprehensive statement of fact in chronological order. It must be relevant to the incident and must not include assumptions or hearsay.

RECOMMENDATION **1.12.30** The report should be signed, followed by a printed name with professional qualifications and date of signing. When referring to other persons in a report it is important always to use their full name and title.

RECOMMENDATION **1.12.31** A well-written statement can be an excellent defence against allegations. Remember the reader may not be a nurse or ODP and may not understand technical information and terms.

Other considerations

RECOMMENDATION **1.12.32** It is recommended that use of electrosurgical equipment should be documented in order to safeguard the user in the situation where a patient may inadvertently experience an electrosurgery burn. Documentation should include electrosurgery settings and the serial number of the electrosurgery unit.

RECOMMENDATION **1.12.33** It is recommended that skin preparation solutions are documented to comply with the Consumer Protection Act 1987. This should include lot/batch number.

RECOMMENDATION **1.12.34** It is recommended that the positioning of the patient, including pressure relieving devices, is recorded. Inadvertent nerve damage and pressure sores are a common source of litigation.

1.13 CARE OF THE DECEASED

STANDARD There is a system in place to ensure that family, legal and religious obligations can be met in the event of a patient's death in the perioperative setting.

There is relatively little information available to perioperative practitioners regarding care of the deceased patient within the perioperative environment. Staff should adhere to the protocols of their particular hospital in the event of patient death. The aim of this section is to outline the general principles concerning care of the deceased patient and to highlight the need to be aware of cultural and religious rites in the perioperative environment.

Advances in surgery and anaesthetic techniques have reduced the incidence of unexpected patient death in this environment. Whenever a patient dies suddenly in the perioperative environment there is a legal requirement to establish the cause of death through a post-mortem examination. With the development of transplant surgery, theatre staff are also caring for deceased patients following organ retrieval. For all patients the general principles of care will apply.

RECOMMENDATIONS FOR LOCAL POLICY

RECOMMENDATION **1.13.1** If death occurs within the perioperative environment the person in charge must ensure the following personnel are informed immediately, in order to comply with legal requirements:

- Operating department manager
- Ward and/or intensive care staff.

It is the responsibility of the medical staff to inform their senior colleagues.

RECOMMENDATION **1.13.2** Local guidelines must include the method of communication in order to ensure that relatives are informed at the earliest opportunity.

RECOMMENDATION **1.13.3** The requirement of differing faiths and religions must be taken into consideration.

RECOMMENDATION **1.13.4** If a death occurs within the perioperative environment:

- all drains must be left in position
- catheters or cannula should be closed with a spigot
- endotracheal or tracheotomy tubes should remain in situ, unless authorised by the coroner/procurator fiscal
- wounds should be covered by a dressing
- a cadaver bag should be used.

These guidelines may vary locally according to the requirements of the coroner in England, Wales and Northern Ireland, or the procurator fiscal in Scotland. It is advisable to ascertain in advance that permission is granted to remove either an endotracheal or tracheotomy tube if the family wish to view the body. This should be agreed when the policy is written or reviewed.

RECOMMENDATION **1.13.5** The care of the deceased patient should be undertaken according to local policy and in accordance with any specific cultural or religious specifications. A brief summary of these should be available as a resource for staff working in the perioperative environment. Trained staff from the patient's previous area of care may be involved in certain situations, for example, unexpected death.

RECOMMENDATION **1.13.6** Staff should ensure that all documents are complete at the time of death. This will include clear identification of the patient.

RECOMMENDATION 1.13.7 Theatre staff must be aware of, and adhere to, the personal and cultural wishes of relatives as to jewellery or artefacts remaining on the patient. The nurse must identify and clearly record these articles.

RECOMMENDATION 1.13.8 It is essential that infection control and good hygiene are practised throughout all stages in this care, including transfer to the mortuary.

RECOMMENDATION 1.13.9 The senior nurse should ensure that the deceased patient is transferred to the mortuary as soon as possible following death. As a mark of respect, it is appropriate for a nurse to escort the deceased to the theatre suite exit.

RECOMMENDATION 1.13.10 The relatives should be given the opportunity to pay their last respects, if this is their preference. The provision of a private waiting area for relatives in the vicinity of the operating department is recommended. A quiet area should be made available to allow them to be alone with the deceased.

RECOMMENDATION 1.13.11 It is essential that operating department staff are given appropriate support following the death of a patient in the area.

1.14 PROCEDURES RELATED TO ORGAN DONATION

STANDARD A system is in place to support perioperative staff who are involved in the UK Transplant Programme, in the retrieval or subsequent transplant of donated organs.

INTRODUCTION

Multi-organ donation has become more frequent with approximately 700 multi-organ donation operations being undertaken each year in the UK. At the end of December 2003, 7,278 people were on the active and temporarily suspended transplant waiting list in the UK (British Medical Association 2004).

The practice of organ donation is now widely accepted by healthcare professionals and the public, and 90% of the public now accept the principle of organ donation. Heart, lung, liver and kidney transplants now have excellent one and five year survival rates; pancreatic and bowel transplantation are also fast developing.

Classically, the potential organ donor is a patient in whom brain stem death has been confirmed, but who still has a beating heart and is maintained on artificial ventilation in an intensive care unit. Over the last few years, due to the increasing demand for organs for transplantation, there has been a revival for non-heart-beating donation. Kidneys and liver are sometimes suitable for donation after asystole in certain circumstances.

In a situation where it is futile to continue to support a patient, a timed withdrawal of treatment offers the relatives of such patients an opportunity for organ donation that would not otherwise be possible. Non-heart-beating donation requires immediate access to the operating theatre within minutes of asystole, making the timing of treatment withdrawal paramount.

IDENTIFICATION AND MANAGEMENT OF POTENTIAL DONORS

The *Code of Practice for the Diagnosis of Brain Stem Death* sets out guidelines for the identification and management of potential organ and tissue donors (DH 1979, 1998).

The criteria for brain stem death clearly outline who can perform brain stem death tests and under what circumstances tests can be undertaken. Regardless of the potential for organ donation, these tests confirm death and thus allow the withdrawal of supportive treatment, resulting in imminent asystole. The time of death is recorded as the time of the first brain stem death tests, indicating that death has been conclusively established, not when ventilation is withdrawn or asystole occurs. In situations where organ donation is offered by the family, supportive treatment is continued in order to preserve organ function up to the time that organ retrieval occurs.

The Human Tissue Act (HMSO 1961) and The Human Tissue Act (Northern Ireland) (HMSO 1962) outline the legal issues relating to consent for donation. The Human Organ Transplants Act (HMSO 1989b) regulates the use of organs for transplantation and makes it illegal to buy, sell or advertise organs in the UK.

The organisation UK Transplant was formed in July 2000 after a five yearly review of its predecessor, the United Kingdom Transplant Support Service Authority (UKTSSA). It is a Special Health Authority and is directly accountable to Health Ministers in Northern Ireland, Scotland and Wales as well as to Parliament through the Department of Health in England.

UK Transplant provides support for transplantation across the UK and is responsible for regulating transplant activity. It is also responsible for maintaining the records of all those who are waiting for transplants as well as maintaining records for those who have had transplants. It provides a 24-hour support service for matching and allocating donor organs and is a focal point for information on transplant issues including an enquiry service.

Prior to the removal of any organ, the following must be established by the regional donor transplant co-ordinator:

- Diagnosis of brain stem death
- Confirmation of a lack of objection to organ donation from the nearest relative
- Screening for hepatitis B and C, HIV, cytomegalovirus and history of malignancy
- Notification to the coroner (procurator fiscal in Scotland) if necessary.

Matching criteria should include:

- compatible blood group
- height and weight
- comparable cytomegalovirus antibody status.

Donor organ procurement is recognised as an emotive subject for perioperative staff. It is therefore imperative that operating departments have a clearly defined policy which outlines the procedures to be followed, thus reducing as far as possible, any confusion and anxiety of the staff involved.

RECOMMENDATIONS FOR LOCAL POLICY

Organ procurement procedures

RECOMMENDATION **1.14.1** The transplant co-ordinator is a key figure in the organisation of organ donation and will advise on the necessary procedures at the time. This individual will liaise with the donor theatre team, transplant teams and the intensive care staff. The overall aim at this point in time is to minimise any difficulties in the procedure so that it may be viewed as a positive experience for the families and personnel involved in the process.

RECOMMENDATION **1.14.2** The timing of organ procurement procedures are usually calculated to co-ordinate with the availability of retrieving surgeons and the recipient procedures. The transplant team will require medical details about the donor, and part of the transplant co-ordinator's role is to provide guidance on the information that may be required for each type of transplant.

RECOMMENDATION **1.14.3** Although the transplant procurement (retrieval) teams are largely self sufficient and bring with them the instruments, drugs and perfusion fluids necessary for their procedure, the donor theatre will need to provide certain items and equipment. This may include but is not limited to:

- trolleys, bowls and stands
- basic general instruments
- gowns, drapes, swabs and sutures
- suction and diathermy
- large quantities of crushed ice
- perioperative personnel.

Considerations for the transplant team

RECOMMENDATION **1.14.4** All procedures during procurement surgery must adhere to the local hospital policies and must meet nationally recognised standards.

RECOMMENDATION **1.14.5** It is important that all procedures are afforded the same professionalism as all other surgical procedures.

RECOMMENDATION **1.14.6** Effective communication and feedback to the donor unit is important to ensure that perioperative staff can identify with the more positive aspects of transplantation surgery and to prevent the feeling of isolation.

Tissue donation

RECOMMENDATION **1.14.7** There are occasions when other tissue will be donated, including heart valves, bone samples and skin. In these situations the transplant co-ordinator will advise on the process of retrieval.

Samples of tissue may also be taken for research but relatives' consent must be obtained in accordance with current legislation. This consent must be clearly recorded in the patient's notes.

RECOMMENDATION **1.14.8** Samples of lymph node tissue and spleen may be taken at the time of kidney retrieval for tissue typing. Again, consent must be obtained from relatives for this routine procedure in transplant surgery.

Last offices

RECOMMENDATION **1.14.9** Once the retrieval is complete and surgeons have closed the abdomen and chest appropriately, last offices can be performed in accordance with the local policy. Wherever possible, the wishes of the donor and their relatives should be respected. It is usual for the transplant co-ordinator to assist the perioperative staff with last offices.

RECOMMENDATION **1.14.10** If a post mortem is required, this should be arranged with the pathologist. The relatives should be assured that this will not affect or delay funeral arrangements.

RECOMMENDATION **1.14.11** Relatives should be encouraged to view the body post-donation, if they wish to do so.

Other considerations for the donor procurement units

RECOMMENDATION **1.14.12** It is helpful to identify a member of staff who will meet the procurement team(s) on arrival and introduce them to the environment. If a member of staff is also available to assist with departure this will streamline the whole process to the advantage of the potential recipients as well as to the donor procurement team.

RECOMMENDATION **1.14.13** Organ procurement is an emotive procedure and perioperative staff involved in the donor phase of the transplant process are often subjected to stressful emotions. It is recommended that consideration is given to the provision of support programmes that staff involved in these procedures can access. Support services such as counselling, peer support and stress management, as well as education on issues around brain stem death and the purpose of donor procurement procedures can all assist perioperative staff to deliver an effective service in this situation. Many hospitals have, or are considering appointing, a donor liaison sister who can provide local support, education and feedback to perioperative staff involved in these procedures, thus enabling them to meet these requirements.

Useful addresses

- **UK Transplant**
  Fox Den Road, Stoke Gifford, Bristol, BS34 8RR
- **UK Transplant Co-ordinators Association**
  UKTCA Secretariat, PO Box 6300, Birmingham, B15 2RN
- **Clinical Ethics and Human Tissue Branch**
  Room 531B, Skipton House, London, SE1 6LH

REFERENCES

Allan v New Mount Sinai Hospital [1980] 109 DLR (3d) 634

Association of Anaesthetists of Great Britain and Ireland 1995 *Risk Management* Hampshire, Alresford Press

Audit Commission 1995 *Setting the Records Straight: a study of hospital medical records* London, Audit Commission

Bolam v Friern Hospital Management Committee [1957] 2 All ER 118

Bolitho v City and Hackney HA [1997] 4 All ER 771

British Medical Association 2004 *Human Tissue and Organs Shortages* London, BMA

Chester v Afshar 2002 The Law Reports [2003] QB356 / EWCA Civ 724

Chilcott J, Hunt A 2001 Nurse Friendly Integrated Care Pathways *Nursing Times* 97 (48) 32–34

Clarke P, Jones J 1998 *Brigden's Operating Department Practice* Edinburgh, Churchill Livingstone

Clarke v MacLennan [1983] 1 All ER 416

Department of Health 1979 *A Code of Practice Including the Diagnosis of Brain Death Cadaveric Organs for Transplantation* London, DH

Department of Health 1998 *A Code of Practice for the Diagnosis of Brain Stem Death* Norwich, The Stationery Office

Department of Health 2001a *Reference Guide to Consent for Examination or Treatment* London, DH. www.dh.gov.uk/consent

Department of Health 2001b *Good Practice in Consent Implementation Guide: consent to examination or treatment* London, DH. www.dh.gov.uk/consent

HMSO 1961 *Human Tissue Act* Norwich, The Stationery Office

HMSO 1962 *Human Tissue Act (Northern Ireland)* Norwich, The Stationery Office

HMSO 1967 *Abortion Act (Scotland, England and Wales)* Norwich, The Stationery Office

HMSO 1969 *Family Law Reforms Act* Norwich, The Stationery Office

HMSO 1980 *The Limitations Act* Norwich, The Stationery Office

HMSO 1982 *The Supply of Goods and Services Act* Norwich, The Stationery Office

HMSO 1983 *The Mental Health Act* Norwich, The Stationery Office

HMSO 1984 *Data Protection Act* Norwich, The Stationery Office

HMSO 1987 *The Consumer Protection Act (Commencement No 1)* Norwich, The Stationery Office

HMSO 1989a *Children Act* Norwich, The Stationery Office

HMSO 1989b *Human Organ Transplantation Act* Norwich, The Stationery Office

HMSO 1990 *The Human Fertilisation and Embryology Act* Norwich, The Stationery Office

HMSO 1998a *The Data Protection Act* Norwich, The Stationery Office

HMSO 1998b *Human Rights Act* Norwich, The Stationery Office

National Association of Theatre Nurses 1998 *Safeguards for Invasive Procedures: the management of risks* Harrogate, NATN

NHS Estates 1997 *Sterilisation* Health Technical Memorandum HTM 2010 and SHTM 2010 (Scotland) London, The Stationery Office. www.knowledge.nhsestates.gov.uk

NHS Executive 1989 *Staffing and Utilisation of Operating Theatres: a study conducted under the guidance of a steering group* (Bevan Report) Leeds, NHS Management Executive VFM Unit

NHS Executive 1999 *Variant Creutzfeldt-Jakob Disease (vCJD): Minimising the Risk of Transmission* HSC 1999/178 Leeds, DH

NHS Executive 2000 *Decontamination of Medical Devices* HSC 2000/032 Leeds, DH

Nursing and Midwifery Council 2002a *Code of Professional Conduct* London, NMC

Nursing and Midwifery Council 2002b *Guidelines for Records and Record Keeping* London, NMC

Perioperative Care Collaborative 2003 The provision of the non-medical perioperative practitioner working as first assistant to the surgeon *British Journal of Perioperative Nursing: supplement* 13 (8)

Rogers WV 1998 *Winfield and Jolowicz on Tort* UK, Sweet and Maxwell

Sidaway v Bethlem RHG [1985] 1 AC 871

United Kingdom Central Council 1992 *Code of Professional Conduct* London, UKCC

Wilsher v Essex AHA [1988] 1 All ER 871

FURTHER READING

Akhtar S 2002 Nursing with Dignity – Islam *Nursing Times* 98 (16) 40–42

Attwood C 1995 Dying with Dignity *Technic* 138 15

Ayrton NA 1982 Last Offices in Cases of Notifiable Disease: the use of cadaver bags in controlling infection *Nursing Times* 78 (19) Supplement 5–6

Baxter C 2002 Nursing with Dignity – Rastafarianism *Nursing Times* 98 (13) 42–43

Bender M 1990 *The Quality of Dying – how to provide good care of the ill and dying patient* Derbyshire, Winslow Press

Blain C, Mackay M 2002 Informed Consent: the global picture *British Journal of Perioperative Nursing* 12 (11) 402–407

Bothamley J 1999 Organ Donation – a review of the literature *British Journal of Theatre Nursing* 9 (11) 521–530

Bothamley J 1999 Organ Donation – consent and patients' rights *British Journal of Theatre Nursing* 9 (12) 573–578

Bothamley J 2000 Organ Donation – brain stem death *British Journal of Perioperative Nursing* 10 (1) 24–29

Bryan S, Holmes S, Postelthwaite D, Carty N 2002 The Role of Integrated Care Pathways in Improving the Patient Experience *Professional Nurse* 18 (2) 77–79

Bryan S, Holmes S, Postlethwaite D, Carty N 2002 A Breast Unit Care Pathway: enhancing the role of the nurse *Professional Nurse* 18 (3) 151–154

Callender S Mathews S 1998 Caring for the Carers During Transplant Surgery *British Journal of Theatre Nursing* 8 (1) 5–12

Chiarella M 1994 Dying With Dignity: recent developments *ACORN Journal* 7 (1) 17–18

Christmas M 2002 Nursing with Dignity – Christianity *Nursing Times* 98 (11) 37–39

Clark A 2003 Protocol-based Care 1: how integrated care pathways work *Professional Nurse* 18 (12) 694–697

Collins A 2002 Nursing with Dignity – Judaism *Nursing Times* 98 (9) 34–35

Cormack K 1998 Audit of Consent Forms *British Journal of Theatre Nursing* 8 (9) 14–16

Currie L, Harvey G 1998 Care Pathways Development and Implementation *Nursing Standard* 12 (30) 35–38

Department of Health 2003 *The Use of Human Organs and Tissue: an interim statement* London, DH

Department of Health 2003 *Essence of Care: patient-focused benchmarking for healthcare practitioners* London, DH

Department of Health, Social Services and Public Safety 2003 *Reference Guide to Consent for Examination, Treatment or Care* Belfast, DH

Descheneaux K 1991 Death Investigations: how you can help *Nursing* 21 (9) 52–55

Dimond B 1990 *Legal Aspects of Nursing* Lancaster, Quay Publishing Ltd

Dimond B 2001 Legal Aspects of Consent 2: the different forms of consent *British Journal of Nursing* 10 (6) 400–401

Dimond B 2001 Legal Aspects of Consent 3: the duty of care to inform *British Journal of Nursing* 10 (7) 466–468

Dimond B 2001 Legal Aspects of Consent 5: duty to inform patients of risks *British Journal of Nursing* 10 (8) 544–545

Dimond B 2001 Legal Aspects of Consent 7: young persons of 16 and 17 years *British Journal of Nursing* 10 (11) 732–733

Dimond B 2001 Legal Aspects of Consent 8: children under the age of 16 *British Journal of Nursing* 10 (12) 797–799

Directory of Operating Theatres & Departments of Surgery 1998 *United Kingdom Transplant Support Service Authority 1–26* Cambridge, CMA Medical Data

Docherty B, McComb J, Simpson S 2003 Protocol-based Care 2: developing pathways with effective teams *Professional Nurse* 19 (2) 97–101

Edwards J 1997 Sudden Death and the Theatre Nurse *British Journal of Theatre Nursing* 6 (12) 11–14

Elliott C, Quinn F 2000 *English Legal System* 3rd ed, Harlow, Longman

Finch J 1994 *Organ Transplants and Disposal of the Human Body. Spellers law relating to hospital* 7th ed, Oxford, Chapman and Hall Medical

Francis R, Johnstone C, Johnston C 2000 *Medical Treatment: decisions and the law* London, Butterworths

Gill BK 2002 Nursing with Dignity – Sikhism *Nursing Times* 98 (14) 39–41

Green J 1992 Death with Dignity – Christianity *Nursing Times* 88 (3) 26–29

Green J 1992 Death with Dignity – Jehovah's Witness *Nursing Times* 88 (5) 36–37

Green J 1992 Death with Dignity – The Mormon Church *Nursing Times* 88 (6) 44–45

Guezo J 2003 Total Abdominal Hysterectomy: development of a patient-centred care pathway *Nursing Standard* 18 (3) 38–42

Hind M, Wicker P 2000 *Principles of Perioperative Practice* London, Churchill Livingstone

Hutchings D 1991 Spirituality in the Face of Death *The Canadian Nurse* 87 (5) 30–31

Jefferies B 1993 Death in the Operating Room *ACORN Journal* 6 (2) 15–18

Jootun D 2002 Nursing with Dignity – Hinduism *Nursing Times* 98 (15) 38–40

Kennedy I, Grubb A 2000 *Medical Law* 3rd ed, London, Butterworths

Ledbetter AK 1995 Trauma Surgery. In Meeker RH, Rothrock JC *Alexander's Care of the Patient* 10th ed, Mosby, St Louis

Lloyd-Jones H, Wheeldon DR, Smith JA, Potter CD, Wallwork J, Large SR 1996 An Approach to the Retrieval of Thoracic Organs for Transplantation *AORN Journal* 63 (2) 416–426

Mallett J, Dougherty L 2000 *The Royal Marsden Hospital Manual of Clinical Nursing Procedures* 5th ed, Oxford, Blackwell Science

Mason JK, McCall Smith RA 1999 *Law and Medical Ethics* 5th ed, London, Butterworths

Meeker MH, Rothrock JC 1995 *Alexander's Care of the Patient* 10th ed, St Louis, Mosby

Montgomery J 2003 *Health Care Law* 2nd ed, Oxford, Oxford University Press

National Association of Theatre Nurses 1999 *Operating Department Records* Harrogate, NATN

National Association of Theatre Nurses 2003 *Staffing for Patients in the Perioperative Setting* Harrogate, NATN

Neuberger J 1994 *Caring for Dying of People of Different Faith* 2nd ed, London, Mosby

NHS Executive 1997 *Caldicott Report on the Review of Patient Identifiable Information* Leeds, DH. www.dh.gov.uk/ipu/confiden/report/caldrep.pdf

Northcott N 2002 Nursing with Dignity – Buddhism *Nursing Times* 98 (10) 36–38

Onslow L, Roberts H, Steiner A, Roberts A, Powell J, Pickering R 2003 An Integrated Care Pathway for Fractured Neck of Femur Patients *Professional Nurse* 18 (5) 265–268

Page S 1996 Responses of Perioperative Nurses to Organ Procurement Surgery *Canadian Operating Room Nursing Journal* 14 (4) 9–11

Papadopoulos I 2002 Nursing with Dignity – Christianity *Nursing Times* 98 (12) 36–37

Patterson D 2002 Day Surgery: an exciting new career pathway *Nursing Times* 98 (14) 44–46

Reid J 2003 Valid Consent to Surgery: dispelling the myth and establishing the evidence *British Journal of Perioperative Nursing* 13 (7) 288–296

Royal College of Nursing 1981 *Verification of Death and the Performances of Last Offices* London, RCN

Shields L, Werder H 2002 *Perioperative Nursing* London, Greenwich Medical Media

Simpson J 2002 Nursing with Dignity – Jehovah's Witnesses *Nursing Times* 98 (17) 36–37

Speck P 1992 Care After Death: cleansing and shrouding the body *Nursing Times* 88 (6) 2–11

Stauch M, Wheat K, Tingle J 2003 *Source Book on Medical Law* 2nd ed, London, Cavendish Publishing

Tingle J, Cribb A 1995 *Nursing Law and Ethics* Oxford, Blackwell Science

United Kingdom Transplant Coordinators Association 1994 *Standards of Practice for Procurement Coordinators* Birmingham, UKTCA

Walsh M 1997 Will Critical Pathways Replace the Nursing Process? *Nursing Standard* 11 (52) 39–42

Whyte A 1997 The Ultimate Gift *Nursing Times* 93 (27) 26–29

Wigfield A, Boon E 1996 Critical Care Pathway Development: the way forward *British Journal of Nursing* 5 (12) 732–735

Wilson J 1997 Integrated Care Management *Nursing Management* 4 (7) 18–19

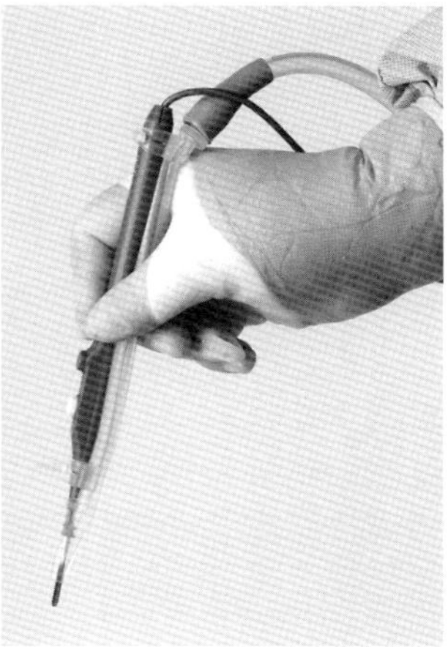

2 RISK MANAGEMENT

2.1 HEALTH AND SAFETY

STANDARD Personnel working in the perioperative setting are aware of their legal and professional obligations for health and safety. There are systems in place to ensure a safe environment for patients, staff and visitors.

INTRODUCTION

Risk management is an integral component both in a clinical governance framework and in the quality assurance process for managing safe patient care. Risk management is particularly important for the perioperative environment because the patient is exposed to many risks whilst undergoing a surgical procedure. Employing organisations must have systems in place which:

- identify risks and hazards
- formulate solutions to reduce the risk where possible
- investigate adverse incidents and near misses so that lessons can be learned
- ensure that mistakes and errors are not repeated
- ensure that staff are risk-aware and proactive in managing risks.

The emphasis should be on preventing adverse incidents by exploring how they happen and what can be done to help prevent them. Policies and procedures must be in place to minimise risk to patients. It is the theatre manager's responsibility to ensure that policies and procedures are adhered to and that audits of compliance with national perioperative standards are undertaken regularly. It is recommended that employing organisations use the NATN *Risk and Quality Management System* (NATN 2002a) as the benchmark audit tool for ensuring that a high standard of care is being delivered to each perioperative patient. This document has been developed in a format that emphasises specific care issues and allows for the identification of good practice, along with the identification of potential shortcomings. Where practice falls below an acceptable standard, the methodology allows for prioritisation for action using a traffic light system.

It is the responsibility of every employer and member of staff to ensure that they are knowledgeable of and comply with health and safety laws that may affect their clinical practice. Risk assessment and risk management is a statutory duty in relation to the management of health and safety in the workplace.

Health and Safety at Work Act 1974

The basic duty of every employer is set out in Section 2 (1) of the Health and Safety at Work Act (HMSO 1974): *'It shall be the duty of every employer to ensure, so far as is reasonably practicable, the health, safety and welfare at work of all its employees.'*

According to this law the employer has to do only what is reasonably practicable. The law however requires the employer to be able to prove, on a balance of probabilities, that it did all that was reasonably practicable to carry out its statutory duty.

The Management of Health and Safety at Work Regulations (HMSO 1992a) introduced more specific requirements to manage health and safety, and required employers to carry out a risk assessment and implement changes as necessary. Employees also have a legal obligation to take reasonable care of their own health and safety, and to follow policies and procedures provided by their employer for their own protection and the protection of colleagues and patients. The regulations were published with an approved code of practice and guidance (ACOP). Hazard is defined in the ACOP as: *'something with the potential to cause harm (this can include articles, substances, plant or machines, methods of work, the working environment and other aspects of work organisation)'* (HMSO 1999a).

HAZARD

A hazard represents the existence of an unsafe system of work, which encompasses a risk to the health and safety of an employee, patient or visitor. A hazard may also involve equipment or fabric of a building which has become unsafe.

RISK

A risk is defined as the potential for harm to arise from a hazard. The extent of the risk will depend on the likelihood of that harm arising.

Employers are expected to use all available information about the risks, such as relevant legislation, controls assurance, medical products and devices manuals, and safety instructions. The risk assessment must be recorded either in writing or electronically and be available for risk managers and visiting inspectorates and auditors.

EMPLOYER

The employer's duty is to provide and maintain systems of work that are, as far as is reasonably practicable, safe and without risks to health. The employer needs to liaise closely with all other departments to fulfil the responsibility to other disciplines using the department. The employer must ensure that all policies relating to health and safety are easily accessible at all times to all members of staff.

EMPLOYEE

The employee's duty is to abide by established systems and to implement the employer's recommendations in order to protect him/herself and his/her work colleagues and clients. In addition, employees must advise their employer of new developments, updates and recommendations of specific dangers that relate to safe practice within the working environment.

RECOMMENDATIONS FOR LOCAL POLICY

Health and safety officer

RECOMMENDATION **2.1.1** A health and safety officer must be appointed in every operating department. It is essential that this officer is trained for and understands his or her role and is allowed to fulfil the necessary duties.

RECOMMENDATION **2.1.2** All members of staff should:

- know who their health and safety officer is
- be aware of the role of the health and safety officer and organisational risk manager
- receive training on the responsibilities of the employer and the employee in relation to health and safety (a record of training should be kept within the department)
- take an active part in, or be aware of the need and necessity for the updating of policies.

RECOMMENDATION **2.1.3** A statutory health and safety law poster should be visibly displayed in a prominent position within the department for the information of all employees.

Identification/documentation of accidents and dangerous occurrences

RECOMMENDATION **2.1.4** All accidents or incidents involving staff and/or equipment and buildings must be reported to the head of department, and the relevant paperwork completed in line with national *Reporting of Injuries, Diseases and Dangerous Occurrences Regulations* (RIDDOR) guidelines (HMSO 1996).

RECOMMENDATION **2.1.5** If necessary, the member of staff should seek medical assessment of any injury sustained. Local reporting protocols should be adhered to. All the documentation should go to an agreed central collecting point and a photocopy kept within the department.

RECOMMENDATION **2.1.6** A manager may initiate an internal enquiry into incidents where a problem has been identified. The use of incident reports is a valuable tool in the development of protocols and procedures.

Preventative maintenance programmes

RECOMMENDATION **2.1.7** The employer has a responsibility for implementing a planned equipment maintenance programme. This is agreed between the estates service department and the users/heads of department, or the company from where the equipment was purchased or leased (possibly with joint responsibility). The programme should cover all types of equipment.

RECOMMENDATION **2.1.8** If maintenance is to be carried out on areas of the perioperative environment and its equipment, written documentation must be completed and signed by the senior member of staff (ie: a permit to work must be given).

RECOMMENDATION **2.1.9** All items for repair must be separated from use, wherever possible being removed from the working environment and clearly labelled for repair.

Medical gases and volatile agents in the perioperative environment

RECOMMENDATION **2.1.10** Employers must have a policy outlining the responsibilities and precautions necessary for the safe storage, handling and incidental exposure to medical gases and volatile agents. The policy should include:

- storage and use of cylinders
- changing of cylinders
- checking procedures after maintenance or repair of equipment used in the delivery of medical gases and vapours
- measures to reduce the occupational exposure to pollutants. These should include scavenging systems which are designed to conduct expired gases and agents away from the occupational environment. Records of the levels of pollutants should be kept.

RECOMMENDATION **2.1.11** There should be clear evidence of risk assessments, a spillage policy, and training for staff dealing with volatile anaesthetic agents.

Noise

RECOMMENDATION **2.1.12** It is the employer's responsibility to reduce, so far as is reasonably practicable, the employees' exposure to noise. Refurbishment programmes, building works and extensions should be undertaken at times when patient care is at a minimum.

Stress

RECOMMENDATION **2.1.13** It is a health and safety requirement for employers to ensure that stress is regarded in the same light as any other health hazard. Working in a perioperative environment can be extremely stressful and the employer should promote a culture that promotes:

- good management with clear objectives and communication
- staff involvement in change with appropriate training and development
- the development of good relationships at work
- training in interpersonal skills
- effective systems for dealing with conflicts, bullying and harassment
- flexible work schedules, with planned and agreed work hours
- good planning, with opportunities for staff to contribute, especially in the organisation of their own job
- clear roles for employees, with support for those with high levels of responsibility for the welfare of people
- appropriate job descriptions with well-defined responsibilities
- proper use of skills and proper hazard controls
- realistic workloads and pace, with reasonable targets.

RECOMMENDATION **2.1.14** There is a potential risk that an employee who works excessively long hours, unsuitable shifts or on calls, may encounter physical or mental ill health, or precipitate fatigue-induced accidents or injury. There is therefore a need for adequate intervals for meals and rest as agreed within local policy.

NB Implementation of the *Working Time Regulations* (HMSO 1998a): workers are entitled to a 20-minute break if they work six hours or more, and this should be taken away from the work station/theatre. Where a rest break cannot be taken, the unused entitlement should be claimed as a period of equivalent compensatory rest within two weeks.

Control of Substances Hazardous to Health (COSHH)

The employer has a duty to comply with *The COSHH Regulations* (HMSO 2002a).

RECOMMENDATION **2.1.15** The employer must ensure that adequate control has been secured by:

- ensuring that all substances are COSHH-assessed in line with local guidelines
- minimising the potential for exposure to hazardous substances by their removal, or by using suitable alternatives
- introducing measures other than personal protective equipment (eg: enclosure of the process)
- using local exhaust ventilation (eg: during the preparation of bone cement).

RECOMMENDATION **2.1.16** It is the employer's responsibility to provide adequate supplies of suitable personal protective equipment (eg: latex gloves, aprons, goggles). The use of latex gloves has increased, as has awareness of the need for the use of standard precautions. Guidelines for the use of latex gloves in terms of latex sensitisation must be adhered to.

RECOMMENDATION **2.1.17** It is the employer's responsibility to ensure that staff have been informed of all hazardous substances within their working environment, and of procedures to control and prevent injury from such substances. This should include methods of use and disposal.

RECOMMENDATION **2.1.18** Employers must ensure that there is a policy for the correct labelling and identification of containers used for hazardous substances.

RECOMMENDATION **2.1.19** Staff must be aware of procedures to be carried out in the event of injury related to such substances, and suitable equipment should be available at all times.

Electrical equipment

RECOMMENDATION **2.1.20** The provision and use of electrical equipment within the perioperative setting should comply within the recommendations of the *Provision and Use of Work Equipment Regulations* (HMSO 1998b) and therefore should:

- be checked by authorised designated personnel on delivery and before use
- be used in accordance with the manufacturer's recommendations
- only be used by employees who have been instructed in its use (eg: monopolar, bi-polar diathermy equipment)
- have a planned preventative maintenance programme including a regular maintenance contract
- ensure that all loan or trial electrical equipment has a current certificate of indemnity and that checks are carried out prior to its use.

Sharps

A policy for the disposal of sharps is recommended.

RECOMMENDATION **2.1.21** Needles, blades and other sharps should be collected and contained safely during surgical procedures.

RECOMMENDATION **2.1.22** Needles should not be re-sheathed.

RECOMMENDATION **2.1.23** Special care should be taken when disposing of needles used to 'draw up' solutions for injections.

RECOMMENDATION **2.1.24** Used needles and syringes should not be parted but placed as a whole in a yellow sharps bin or other recommended container in accordance with Health Service Circular (HSC) specifications.

- Sharps bins should be available at all times and located at the most suitable place.
- Sharps containers must conform to the British Standard (BS) 7320 which specifies that they must: be leak-proof, have a handle which does not interfere with the disposal process, have a suitable aperture, be sealable, have a line showing when the container is three quarters full, be able to be incinerated, be yellow and clearly marked 'Danger, contaminated sharps only, destroy by incineration'.
- Sharps bins are to be sealed and sent for incineration when they are three quarters full.

RECOMMENDATION **2.1.25** All staff should be made aware of the protocols to be followed in the event of a sharps injury.

RECOMMENDATION **2.1.26** The number, frequency and types of sharps injuries should be reviewed periodically.

Floors

RECOMMENDATION **2.1.27** All floors must be kept clear of loose materials and prevented from becoming slippery. All reasonably practicable steps must be taken. Specific dangers are:

- spillage of water around scrub up area
- water spillage from autoclaves
- cables trailing on floors. These should be avoided, but where this is unavoidable they should be orange in colour and easily visible.

RECOMMENDATION **2.1.28** Aisles, corridors and exit areas should be kept free from refuse and obstructions so that evacuation can be carried out without danger.

RECOMMENDATION **2.1.29** Approved notices should be in place which identify potential hazards (eg: floor cleaning or spillages).

Catering

RECOMMENDATION **2.1.30** If catering is available within the perioperative environment, it is essential that the requirements of the Food Safety Act (HMSO 1990a) and Food Standards Act (HMSO 1999c) are complied with. Food and drink should not be brought into clinical areas and should only be consumed in designated rest areas.

2.2 FIRE PREVENTION

STANDARD Statutory and local fire precaution policies are provided and observed. A system is in place for the assessment of potential fire hazards within the perioperative setting.

INTRODUCTION

Legislation covering fire safety within the UK is currently being reviewed. The Fire Precautions Act (HMSO 1971) and the Fire Precautions (Workplace) Regulations Act (HMSO 1997) are to be repealed and replaced by the Regulatory Reform (Fire Safety) Order which is to become law in early 2005. The new regulations are also based on the *Dangerous Substances and Explosive Atmosphere Regulations* (DSEAR) (HMSO 2002b). The fire risk assessment element of the previous regulations will remain, and additional duties will be imposed, such as a duty to:

- prevent fire spread
- monitor and maintain building regulation standards
- appoint one or more employees to assist in ensuring compliance with the regulations.

The responsible person will need to demonstrate that they did everything 'reasonably practicable' to prevent injury, and there will be a civil liability if a breach of duty causes harm.

POLICY AND PROCEDURE

All operating theatre departments must demonstrate a commitment to the Health and Safety at Work Act (HMSO 1974) by having clearly defined up-to-date policies and procedures relating to fire prevention. Almost all fires in the perioperative setting are preventable and it is essential that personnel are aware of the potential hazards and how to respond to a surgical fire.

Risk management requires commitment from all staff. Staff must be aware, for example, of the necessity of keeping fire exits clear, fire doors closed, flammable products stored safely in compliance with regulations, and of having a program of checking fire alarms and fire appliances by a nominated person. The potential for fire requires constant consideration and demands appropriate action planning to ensure a safe working environment. Potential ignition sources include electrocautery units, surgical lasers, high speed drills and fibreoptic light sources.

All personnel should receive education on the importance of managing heat sources by following laser and electrosurgery safety practices, and by establishing guidelines for minimising oxygen concentration under surgical drapes.

It is recommended that policies and procedures are considered in conjunction with the *NATN Risk and Quality Management System* (NATN 2002a).

RECOMMENDATIONS FOR LOCAL POLICY

Fire precautions

RECOMMENDATION **2.2.1** When planning a new complex or refurbishment of a theatre suite the project team should consult with the specialist personnel.

At appropriate stages of the design process the architect and engineer should discuss and verify their proposals with the relevant fire authority, and should ensure that the project team and all other planning staff are fully acquainted with the fire safety strategy for the design of operating facilities.

RECOMMENDATION **2.2.2** All units must take sensible precautions against fire, in consultation with a fire safety officer or specialist fire prevention officer.

RECOMMENDATION **2.2.3** The advice of the chief fire officer of the local fire authority should be sought when defining policies and procedures in hospitals and other health premises.

RECOMMENDATION **2.2.4** A fire policy must be available in the department and understood by all staff.

RECOMMENDATION **2.2.5** There must be a nominated fire officer within the department.

RECOMMENDATION **2.2.6** Policies should stipulate that all staff attend a mandatory fire lecture at least once a year. There should be a register of attendance, signed by participants.

RECOMMENDATION **2.2.7** Alarm testing should be carried out weekly in line with local policy.

RECOMMENDATION **2.2.8** There must be a well-developed procedure for evacuation and this should be part of the induction course for newly appointed staff. The evacuation procedure should be displayed within the department.

Evacuation procedures for patients and staff should be practised not less than once per year.

Potential fire hazards

ALCOHOL SKIN PREPARATION

RECOMMENDATION **2.2.9** Alcohol-based skin preparations are known to be flammable (MDA 2000, HMSO 2002a). A risk assessment should be undertaken for the use and application of alcohol-based skin preparations.

RECOMMENDATION **2.2.10** The quantity of flammable fluid used to prepare the skin should be kept to a minimum in order to avoid run-off and pooling, either on or around the patient. Precautions should be taken to prevent pooling underneath drapes or in the patient's umbilicus.

RECOMMENDATION **2.2.11** The size of sponge applicators used for painting the skin should be reviewed. Some sponges can absorb up to 250–300ml. Use of this volume will almost certainly lead to run-off.

RECOMMENDATION **2.2.12** Any run-off that occurs should be contained by absorbent material placed around the patient which is removed before the drapes are applied.

RECOMMENDATION **2.2.13** Time should be allowed for the alcohol to evaporate and disperse prior to applying the drapes.

RECOMMENDATION 2.2.14 Care should be taken in using sprays with flammable propellants such as butane when electrosurgery is planned.

MONOPOLAR ELECTROCAUTERY

Electrosurgery units use a high frequency alternating electrical current for cutting and coagulation. They are the main potential ignition source for a fire.

RECOMMENDATION 2.2.15 Electrosurgery can produce a high temperature electrical arc if carbonised tissue is allowed to build up on the tip of the electrosurgery device. It is recommended that an electrocautery tip cleaner is applied to remove the build-up of carbonised tissue.

- The active electrode should be stored securely in a non-conductive container when not in use.
- The active electrode should be activated only by the person holding the device.
- Active electrodes should not be used in the presence of flammable substances, including antimicrobial skin preparations, and tinctures.
- The active electrode should not be used in the presence of intestinal gases, as these contain hydrogen and methane which are highly flammable.

RECOMMENDATION 2.2.16 A risk assessment should be undertaken for head and neck operations, where there may be an oxygen enriched atmosphere underneath the drapes. The use of electrodiathermy with tracheostomy may cause a fire hazard. In this procedure diathermy is best avoided, as recommended by the British Association of Otorhinolaryngologists.

RECOMMENDATION 2.2.17 Theatre staff should be aware that an airway fire may occur during tracheostomy. It is recommended that a bowl of saline is available on the surgical instrument trolley at all times and a carbon dioxide fire extinguisher is available.

RECOMMENDATION 2.2.18 The power setting for the electrosurgery unit should be verbally confirmed between the operator and the user prior to activation.

LASER

All lasers currently used in surgery are thermal lasers which create a very high temperature to vaporise tissue. Adequate precautions are therefore essential to prevent the risk of fire.

RECOMMENDATION 2.2.19 A carbon dioxide fire extinguisher must be available in theatre at all times and staff must have received training in its use.

RECOMMENDATION 2.2.20 Prior to the surgical procedure, the laser should be tested to ensure that the aiming of the beams are aligned.

RECOMMENDATION 2.2.21 Anaesthetic gases will support combustion, therefore an effective anaesthetic scavenging system must be in place. Non-flammable endotracheal intubation tubes should be used where there is a risk of damage from laser radiation (BSI 1995). Such tubes should be considered mandatory for head and neck surgery.

RECOMMENDATION 2.2.22 Non-flammable skin preparation fluids must be used. (Betadine, whilst non-flammable, will give off toxic fumes if the laser is fired into a pool of solution.)

- Particular care must be taken as there is potential risk of setting fire to the surgical drapes. Close observation of clinical drapes during the laser procedure is critical. Draping materials should have non-flammable properties.

FIBREOPTIC LIGHT SOURCES OR CABLES

RECOMMENDATION **2.2.23** Light sources can generate sufficient energy to melt, scorch or become an ignition source, especially when placed on patient drapes.

- The light cable should be contained securely, away from the patient's drapes whenever reasonably practicable.
- The light source should be placed on standby mode when not in use.

2.3 MANAGEMENT OF CLINICAL WASTE

STANDARD All clinical and non-clinical waste generated within the perioperative setting is managed safely. Waste is segregated and disposed of in accordance with local policy. Policy reflects the requirements of all government agencies that are involved in co-ordinating the safe and effective management of clinical waste disposal.

INTRODUCTION

A large quantity of both clinical and non-clinical waste is generated on a regular basis within the perioperative setting. This in turn has environmental and financial implications in relation to the need for safe and effective disposal, although most clinical waste is disposed of by incineration in specifically designated sites. There are a number of government bodies that have an input into clinical waste disposal. These are the Health and Safety Executive (HSE), the Environment Agency and, in Scotland, the Scottish Environment Protection Agency (SEPA). These agencies enforce and regulate the different laws that apply to the disposal of clinical waste.

Clinical waste is defined under the *Controlled Waste Regulations* (HMSO 1992b) as any waste which consists wholly or partly of:

- human or animal tissue
- blood or other body fluids
- excretions
- drugs or other pharmaceutical products
- swabs or dressings
- syringes, needles or other sharp instruments

which, unless rendered safe, may prove hazardous to any person coming into contact with it.

It could also be any other waste arising from medical, nursing, dental, veterinary, pharmaceutical or similar practice, investigation, treatment, care, teaching or research, or the collection of blood for transfusion, being waste which may cause infection to any person coming into contact with it.

Clinical waste is divided into five categories.

- **Category A** Identifiable human tissue, blood, and other tissue from hospitals or laboratories, surgical dressings or swabs or other similar soiled waste, and other waste such as that generated in infectious cases and not covered in categories B–E.
- **Category B** Contaminated sharp instruments or items such as broken glass, discarded syringes and needles.
- **Category C** Potentially infected waste such as microbiological waste from pathology or other laboratories.
- **Category D** Pharmaceutical products including drugs.
- **Category E** Any items which are used to dispose of urine, faeces and other body fluids that are not included in Category A, such as disposable bedpans, liners, incontinence pads, stoma bags and urine containers.

Waste can be segregated into different coloured bags and containers as follows:

- **Yellow bags** can be used for Category A waste. However, some areas (particularly in Scotland) use orange bags for waste that is sent for heat treatment prior to disposal.
- **Yellow bags with black stripes** can be used for Category E waste that is suitable for landfill disposal.
- **Blue bags** or bags with blue writing can be used for waste that requires autoclaving prior to disposal.
- **Black bags** can be used for non-clinical and household waste.

Aerosol sprays and other types of pressurised containers also need to be considered as clinical waste. Due to the potential risks of explosion and subsequent leakage of contents such as flammable liquids or prescription drugs, they cannot be incinerated. Therefore, a separate container specifically for aerosols needs to be available and an alternative method of disposal found.

Clinical waste from the perioperative setting can potentially contain all of the above categories of waste, therefore robust waste management policies and risk assessment policies need to be in place in order to comply with legislation.

RISK ASSESSMENT AND HEALTH AND SAFETY LEGISLATION

As a result of the Health and Safety at Work Act (HMSO 1974) employers are required to have safe systems of work. Risk assessment is part of this process, the purpose of which is to identify and address actual or potential risks in order to minimise risk within the workplace. This may include the provision of personal protective equipment or clothing which is intended to reduce the potential for contamination of any individual who handles waste from the perioperative setting.

Recommendations from the risk assessment process should be incorporated into the waste management policy. This in turn can be identified as the provision of a safe system of work. All staff who dispose of waste have a responsibility to ensure that their actions are in accordance with the waste management policy.

RECOMMENDATIONS FOR LOCAL POLICY

RECOMMENDATION **2.3.1** Clinical waste, other than sharps and fluids, should be placed in yellow bags, and clearly labelled as 'clinical waste for incineration'. These bags must conform to the NHS supplies standard. The waste should then be placed in suitable rigid containers. These containers need to store waste without spillage and, if they are a reusable item, it must be possible to adequately clean and if necessary disinfect these containers. These containers should also incorporate a facility where the lid can be opened without the need to lift it by hand.

RECOMMENDATION **2.3.2** Clinical waste bags should only be filled to three quarters of capacity, to ensure each bag can be adequately closed. The neck of the bag should be gathered and then twisted prior to being turned over and sealed with a cable tie, a process identified as 'swan neck'. Alternatively, a specific heat sealing device designated for clinical waste may be used. Staples are not a suitable closure for clinical waste bags.

All clinical waste should be clearly labelled with its point of origin.

RECOMMENDATION **2.3.3** All sharps containers should conform to the British Standard (BS) 7320. Faulty collection containers must be identified and removed from service until the fault has been rectified.

Sharps disposal boxes should be placed in suitable positions to ensure easy placement of contaminated items. Sharps containers should not be placed in an area where visitors (particularly young visitors) can access the contents.

Sharps disposal boxes should not be filled more than three quarters full and should be of a design that allows them to be locked after sealing. In the event that it may take some time for the container to be filled quickly, advice should be sought from the infection control nurse regarding the potential infection risks from the container.

RECOMMENDATION **2.3.4** Body fluids should not be tipped into clinical waste bags. They should be sealed in leak proof containers and placed in rigid boxes that are clearly marked as clinical waste.

Some perioperative settings allow black bags to be used for non-clinical waste such as tray wrappings and other types of product packaging, providing that the bag is removed from the preparation area prior to the start of a case. This is to ensure that the bag cannot become contaminated.

RECOMMENDATION **2.3.5** There should be adequate waste containers in a designated 'dirty' area. This area must be kept locked at all times in order to prevent unauthorised access to contaminated substances. Waste from a perioperative setting should be removed without being transported through clean areas. The design and layout of theatres should incorporate this requirement.

RECOMMENDATION **2.3.6** Consideration needs to be given to the number of times that waste is uplifted from these containers. Personnel involved in this process must be provided with suitable training and personal protective equipment or clothing.

RECOMMENDATION **2.3.7** Waste contractors should collect clinical waste from the main waste storage areas and transport it to the designated incinerators in accordance with the relevant legislation.

2.4 CONTROL OF WASTE ANAESTHETIC GASES

STANDARD Statutory recommendations and guidance as provided by the *Control of Substances Hazardous to Health Regulations* are observed. The potential risks of waste and anaesthetic gases in the perioperative setting are assessed and managed.

INTRODUCTION

All employers and health workers have responsibilities under the regulations relating to the control of substances hazardous to health (HMSO 2002a, Health and Safety Commission 1999, 2002). The perioperative practitioner should be specifically alert to the statutory need to ensure that the regulations are implemented and adhered to within the perioperative setting.

Occupational exposure limits

What are the waste anaesthetic gases and the current occupational exposure limits (OELs)?

- Nitrous oxide = 100 parts per million (ppm)
- Enflurane = 50ppm
- Isoflurane = 50ppm
- Halothane = 10ppm

Currently there are no OELs for sevoflurane or desflurane.

Research by Hoerauf et al (1999) suggests that:

- exposure to even low concentrations of waste anaesthetic gases may increase the risk of foetal genetic damage by an amount comparable to smoking 11–20 cigarettes a day – whether this may lead to increased morbidity remains unclear
- the highest levels of pollution in paediatric anaesthesia occur at induction, but with good air conditioning the OEL levels quickly return to normal
- using a laryngeal mask airway in patients undergoing ventilation is not necessarily associated with high concentrations of waste gases, providing the air conditioning is running at 20 air changes per hour
- during cardiopulmonary bypass, where gas outlet ports on membrane oxygenators are not routinely connected to exhaust systems, the routine use of scavenging is recommended.

RECOMMENDATIONS FOR LOCAL POLICY

Risk assessment

RECOMMENDATION **2.4.1** Every theatre department should undertake a comprehensive risk assessment, under COSHH regulations, for anaesthetic gases.

RECOMMENDATION **2.4.2** A COSHH safety co-ordinator should be appointed within the department to co-ordinate the risk assessment. The employer is responsible for ensuring the co-ordinator receives appropriate training for this role.

RECOMMENDATION **2.4.3** Samples from the employees' breathing zones must be checked to ensure that occupational exposure limits are not exceeded (*Approved Code of Practice*, Regulation 10 – HSC 1999).

Annual review is required even if significant changes in practice are made.

Ventilation and gas scavenging

RECOMMENDATION **2.4.4** Ventilation and anaesthetic gas scavenging systems should be implemented to ensure a safer environment for staff.

RECOMMENDATION **2.4.5** Requirements are laid down in *Health Technical Memorandum* (HTM) *2025* (NHS Estates 2000). Air must be filtered through a series of filters in the ductwork and delivered, under positive pressure, to the theatres at a suitable temperature and humidity.

The estates department should be contacted if the theatre temperature or humidity reading is incorrect.

RECOMMENDATION **2.4.6** Routine inspection and maintenance is required at least every half year and annual bacteriological sampling is required for ultra-clean ventilated theatres.

RECOMMENDATION **2.4.7** Successful ventilation relies on having theatre doors closed, so if the doors are propped open the system cannot work. The baffles in theatres are in place to balance the air pressures and ensure correct air flows, with air moving from the cleanest areas (prep room and theatre) to the outside areas.

RECOMMENDATION **2.4.8** The scavenging systems must be checked at least every 14 months.

RECOMMENDATION **2.4.9** The system must conform to BS 6834 (1987) and must be in situ wherever nitrous oxide is used in anaesthetic procedures. Both require proper records to be maintained.

Managing the risk

RECOMMENDATION **2.4.10** The Occupational Safety and Health Administration (OSHA) in the USA states that the symptoms of exposure to waste anaesthetic gases include nausea, dizziness, headaches, fatigue and irritability. If a staff member reports any of these symptoms they should be referred to the occupational health department immediately.

RECOMMENDATION **2.4.11** A fume cupboard should be used to refill vaporisers, and this should be done at the end of the operating list.

RECOMMENDATION **2.4.12** There should be a planned service routine for vaporisers.

RECOMMENDATION **2.4.13** Anaesthetic equipment should fit the patient correctly (eg: face masks for children).

RECOMMENDATION **2.4.14** Gases should only be operated during anaesthesia. Gases should be turned on before induction and turned off on the completion of anaesthetic.

RECOMMENDATION **2.4.15** The connection of the scavenging system should be checked prior to any anaesthetic administration to ensure that it is correct.

RECOMMENDATION **2.4.16** A system should be in place for monitoring potential pollution from waste anaesthetic gases. There are two methods:

- Infrared spectrophotometry which measures concentrations of pollution and leaks in scavenging systems
- Personal sampling for staff (ie: monitors worn by those most at risk).

RECOMMENDATION **2.4.17** Staff should be educated about the risks of anaesthetic gases and must be familiar with the manufacturer's medical gas data sheets.

Post-anaesthetic care

Anaesthetic gases are exhaled by patients in the recovery area. The gases are virtually unchanged and initially are at very high levels. Recovery staff work in close proximity to the patients' heads, and gas concentrations can exceed those found in scavenged theatre areas.

RECOMMENDATION **2.4.18** It is recommended that recovery staff are aware of:

- the importance of ventilation systems being in proper working order
- the importance of education programmes
- the need to perform air sampling accurately and during an operating list (not during a non-working period).

RECOMMENDATION **2.4.19** It is also recommended that recovery staff review regularly:

- new systems for recovery scavenging
- the sampling methodology, to ensure that waste anaesthetic gas levels are measured accurately at the point representing the breathing zone of the carer
- the use of personal monitoring devices
- staff rotation methods.

Websites to visit

You may find these websites useful:

- gasnet.med.yale.edu
- www.itl.co.uk
- www.piezoptic
- www.osha-slc.gov/SLTC/wasteanestheticgases
- www.shawcity.co.uk

2.5 DISPOSAL OF SURGICALLY EXPLANTED ITEMS

STANDARD There is a written policy outlining the disposal of human tissue and explanted items.

Returning surgically removed human tissue, such as gallstones and calculi and explanted items, to the patient following surgery has been common practice in most operating departments throughout the UK. The items are usually decontaminated by manual cleaning. Explanted items such as plates and screws are sterilised in a bench top steriliser within the theatre department, or are sent to the central sterile supplies unit for decontamination, before being returned to the patient. This practice raises health and safety issues that a hospital organisation must address by having a written policy detailing the management of the disposal of surgically removed human tissue and explanted items.

Surgically removed human tissue and explanted items include:

- bone fragments
- foreign bodies
- Kirschner wires and pins
- nails, plates and screws
- stones and calculi
- teeth.

RECOMMENDATIONS FOR LOCAL POLICY

RECOMMENDATION **2.5.1** A written policy should be formulated detailing how the operating department manages the disposal of human tissue and explanted items safely. The policy must minimise the risk of contamination arising from ineffective decontamination processes.

RECOMMENDATION **2.5.2** Advice should be taken from the risk manager, infection control nurse, sterile services manager, trust legal team and the organisations decontamination lead.

RECOMMENDATION **2.5.3** The policy should identify how human tissue and explanted items should be handled in the perioperative setting.

RECOMMENDATION **2.5.4** A risk assessment must be undertaken on each individual prosthesis to be returned to the patient. This includes Kirschner wires, pins, or interlocking nails which are particularly hazardous sharp devices and present a risk to the practitioner undertaking the decontamination process. It is recommended that these devices are disposed of in a suitable clinical waste container in accordance with local clinical waste policy.

RECOMMENDATION **2.5.5** The risk assessment should determine whether the prosthesis could be decontaminated effectively and any bio-burden effectively removed. This may prove very difficult with implants that have become impacted with bone tissue (eg: internal fixation plates). The presence of any organic material will inhibit the sterilisation process. If material cannot be removed then effective decontamination and sterility cannot be guaranteed. Due to the potential risk of contamination such devices should not be returned to the patient.

RECOMMENDATION **2.5.6** Guidance from the Department of Health (NHS Estates 2001) is that local decontamination is no longer acceptable. Explanted items should be decontaminated through an automated washing method rather than a manual cleaning process. This will protect the worker from potential exposure to harmful microorganisms and aerosol contamination, which may occur as a direct result of manual cleaning. It is therefore recommended that such devices should be sent to a central sterile supplies unit for decontamination.

RECOMMENDATION **2.5.7** Where bench top sterilisers are still in operation within the theatre department it is important that a risk assessment is undertaken to identify the type of prosthesis which is suitable for this sterilisation process. Non-vacuum bench top sterilisers in which air is passively displaced by steam are suitable only for processing devices that are not wrapped or hollow. This method of decontamination should not be used for prosthesis with contain lumens such as cannulated screws, as sterility is not guaranteed. Porous load sterilisers located in the central sterile supplies unit achieve sterilisation by dry saturated steam under pressure and are therefore suitable for the decontamination of explanted items such as prosthesis, which contain a lumen.

RECOMMENDATION **2.5.8** There must be a documented system in place for identifying that the explanted item has been decontaminated and sterilised appropriately. One of the implications of the Consumer Protection Act (HMSO 1987) for re-processing is that hospital organisations must be able to demonstrate how the device was processed, which method was used, and who was responsible for managing the process. This is so that the patient is not supplied with a contaminated device which might pose a potential risk.

RECOMMENDATION **2.5.9** The policy should identify the method of containment for human tissue and explanted items.

RECOMMENDATION **2.5.10** It is recommended that, in the absence of an adequate tracking and traceability system, explanted items should not be returned to the patient. *Health Technical Memorandum 2010* (NHS Estates 1994) explains the specific responsibilities of the user of the steriliser, and this includes management of a tracking system for processed devices.

RECOMMENDATION **2.5.11** The patient should sign a disclaimer accepting responsibility when human tissue and explanted items are returned. Both human tissue and explanted items would be classed as clinical waste and therefore should be disposed of appropriately as according to the recommendations of the Environment Protection Act (HMSO 1990b). The disclaimer should indicate that the patient will adhere to the regulations of the Environment Protection Act and remove the liability of the hospital.

2.6 LASERS

STANDARD There is a system in place for the management of laser safety to minimise the risks to patients and staff within the perioperative setting.

INTRODUCTION

The development of medical lasers has revolutionised surgery. Many different types of lasers are used routinely in the operating department for a wide range of procedures. Since the Medical Devices Agency *Guidelines on Laser Safety* (MDA 1996), more sophisticated lasers have been introduced. However the guidelines on the safety aspects have not changed. The technical detail on classification has changed, but this is not relevant to the user. Each laser may require different operational techniques and the associated hazards may vary. It is therefore essential that the particular manufacturer's instructions and recommendations are adhered to at all times. Policies and procedures must be developed in conjunction with the *Risk and Quality Management System* (NATN 2002a).

What is a laser?

The word **LASER** is an acronym of the process in which high energy light is created.

Light

Amplification (by)

Stimulated

Emission (of)

Radiation

In this instance, the term radiation applies to light energy only (non-ionising radiation). Laser light is formed when an electron in a lasting medium (usually gas or crystal) is stimulated to produce particles of light. This stimulation is brought about by the application of energy.

THE PROPERTIES OF LASERS

A laser beam is collimated, spatially coherent and monochromatic.

Collimation

Laser light can be thought of as a parallel beam of light which is highly directional. This property makes lasers very accurate aiming devices. In theory the collimated laser light travels into infinity, and this demands safety precautions to prevent accidents and injury.

Spatial coherence

Ordinary light travels in random waves. In contrast, laser light features waves that are in harmony (in phase). Particles of laser light leave the source and travel in harmonised wave forms, arriving at the target tissue at the same moment. This produces a more concentrated form of light than ordinary light.

Monochromatic light

Lasers usually produce light of one colour. Some lasers produce a single green laser light while carbon dioxide lasers produce a single band of infrared light. It is important to remember that laser light is not always visible and care should be taken accordingly. The exception to this rule of monochromatic light is the argon laser which may have up to eleven different colours. In the surgical argon laser there are two bands – blue and green.

Laser classification

Lasers and laser systems are assigned one of the four broad classes (1 to 4) depending on the potential for causing damage.

- **Class 1:** 'Safe' if not disassembled (eg: laser printers, CD-ROM players/drives).
- **Class 2:** May exceed class 1 exposure limits if viewed for more than 0.25 seconds (aversion respond time), but still does not pose a significant eye hazard (eg: supermarket scanners).
- **Class 3a:** Eye hazard if viewed using collecting optics (eg: telescopes, microscopes, or binoculars).
- **Class 3b:** Eye hazards if beams are viewed directly or specular reflections are viewed.
- **Class 4:** Eye hazards if beams are viewed directly or specular reflections – and sometimes even diffuse reflections – are viewed. Also skin burns from direct beam exposure.

Most surgical lasers are in class 3B or 4 (0.5W to 100W power output).

RECOMMENDATIONS FOR LOCAL POLICY

Potential hazards associated with lasers

EYE HAZARDS

RECOMMENDATION **2.6.1** Laser light can strike the cornea of the eye causing vaporisation and possible destruction to the outer layer. Laser light may also pass through the cornea, be focused by the lens and destroy the retina. When lasers are in use, laser safety eyewear must be worn. Protective eyewear is laser specific, and it must be of the appropriate optical density and wavelength. It is essential therefore that the correct eye protection is used by staff and patients at all times. Eyewear must be labelled with the appropriate optical density.

RECOMMENDATION **2.6.2** Surgical instruments should have a non-reflective surface and should be blackened to reduce the potential risk of reflection of the laser beam. Such instruments should be inspected regularly to ensure the integrity of the coating.

RECOMMENDATION **2.6.3** Personal protective equipment (PPE) regulations (HMSO 1992c) state that the correct goggles/glasses must be used for protection. The glasses will state which type of wavelength and optical density they are designed to filter out. One pair of eye protectors cannot be used for all lasers, the glasses are specific to each type of laser.

SKIN HAZARDS – HANDS AND FACE

RECOMMENDATION **2.6.4** Exposure to ultra violet light can cause pathological effects such as erythema, skin aging, pigmentation, photosensitive reactions, and risks of carcinoma. To avoid accidental injury it is essential that clear communication is maintained at all times between the surgeon and the team when lasers are in use. There should therefore be a strict procedure for communicating with the laser operator (surgeon), via the scrub practitioner, which must be adhered to at all times.

CHEMICAL HAZARDS

Chemical hazards from lasers include infective agents in laser plume (smoke). All thermal instruments used in surgery produce smoke. It is possible that infective agents can be present in the laser plume. These may be a potential risk to staff.

RECOMMENDATION **2.6.5** Dedicated smoke evacuation machines must be used to remove the smoke, and the smoke evacuation filters should be checked and changed as per the manufacturer's recommendations. The collection device should be placed as near as possible to the point where the plume is produced.

RECOMMENDATION **2.6.6** Piped hospital suction apparatus must not be used for smoke evacuation, and portable suction units are not suitable.

RECOMMENDATION **2.6.7** High-filtration surgical masks for laser use should be worn during procedures that produce plume to minimise inhalation of the larger carbonaceous particles.

ELECTRICAL HAZARDS

RECOMMENDATION **2.6.8** All laser equipment should adhere to British Safety standard BS EN 60825-1 (BSI 1994a) and where relevant BS EN 60601-2-22 (BSI 1993). If manufactured after June 1996, the equipment should have the European manufacturing standard CE mark on it.

RECOMMENDATION **2.6.9** Inspection should be carried out by the organisation's nominated medical electronics officer, prior to planning and installation.

EXPLOSION AND FIRE HAZARDS

RECOMMENDATION **2.6.10** Flask tube beam systems can shatter or explode if dropped or accidentally hit. Gas tubing carrying inflammable gases must be protected from the laser light.

RECOMMENDATION **2.6.11** Patient airways such as endotracheal tubes need to be protected by metallised taping or the use of metal tube.

General standards to protect patients and staff

PATIENT SAFETY ISSUES

RECOMMENDATION **2.6.12** Laser procedures and precautions should be explained to patients preoperatively and the details recorded in the patient care plan.

RECOMMENDATION **2.6.13** When thermally intensive lasers are being used, exposed tissues around the surgical site should be protected with saline-saturated or water-saturated materials. These materials should be remoistened periodically to ensure that they do not dry out and become a source for ignition.

RECOMMENDATION **2.6.14** Appropriate guards should be used during laser surgery to prevent the laser beam from marking normal tissue.

RECOMMENDATION **2.6.15** During local anaesthetic, a patient's eyes and eyelids must be protected from the laser beam by goggles designated for the type of laser being used. During a general anaesthetic, wet eye pads or laser specific corneal eye shields should be used (BS EN 207 and 208) (BSI 1994b).

STAFF SAFETY ISSUES

RECOMMENDATION **2.6.16** Any staff member who will be involved in surgical procedures involving a laser must have undertaken a training programme and have been assessed as having the knowledge and skills to participate in the use of the equipment. The individual practitioner must acknowledge their competence to participate and this should be recorded in their personal portfolio/personnel file.

RECOMMENDATION **2.6.17** For each specific laser in an operating department, authorised operators and safety officers must be clearly identified within the local policy. These individuals will carry total responsibility for security of the laser keys and safe practice for that area of care. Where the laser is to be used it is essential to have a 'laser controlled area'.

RECOMMENDATION **2.6.18** When the laser is in use it is essential to:

- restrict access to the laser theatre
- reduce the number of people present in the theatre
- use warning signs and lights as indications of laser in use.

These should be used at all entrances to laser treatment areas when in use.

RECOMMENDATION **2.6.19** The laser foot switch should be placed in a position convenient to the operator, thereby reducing unintended activation of the laser beam and potential injury to the patient, operator or staff.

RECOMMENDATION **2.6.20** Window coverings must be non-flammable and should reduce transmission to below the maximum permissible exposure. When class 3B and 4 lasers are in use a remote interlock facility (BS EN 60825-1) should be incorporated. When not in active use, lasers should be placed in a standby mode. This is not always possible however, reinforcing the need for restricted access.

MAINTENANCE AND INSPECTION

RECOMMENDATION **2.6.21** There should be a planned preventative maintenance programme in place for all laser equipment. This should include calibration of power output checks.

RECOMMENDATION **2.6.22** Before use, the operator should perform a visual inspection of the integrity of all electrical components, including mains, foot switch connector and power cable prior to activating the laser system.

RECOMMENDATION **2.6.23** When not in use, the laser must be kept in a secure place. The keys should be kept in a locked cupboard. A register of the laser key issue must be maintained. Only recognised operators and user staff are allowed access to the key. A laser log book must be updated each time the laser is used with specific records of laser operations, surgical procedure and personnel present in the area of care. This information should also be entered into the patient's notes.

RECOMMENDATION **2.6.24** All laser incidents/accidents should be recorded on a special incident/accident form and reported to the unit laser safety officer/supervisor, who in turn will notify the regional laser safety protection advisor. Laser incidents must also be reported in accordance with local incident/accident policies.

RECOMMENDATION **2.6.25** Occupational health and surveillance, in particular ophthalmic examination of personnel participating in the use of lasers, is recommended (BS EN 60825-1).

Obligation of the employer with regard to health and safety at work

RECOMMENDATION **2.6.26** The legislation identified in the Health and Safety at Work Act (HMSO 1974) places a duty on the employers to maintain a working environment for employees that is as safe as is reasonably practicable. This duty extends to incorporate the environment, safe equipment, and safe systems of work as well as providing the necessary education, training and supervision to ensure safe working practices.

RECOMMENDATION **2.6.27** A duty of care is also to be extended to visitors and patients. It is recommended that a laser safety committee is in operation to audit standards for effective laser use. The laser committee should include:

- the laser safety officer/supervisor
- operating manager
- laser surgeon
- anaesthetist
- occupational health representative
- biomedical/medical physics engineer.

RECOMMENDATION **2.6.28** There should be a register of authorised users (for class 3B and 4 lasers) which should be maintained by the designated laser protection advisor. The laser protection advisor is responsible for undertaking risk assessments and ensuring that policy is being complied with.

RECOMMENDATION **2.6.29** Employees have a duty to consider their own role and contribution in maintaining a safe working environment, and are required to exercise reasonable care in maintaining the safety of the working environment, for themselves and for those who may be affected by their practice (colleagues, visitors and patients).

RECOMMENDATION **2.6.30** Employees are also required to co-operate with the reasonable instructions of their employer to secure and maintain a safe working environment.

2.7 MOBILE PHONES

STANDARD There is a system in place that prevents the use of mobile phones within the perioperative setting.

There is considerable evidence to suggest that a mobile or cell phone increases the potential for electromagnetic interference with medical devices, especially at short range, thereby placing patients at risk. This risk exists because mobile phones are low power devices that emit and receive radio waves which connect each phone to a network of base stations, so that users can make and receive calls. Radio signals emitted by mobile phone systems can interfere with sensitive electronic equipment such as monitors, ventilators, infusion pumps, pulse oximeters and defibrillators.

The Medical Devices Agency (MDA) discovered that 4% of medical devices suffered electromagnetic interference from digital mobile phones at a distance of one metre. This was confirmed by research undertaken in the USA by Tri et al (2001) which indicated that mobile phones interfered with the signal on monitors such as electrocardiographs. It was due to this research that the MDA issued two safety notices, MDA SN 9706 and MDA DB 9702 (MDA 1997a, b), giving clear guidance on how to reduce the risks.

RECOMMENDATIONS FOR LOCAL POLICY

RECOMMENDATION **2.7.1** In the interests of patient safety it is recommended that mobile phones are not used in the perioperative environment.

RECOMMENDATION **2.7.2** Signage indicating that mobile phones are not permitted should be placed at all key entrances to the operating department.

RECOMMENDATION **2.7.3** Mobile phones should be switched off and not left on standby or silent mode.

RECOMMENDATION **2.7.4** Perioperative personnel should be made aware of the risks of electromagnetic interference with medical devices.

RECOMMENDATION **2.7.5** An organisational policy should be in place for mobile phone use. The policy should designate a safe area for the use of mobile phones, such as a non-clinical area where clinical activity does not take place and where there is little likelihood of interference with medical devices.

In the formulation of a policy, advice should be taken from the health and safety officer or risk manager and the telecommunications advisor.

2.8 HANDLING OF PATIENTS WITH BODY PIERCING

STANDARD There is a system in place for the safe handling and management of surgical patients with body piercing. Staff are aware of different types of body piercing and safe techniques for removal.

Body piercing has become increasingly popular in recent years, particularly amongst young adults and adolescents. It is essential that all perioperative personnel have an understanding of the principles of safe practice for surgical patients with body piercing.

RECOMMENDATIONS FOR LOCAL POLICY

General considerations

The following considerations will give perioperative staff guidelines for the handling of the issue of body piercing for both elective and emergency surgery.

RECOMMENDATION **2.8.1** Pieces of jewellery are often different in construction and content. Each patient must therefore be assessed accordingly with reference to the type of anaesthetic to be administered and the type of surgery to be performed.

RECOMMENDATION **2.8.2** Piercings are a form of self expression and it is the responsibility of all perioperative staff not to criticise or pass any judgement on this issue.

RECOMMENDATION **2.8.3** If it cannot be removed, then the jewellery must be taped, especially if the piercing is at risk of being caught or ripped out by ECG leads, surgical drapes, surgical instruments or towel clips.

RECOMMENDATION **2.8.4** The jewellery must be removed, or covered and secured with tape, if the piercing causes any risk of pressure. For example, chin or lip piercing may cause damage to soft tissue from the pressure of an anaesthetic mask, or nipple piercing may cause pressure if the patient is to lie prone.

RECOMMENDATION **2.8.5** The piercing must be removed if it is in close proximity to the surgical site or any other associated procedure (Faulkner 1999).

RECOMMENDATION **2.8.6** If part of the piercing remains within the body tissue, antiseptic cover cannot be guaranteed.

Tongue and lip piercing

RECOMMENDATION **2.8.7** All tongue and lip jewellery should be removed before a general anaesthetic. Tongue barbells may cause obstruction of the airway during induction and maintenance of general anaesthesia. Tongue labrets can contain a gemstone which is at risk of falling out and entering the airway, as gemstones are only glued in. If the patient refuses to remove the piercing this should be documented in the patient's notes.

Other body areas

RECOMMENDATION **2.8.8** Other areas of the body where jewellery and piercing must be removed include the nasal septum, nose or ear piercing for ENT surgery.

RECOMMENDATION **2.8.9** Navel piercing should be removed for laparoscopic surgery. This can be achieved by pushing the ball out to remove the ring.

RECOMMENDATION **2.8.10** Genital piercing does not have to be removed if the surgical procedure is elsewhere on the body.

- **Male genital piercing** Penile piercing can be pulled to one side if the patient requires a urinary catheter and therefore does not need to be removed.
- **Female genital piercing** The site of the piercing should be assessed for surgical access and removed if it is likely to hinder the type of surgery to be performed.

RECOMMENDATION **2.8.11** If there are signs of infected inflammation around the piercing site the jewellery should be removed as it is a focus for infection and may require appropriate treatment before surgery takes place.

Security

RECOMMENDATION **2.8.12** If a body piercing is removed whilst in the operating theatre it must be placed in a property envelope and held in a secure place as per local policy. The envelope should be checked and witnessed by two practitioners and either returned to the ward or the department where the patient came from. If out of hours, the envelope should be placed in the hospital's general office safe for safe keeping.

RECOMMENDATION **2.8.13** Jewellery must not be taped to the patient's clothing or kept within the department when the patient has returned to the ward area.

Body piercing remaining in situ

RECOMMENDATION **2.8.14** The site and type of body piercing should be documented on the preoperative checklist by the ward staff and on the theatre care plan by the theatre practitioner checking the patient into theatre.

RECOMMENDATION **2.8.15** Depending on the location of the piercing, a check must be made postoperatively to ensure that the body piercing is still in situ and is documented as such on the anaesthetic chart and the theatre care plan.

RECOMMENDATION **2.8.16** The electrical conductivity of jewellery poses no significant increase in alternative site burns (ie: those away from the return electrode). The patient's rights must therefore be taken into consideration if they do not wish to remove the body piercing.

2.9 RADIATION PROTECTION

STANDARD Radiation exposure within the perioperative setting is assessed and managed in a way that minimises risk to patients and staff.

Radiation is the propagation of energy through space or matter in the form of waves or particles. In general there are two types of radiation: background or natural radiation and man-made radiation. Medical radiation exposure arises from two classes of radiation: ionising and non-ionising.

Ionising radiation is used in diagnostic radiology, nuclear medicine CT and radiation therapy. Recent developments in radiology have facilitated non-invasive surgical procedures in many specialities. The increase in the number of intraoperative x-rays has raised the potential risk to perioperative staff.

Technological refinements have improved the safety aspects of radiation equipment. In general, most staff are exposed to very low radiation doses. Theatre staff must however be aware that radiation exposure carries a risk and it is essential that staff adhere to the national radiation regulations and policy at all times.

Each hospital should appoint a local radiation protection advisor who must be consulted when a local policy is developed, as well as a local radiation protection officer who will take responsibility within the operating department.

RECOMMENDATIONS FOR LOCAL POLICY

Use of radiation as a method of diagnosis and an aid to surgery

RECOMMENDATION **2.9.1** The employer must ensure that written protocols are in place for every type of standard radiological practice required in the operating theatre.

RECOMMENDATION **2.9.2** All staff have a responsibility to protect themselves and others. They should not knowingly expose themselves or others to radiation more than is necessary. Staff must not stand in the direct primary beam and must maintain a desired distance from the beam, consistent with relevant duties.

RECOMMENDATION **2.9.3** Radiation monitoring should be carried out considering the following:

- Any incident which may have resulted in unforeseen exposure must be reported immediately to the radiation protection officer. A record of persons involved must be documented and the incident outlined. An adverse incident report should be submitted.
- Any defect identified in monitoring equipment must be reported to the radiation protection officer. The equipment must be taken out of circulation and labelled as defective and only returned to circulation after it has been recommissioned.
- Staff working routinely in controlled areas may be issued with personal dose-meters on the advice of the radiation protection officer.
- A single film badge is used to measure the whole body dose. It should be worn on the trunk, at the chest or waist level, underneath protective clothing.
- Where dose-meters are used they should be monitored monthly and documented.
- The results of personal monitoring should be kept at local level by the radiation protection officer and may be inspected by any individual worker before the results are forwarded to the radiation protection advisor.

DOSE

RECOMMENDATION **2.9.4** The radiation dose to patients should be kept as low as is reasonably practicable whilst still providing diagnostic information.

RECOMMENDATION **2.9.5** All exposures should be in accordance with accepted practices, and additional protection should be considered (eg: thyroid, gonadal and ovarian shielding).

A SAFE ENVIRONMENT

RECOMMENDATION **2.9.6** Only authorised personnel who are trained and assessed may use x-ray equipment. It is their responsibility to ensure a safe environment for all patients and staff.

RECOMMENDATION 2.9.7 Any faults identified in the x-ray equipment or safety systems must be documented and reported to the radiation protection officer.

RECOMMENDATION 2.9.8 *'If an employer knows or has reason to believe that an incident has or may have occurred in which a person, while undergoing a medical exposure was, otherwise than as a result of a malfunction or defect in equipment, exposed to ionising radiation to an extent much greater than intended, he shall make an immediate preliminary investigation of the incident and, unless that investigation shows beyond a reasonable doubt that no such overexposure has occurred, he shall forthwith notify the appropriate authority and make or arrange for a detailed investigation of the circumstances of the exposure and an assessment of the dose received'* (HMSO 1999c).

RECOMMENDATION 2.9.9 Following its commissioning, all radiation equipment must be subjected to a planned preventative work programme for which clear documentation is maintained.

PROTECTIVE CLOTHING

RECOMMENDATION 2.9.10 Protective garments, for example lead aprons or gloves, should be:

- uniquely identified with a code in order that faulty equipment may be withdrawn from use
- safeguarded from damage and cleaned after use – it is the responsibility of the user to return the garment in a clean condition and store appropriately
- examined visually at frequent intervals to ensure they remain undamaged. Storage facilities must be available which allow lead aprons to hang freely and singly on appropriate racking. Such garments should not be folded or left on the operating theatre floor. Lead aprons are susceptible to cracking which can reduce the effectiveness as a shielding barrier.

RECOMMENDATION 2.9.11 The radiation protection officer should arrange tests of each protective garment not less than once each year and maintain records accordingly.

RECOMMENDATION 2.9.12 Staff who are required physically to support a patient having radiological investigation must wear specialised protective clothing, for example lead gloves. Discretion is required in assessing the degree of risk to staff when maintaining patient safety and providing support.

RECOMMENDATION 2.9.13 Protective garments should be available and used to prevent undue exposure to harmful rays.

RECOMMENDATION 2.9.14 X-rays to the abdomen and pelvis of patients who are pregnant or may be pregnant should be avoided if possible. A lead shield should be used to protect the foetus when other areas of the body are x-rayed.

PREGNANCY

RECOMMENDATION 2.9.15 Staff who become pregnant must inform their head of department as soon as their pregnancy is known, and should seek advice from the radiation protection officer concerning radiation exposure in controlled areas.

RECOMMENDATION 2.9.16 When x-ray is in use, there is an absolute need to ensure that:

- notices are displayed to inform people that x-ray equipment is in use, thus restricting access to the area
- the theatre team is aware that x-ray procedures are required in order that all relevant equipment is available (eg: x-ray tables and protective clothing)

- leaded shielding is available to personnel who are unable to leave the operating theatre, or who cannot stand more than approximately two metres away from the x-ray source – where lead protective aprons are not available, portable leaded shielding should be available
- personnel are positioned out of the direct line of the primary beam – personnel with protective lead aprons should position themselves behind or to the side of, as far away as possible from, the radiation beam
- personnel do not hold the patient unless absolute necessary – traction devices and sandbags should be available and used to maintain the patient position during radiation exposure
- asepsis is actively promoted when equipment is used in close proximity to the surgical wound
- a safe environment is maintained at all times
- the allergy status of a patient is identified if they are to undergo an x-ray investigation where a radio-opaque contrast medium is used – iodine allergy is potentially life-threatening and resuscitation equipment must be available
- perioperative nursing documentation includes the type of patient protection and the areas protected.

Use of radioactive sources as a method of treatment

RECOMMENDATION **2.9.17** Operating department staff involved in caring for patients who are undergoing treatment using radioactive sources must receive training in these specialist practices and be assessed accordingly.

RECOMMENDATION **2.9.18** A local policy must be in place which identifies the designated individuals with responsibility for safe practice. It is essential to ensure that advice regarding particular incidents is forthcoming immediately (eg: decontamination procedures). Contact telephone numbers of key staff are essential. It is strongly recommended that surgery involving radioactive sources is only undertaken when the radiation protection officer is available.

RECOMMENDATION **2.9.19** Contingency plans should be in place in case the following incidents occur when radioactive sources are in use:

- A patient dies in theatre
- An outbreak of fire
- A loss of, suspected loss of or damage to radioactive sources.

RECOMMENDATION **2.9.20** Since active iridium and gold treatments are infrequently used in theatre, it is recommended that a physicist is present to supervise their use.

DURING SURGERY

RECOMMENDATION **2.9.21** When unsealed radioactive sources are used in surgery, it is recommended that two pairs of surgical gloves are worn to give some protection to the hands.

RECOMMENDATION **2.9.22** If surgical gloves are torn and injury occurs to the hands of the scrubbed person, the injury should be irrigated immediately with tap water, taking care not to wash the contamination into the wound or spread contamination to other areas of the body. The incident should be recorded and the radiation protection officer contacted immediately.

RECOVERY

RECOMMENDATION **2.9.23** Where patients are receiving treatment in recovery with active implants, their beds should be placed a minimum of two metres away from occupied beds. Alternatively the patient may be isolated in a partitioned area away from other patients.

RECOMMENDATION **2.9.24** A notice should be displayed which informs personnel that the patient is receiving treatment with radioactive implants.

RECOMMENDATION **2.9.25** Depending on the radioactivity of implants used, no one practitioner should stay with the patient for more than 30 minutes.

RECOMMENDATION **2.9.26** Staff should seek advice from the regional protection advisor when planning and implementing care of such patients.

MONITORING

RECOMMENDATION **2.9.27** At the end of the operation, staff and equipment (which includes the operating tables and instruments etc), the theatre and the recovery room should be monitored for radioactivity.

Radiological equipment safety

RECOMMENDATION **2.9.28** At each radiological installation the employer should draw up, keep up to date and preserve an inventory of radiological equipment.

The inventory should contain:

- name of manufacturer
- model number
- serial number or other unique identifier
- year of manufacture
- year of installation.

2.10 RISKS TO EXPECTANT MOTHERS

STANDARD The potential risks to the expectant mother in the perioperative setting are assessed and managed.

There are many potential risks to the expectant mother whilst working in the perioperative environment especially within anaesthetics and recovery settings. Hazards include fatigue, manual handling of loads, extremes of temperature, ionising radiation, chemicals, biological hazards, as well as exposure to anaesthetic waste agents.

The evidence of whether exposure to anaesthetic gases can create a risk to health is open to debate, but clinical evidence does indicate a risk to expectant mothers. Early research by

Harrington (1987), Spence (1987) and Monson (1990) found connections between occupational exposure to nitrous oxide and increased rates of spontaneous abortions, low birth weight and congenital defects in operating staff and their offspring. Harrington noted an increased risk for staff working particularly in obstetrics and delivery suites, where higher levels of waste gases were recorded. Hoerauf et al (1997) suggest that:

- exposure to even low concentrations of waste anaesthetic gases may result in an increased risk of foetal genetic damage comparable to smoking 11–20 cigarettes a day – whether this may lead to increased morbidity remains unclear
- the highest levels of pollution in paediatric anaesthesia occur at induction but, with good air conditioning, the occupational exposure limits levels quickly return to normal
- using a laryngeal mask airway in patients undergoing ventilation is not necessarily associated with high concentrations of waste gases, providing the air conditioning is running at 20 air changes per hour
- during cardiopulmonary bypass, where gas outlet ports on membrane oxygenators are not routinely connected to exhaust systems, the routine use of scavenging is recommended.

In 1996 the Department of Health (NHS Executive 1996) published advice on the exposure standards for anaesthetic agents. In certain clinical situations (eg: paediatric, ear, nose and throat procedures), and for the recovery practitioner working close to the patient, exposure levels will be higher. A risk assessment should ensure that the expectant mother is removed from the clinical area in these situations.

RECOMMENDATIONS FOR LOCAL POLICY

Duty of the employee

RECOMMENDATION **2.10.1** As soon as is reasonably practicable, the employee who is an expectant mother has a duty to inform her line manager and occupational health department. This should be confirmed in writing so that the employer can make provision for maternity leave.

Duty of the employer

RECOMMENDATION **2.10.2** The line manager has a responsibility to ensure that potential hazards are assessed by a risk assessment, undertaken in conjunction with the risk manager and the occupational health department. Once the risks are identified, a plan of action must be formulated to ensure that the expectant mother is not exposed to any risks within the workplace. The action plan should be evaluated at frequent intervals to ensure that the working environment is safe. This is a legal requirement (HMSO 1994).

The risk assessment must be specific to the workplace environment where the expectant mother is required to work.

The risk assessment should identify any concerns about potential hazards to which the expectant mother may be exposed, including potential exposure to waste anaesthetic agents.

RECOMMENDATION **2.10.3** If the level of risk is high and cannot be avoided, the employer is legally obliged to provide the expectant mother with suitable alternative work away from any hazards.

RECOMMENDATION **2.10.4** It is recommended that advice is obtained from the local Control of Substances Hazardous to Health (COSHH) advisor as this person will have a record of manufacturing safety data sheets for anaesthetic agents used within the clinical area which are known to be of risk to expectant mothers.

RECOMMENDATION **2.10.5** The Department of Health advise that if scavenging equipment is effective, and concentration levels are contained within recommended levels, then the risk to the pregnant worker is low. It is therefore recommended that all theatres should have local scavenging systems to recover anaesthetic agents, and ventilation systems should be in place to help prevent atmospheric pollution at all times.

RECOMMENDATION **2.10.6** Exposure to waste anaesthetic gases should be avoided, particularly in the first 12 weeks of pregnancy. The available clinical evidence indicates that there is a risk during this period.

Managing the risk

The management of waste anaesthetic gases and exposure to personnel comes under the remit of the *Control of Substances Hazardous to Health Regulations* (HMSO 2002a) which clearly state that employers have a legal obligation to monitor the exposure of employees to substances hazardous to health. *'The employer shall ensure that the exposure of employees to substances hazardous to health is monitored in accordance with a suitable procedure'* (Regulation 10b).

RECOMMENDATION **2.10.7** It is recommended that the risk of leaks of anaesthetic agents can be minimised:

- Use a fume cupboard to refill vaporisers. It is recommended that this is done at the end of the day.
- Ensure that there is a planned service routine for vaporisers.
- Ensure that anaesthetic equipment fits the patient correctly (eg: face masks for children).
- Ensure that gases only flow during anaesthesia, and are turned on before induction and turned off on completion of anaesthetic.
- Check the scavenging system for correct connection prior to anaesthetic administration.

RECOMMENDATION **2.10.8** A system should be in place for monitoring potential pollution from waste anaesthetic gases. There are two methods: infrared spectrophotometry measures concentrations of pollution and leaks in scavenging systems; and personal sampling for staff (ie: monitors worn by those most at risk).

RECOMMENDATION **2.10.9** Anaesthetic gases are exhaled by patients in the recovery area. The gases are virtually unchanged and initially are at very high levels. Recovery staff work in close proximity to the patients' heads and gas concentrations can exceed those found in scavenged theatre areas.

It is recommended that recovery staff are aware of:

- the importance of ventilation systems being in proper working order
- the need to perform air sampling accurately and during an operating list (not during a non-working period) and review regularly
- new systems for recovery scavenging
- the sampling methodology, to ensure that waste anaesthetic gas levels are measured accurately at the point representing the breathing zone of the carer
- the use of personal monitoring devices
- staff rotation methods.

2.11 SAFE HANDLING AND POSITIONING OF PATIENTS

STANDARD There is a system in place for the assessment of safe positioning of the patient in the perioperative setting. The patient's position provides optimum exposure for the operative procedure, access to intravenous lines and access to monitoring devices. Careful attention is given to patient comfort, dignity and safety with regards to circulatory, respiratory, musculoskeletal and neurological structures at all times.

The Health and Safety at Work Act (1974), *Management of Health and Safety at Work Regulations* (HMSO 1992a) and the *Manual Handling Operations Regulations* (HMSO 1992d) impose specific requirements on both employers and employees to avoid, assess and reduce manual handling risks in the workplace.

Manual handling operations have been defined by the Health and Safety Executive (1998a) as *'any transporting or supporting of a load (including the lifting, putting down, pushing, pulling, carrying or moving thereof) by hand or bodily force'.*

In response to the Manual Handling Operations Regulations and subsequent guidance (Health and Safety Executive 1998b), manual handling advisors are now employed by most hospitals, and risk assessments have been performed for most situations. Training in moving and handling is statutory and, over the last few years, great headway has been made in training and a greater emphasis placed on safer handling. Managers and staff have to consider the working environment and plans should be in place for dealing with manual handling situations. Although the principles for moving heavy patients are the same, hospitals should have a policy which takes into account the increased risk.

TILE assessment method

The employer must ensure that an assessment of the task is undertaken with a view to identifying manual handling risks. The **TILE** format can be adapted to suit each individual situation. It considers the safe positioning, limb prepping, equipment moving, handling, and transferring of patients.

TASK – Is it essential? What do you want to achieve? Does it require loads to be held away from the trunk? Does it lead to unnatural positions? Does it involve excessive pushing or pulling? Does it require excessive reaching? Are there sufficient rest or recovery periods?

INDIVIDUAL – including their strength, height, experience, capability and any training required.

LOAD – including the weight, temperature, ease of lifting, stability, attachments, manoeuvrability and any inherent danger.

ENVIRONMENT AND WORK PRACTICES – including space constraints, unstable floors, poor lighting, complex procedures, staff availability and levels of responsibility for change in practice.

It is a legal requirement for employers to undertake a risk assessment. Following an assessment, the employer must take steps to reduce the risk of injury to the lowest level that is reasonably practicable. It may not be possible to eliminate risks entirely within the perioperative setting but the employer and employee must reduce the risks to an acceptable level through the use of aids and by changing practices. For example, if limbs need to be raised for skin preparation, this should be done at the last moment possible.

The Royal College of Nursing introduced a *Code of Practice* (RCN 1993) which recommended that nurses should not lift more than 30kg alone, or 50kg if working in pairs. The *Code of Practice* provides guidelines for positioning the patient in the perioperative setting. The operative procedure, the surgeon's preference and the patient's medical condition will determine the equipment that is required for positioning the patient safely.

The manual handling of patients is a potentially hazardous procedure to both patients and staff. The incidence of manual handling accidents is higher in the health service than in the rest of the working population. Safe patient positioning requires competent skills and an underpinning knowledge of the physiological implications of the patient's position. Therefore no member of the perioperative team, regardless of their designation, should be allowed to take part unsupervised in the positioning of patients until they have received instruction, and have been assessed as proficient in the techniques involved. A record of proficiency in manual handling techniques should be maintained, kept on the individual employee training file and updated annually.

The operating surgeon is ultimately responsible for the safe positioning of the patient and should take an active role in positioning the patient to facilitate the operation.

Safe and appropriate positioning requires teamwork, effective communication and the anticipation of a patient's needs. Subsequent planning will ensure safe and secure positioning with optimal comfort for the patient. Co-ordinated, successful and competent positioning will maximise the safety of the patient, allow adequate exposure of the operating site, and will prevent unnecessary postoperative complications.

RECOMMENDATIONS FOR LOCAL POLICY

Risk assessment for all positioning should be undertaken and understood by all members of the multidisciplinary team.

Preoperative assessment of individual patient needs

RECOMMENDATION **2.11.1** The clinical history of each patient should be known before any positioning takes place, thus allowing individual consideration to be given to:

- the physical condition of the patient, including age, height and weight, skin condition and integrity, nutritional status, pre-existing conditions, physical mobility impairments (prosthesis, implants, range of motion), pressure area risk score – it may be necessary to seek specialist advice, for example from the physiotherapy department
- patient tolerance to the planned position, including the type of anaesthesia and the length of the surgery
- the nature of surgical intervention. This assessment should include the position required in order to optimise exposure of the surgical site for surgery.

RECOMMENDATION 2.11.2 When positioning patients with physical abnormalities, careful consideration is required. For example, no patient should have his or her limbs forced into position; rather a compromise position should be sought.

RECOMMENDATION 2.11.3 It is essential that sufficient members of staff are made available to ensure the safe positioning of individual patients. An inadequate number of personnel can result in patient injury and also may put the employee at risk of injury.

Patient safeguards

RECOMMENDATION 2.11.4 Prior to patient transfer (ideally prior to the patient entering the anaesthetic room) the surgeon, anaesthetist and anaesthetic assistant should be familiar with the operating table and should be happy that it is set up correctly. This is especially important with orthopaedic traction tables.

RECOMMENDATION 2.11.5 It is recommended that patients are anaesthetised prior to positioning to facilitate airway management. Anaesthetised patients must only be moved with the anaesthetist's permission.

RECOMMENDATION 2.11.6 The team leader or scrub practitioner should check with the operating surgeon about the position and positioning equipment required.

RECOMMENDATION 2.11.7 The patient's correct body alignment must be maintained and their extremities and joints supported when moving them, in order to minimise the risk of patient injury. Transfer onto the operating table should be co-ordinated, ensuring that no attachments such as catheters or intravenous drip tubing are caught up. Urinary catheters should be secured and positioned out of the way of the surgical field but available for the anaesthetist to monitor urinary output.

RECOMMENDATION 2.11.8 There should be one person in charge of the transfer, usually the anaesthetist. Transfer should begin on a pre-agreed count or by saying *'ready, steady, move'*.

RECOMMENDATION 2.11.9 Care must be taken at all times during the positioning procedure to avoid friction burns, damage to soft tissue (eg: genitals of males and breasts of females), damage to eyes from intraocular pressure and corneal abrasions, pressure on ears, and nerve damage.

RECOMMENDATION 2.11.10 The required equipment should be in the operating theatre prior to the commencement of patient positioning.

RECOMMENDATION 2.11.11 The patient must be carefully positioned over the operating table breaks, prior to adjustment of the table.

RECOMMENDATION 2.11.12 The patient must not come into contact with any metal part of the operating table in order to reduce the risk of diathermy burns.

RECOMMENDATION 2.11.13 Correct and appropriate padding must be used to protect the patient's veins, nerves and bony prominences from pressure. Local pressure on the globe of the eye should be avoided at all times as raised pressure or globe injury can result in retinal ischaemia or blindness. Corneas should be protected by keeping the eyelids closed using eye pads fit for the purpose and lubricated as necessary. The practice of using tape is not recommended, with the exception of securing an eyepad.

RECOMMENDATION **2.11.14** Patient's limbs, joints and spinal lordoses must be supported with appropriate equipment in order to reduce the risk of postoperative pain.

RECOMMENDATION **2.11.15** At all times the patient's anatomical position must be maintained in order to prevent injury from hyperextension of joints.

RECOMMENDATION **2.11.16** Preventative measures must be taken to reduce the risk of veno-stasis.

RECOMMENDATION **2.11.17** The patient should not be unduly exposed during positioning, to avoid heat loss and to maintain patient dignity.

RECOMMENDATION **2.11.18** Members of the scrub team must avoid leaning against the patient's body/limbs at all times in order to prevent injury to the patient.

RECOMMENDATION **2.11.19** The surgeon should be comfortable during surgery. The operating table should be at the correct height for the surgeon when standing or low enough if operating sitting down.

RECOMMENDATION **2.11.20** Clinical evidence indicates that procedures longer than two to three hours significantly increase the risk for pressure ulcer formation. Consideration should be given to the circulation of the limbs to reduce the risk of thromboembolism, ischaemia or compartment syndrome. External pressure exceeding normal capillary interface pressure (ie: 23–32mm Hg) can cause occlusion that will restrict or block blood flow causing tissue breakdown. In such situations it is recommended that limbs are either moved or massaged during the operation. This particularly applies to patients with their legs raised or compressed by the surgical position such as Lloyd Davies stirrups. Compression stockings or pneumatic compression pumps can be used in thromboembolic prophylaxis.

RECOMMENDATION **2.11.21** The condition of a patient's skin should also be checked following surgery and any changes in condition documented and action taken as required.

Specific considerations for individual positions

The following information should be considered in addition to the recommendations made above.

LITHOTOMY POSITION

RECOMMENDATION **2.11.22** The lithotomy position is used for urological procedures, gynecological procedures involving the perineum and lower gastrointestinal surgery involving the rectum and the anus. The position is often combined with head down tilt to aid surgical access.

- The end of the table is removed.
- The patient is moved to the lower end of the operating table with the legs supported by an assistant.
- The anterior superior iliac spine should be positioned at the level of the break in the table. Care should be taken to avoid overhanging buttocks at the end of the operating table. The lower back should be supported to maintain normal lumbar lordosis.
- Flexion of the knees and hips to more than 90 degrees should be avoided to protect the sciatic, femoral and obturator nerves.
- The legs are held before being placed in the stirrups.
- The legs are placed outside of the poles to avoid pressure on the common peroneal nerve.
- The patient's hands should be comfortably protected to avoid injury when the operating table is adjusted. Arms should be kept away from the chest to facilitate respiration.

- Arms should be positioned on arm boards at less than 90 degrees or over abdomen.
- The stirrups should be placed at an even height.
- Lateral or posterior knees and ankles should be padded to prevent pressure and contact with a metal surface.

RECOMMENDATION **2.11.23** At the beginning and end of surgery the patient's legs must be moved simultaneously and with care to prevent pelvic injury and sudden hypertension. Pedal pulses should be checked and calves massaged.

PRONE POSITION

RECOMMENDATION **2.11.24** The prone position is used for spinal surgery, neurosurgery involving the posterior cranial fossa, surgery to the buttocks, natal clefts or heels and varicose vein surgery involving the short saphenous vein.

- Cervical neck alignment must be maintained.
- A reinforced tracheal tube is recommended and should be well secured. If a laryngeal mask is used to maintain the patient's airway this should be used by an experienced anaesthetist.
- Staffing of the theatre should be appropriate to allow for the patient to be rolled.
- The position of the tube should be checked after turning the patient.
- The forehead, eyes and chin must be adequately protected. The neck should be protected from hyperextension and excessive rotation. The face should be protected evenly on a cushioned horseshoe support and appropriate single use support, taking care to avoid pressure on the eyes.
- Breasts and male genitalia must be kept free from torsion.
- Legs should be padded with a pillow, from the knees to the feet.
- Spinal alignment must be maintained during turning.
- The arms should be moved simultaneously and symmetrically. Abduction or flexion to more than 90 degrees should be avoided.

LATERAL POSITION

RECOMMENDATION **2.11.25** Spinal alignment must be maintained during turning.

RECOMMENDATION **2.11.26** A padded restraint should be placed around the operating table and pelvis to secure the patient.

RECOMMENDATION **2.11.27** Precautions should be taken against heat loss as this is a particular hazard for patients in this position.

RECOMMENDATION **2.11.28** The operating table must be adjusted gradually to allow the anaesthetist to monitor the patient's blood pressure throughout the manoeuvre.

SUPINE POSITION

RECOMMENDATION **2.11.29** This is the standard position for most surgical procedures. Pressure areas to be protected include the occiput, elbows, knees, sacrum, greater trochanter of the femur and the heels.

- The hips and spinal column must be in alignment, with legs parallel and ankles uncrossed.
- The head should be positioned in a neutral position.
- Arm boards should be placed at less than 90 degrees. Abduction of the arm above 90 degrees can result in brachial plexus injury and ulnar nerve palsy.

RECOMMENDATION **2.11.30** Pregnant patients may become hypotensive when supine as a result of pressure on the inferior vena cava from the pregnant uterus. A 20 degree right-sided tilt will help relieve the pressure.

RECOMMENDATION **2.11.31** Traction tables may pose specific problems to patient positioning. Counter traction may be provided by a perineal post. The post should be well padded and should rest against the pubic rami on the operative side. It should not press against the external genitalia or the pudendal nerve.

TRENDELENBURG (HEAD DOWN) POSITION

RECOMMENDATION **2.11.32** The Trendelenburg position is used for pelvic surgery and central venous line insertion.

- A non-slip mattress should be used to prevent the patient from moving.
- Most head down positions are limited to a maximum of 20 degrees.

RECOMMENDATION **2.11.33** In patients with a head injury, the head down position should be limited to the absolute minimum.

REVERSE TRENDELENBURG (HEAD UP) POSITION

RECOMMENDATION **2.11.34** The reverse Trendelenburg position is used for surgery to the head and neck (eg: thyroid surgery) because it improves venous drainage. It is used for surgery to the upper gastrointestinal tract and the gallbladder and for shoulder operations.

- A tilt of 15–20 degrees is usually sufficient.
- The patient must be normo-volaemic and well secured.

Equipment and safeguards

RECOMMENDATION **2.11.35** The operating table and its accessories to enhance safe patient positioning must always be used according to the manufacturer's instructions. The operating table and all related equipment should be checked for effective function, size and cleanliness before patient use.

RECOMMENDATION **2.11.36** The operating table should have the following essential characteristics:

- Stable – usually achieved by a heavy base.
- Easily manageable – with some form of lockable castor system.
- Highly adjustable – by use of ether electrohydraulic or hand operated controls. Adjustments should be possible to the height, lateral tilt, head down (Trendelenburg) and head up reverse tilt, and central break (sitting and jack-knife positions).
- Adaptable – with the possibility of attaching a variety of supports, rests and traction extensions. One half of the table should be removable.
- Comfortable – cushions should be removable and easily cleaned.
- Radiolucent – to allow x-ray films or an image intensifier to be used.

The modern operating table is a complex medical device which must be serviced regularly under a planned preventative maintenance programme in order to ensure optimal patient safety during surgical interventions.

RECOMMENDATION **2.11.37** All controls, brakes and accessories on operating tables must be checked daily prior to use, in order to ensure that they are clean, in good repair and in working order. All accessories must be correctly and appropriately padded to prevent injury to the patient.

RECOMMENDATION **2.11.38** Table mattresses should be clean and inspected regularly for any damage and should conform to British Standard recommendations.

RECOMMENDATION **2.11.39** Any equipment which is damaged will compromise patient safety and infection control. It must therefore be immediately taken out of use and labelled for repair.

RECOMMENDATION **2.11.40** Patient positioning devices should be available for each surgical position; the choice of the appropriate device should take into account cross infection and tissue viability issues.

RECOMMENDATION **2.11.41** It is recommended that a tissue viability nurse should advise on the purchase of appropriate positioning devices.

RECOMMENDATION **2.11.42** Positioning devices should maintain intraoperative positions and should minimise potential tissue injuries by absorbing compression forces by gel pads, redistributing pressure and preventing excessive stretching.

RECOMMENDATION **2.11.43** Selection criteria for positioning equipment include:

- the ability to maintain a normal capillary interface pressure of 32mm Hg or less
- resistance to moisture and fluids
- radiolucency
- fire resistant
- non-allergic to the patient (latex free)
- easy to use
- easy to clean and disinfect if not disposable
- easy to handle and store
- cost-effective.

Documentation

RECOMMENDATION **2.11.44** Documentation should include:

- a preoperative assessment
- skin integrity before and after the procedure
- the type and location of positioning, including pressure relieving devices used
- names and designation of staff members positioning the patient
- postoperative outcome.

2.12 VISITORS/EXTERNAL CONTRACTORS

STANDARD A patient's right to privacy is adhered to at all times and consent obtained for the presence of a visitor/external contractor during the patient's surgical care pathway. A policy is in place for the management of visitors/external contractors to the perioperative setting.

The Human Rights Act (HMSO 1998c) came into force in October 2000. Article 8 states: *'Everyone has the right for his private and family life, his home and correspondence, to be private unless it is in the interests of national security, public safety or the protection of others'.*

This raises the issue of the importance of maintaining confidentiality and privacy for perioperative patients, and endorses the requirement for patients to be informed and their consent obtained for the presence of any visitors during their care.

Visitors/external contractors approach the perioperative environment for various reasons and there is often pressure for access to be given. Visitors/external contractors may include medical device representatives, student nurses and observation students. The paramount aim of perioperative practice is that perioperative personnel must act in a way that justifies patients' trust and confidence.

Patients have the right to confidentiality unless they have consented to have information divulged. Patients have the right to refuse the presence of visitors during their perioperative phase. Only visitors who have obtained permission for definite supportive and/or educational reasons should be allowed into the perioperative environment during a patient's surgical care pathway. The number of visitors permitted to the perioperative environment should be kept to a minimum.

RECOMMENDATIONS FOR LOCAL POLICY

General considerations

RECOMMENDATION **2.12.1** Each department should have a written policy stating the correct protocol for visitors/external contractors to the environment and all staff should be aware of the policy. The number of visitors/external contractors/medical device representatives should be limited.

RECOMMENDATION **2.12.2** All visitors/external contractors should gain permission prior to their visit to enter the perioperative environment. On arrival visitors/external contractors should report their presence to the appointed person.

RECOMMENDATION **2.12.3** There must be a control mechanism to authorise people visiting the perioperative environment. This should include documentation of their arrival and departure in a specific register.

RECOMMENDATION **2.12.4** All visitors/external contractors must be provided with the necessary theatre attire and understand how it is worn. Visitors/external contractors should be clearly identified as such (ie: with a visitor identity badge).

RECOMMENDATION **2.12.5** Visitors/external contractors must be made aware that all procedures within the perioperative environment are confidential, and that any information, discussions, technical details or documentation data must be treated confidentially.

RECOMMENDATION **2.12.6** Visitors/external contractors should be made aware of perioperative etiquette and, if they are observing clinical procedures, they should be introduced to the staff in the area.

RECOMMENDATION **2.12.7** Visitors/external contractors should be chaperoned by an assigned staff member at all times.

RECOMMENDATION **2.12.8** The presence of a visitor should be recorded in the operating register or computerised theatre record. This includes students, medical device representatives and observers.

RECOMMENDATION **2.12.9** Visitors/external contractors/medical device representatives must be advised of the correct procedure should they feel faint or unwell during their visit.

RECOMMENDATION **2.12.10** Medical, nursing and technical personnel who are not designated employees of the hospital, but who wish to participate during their visit, must have their professional qualification(s) and health status endorsed by the theatre manager or a designated deputy prior to their visit.

Special considerations

THE PATIENT

RECOMMENDATION **2.12.11** The patient must be informed of why the visitor will be in attendance, and the patient should be asked whether they find this acceptable. If the patient refuses to give consent for a visitor to be in attendance, their decision should be respected. Any objection should be documented in the patient's notes or theatre register to ensure that it is well recorded.

RELATIVES, FRIENDS AND STAFF ACCOMPANYING PATIENTS

RECOMMENDATION **2.12.12** It is recommended that patients with special needs or requirements are accompanied into the perioperative environment by a support person.

RECOMMENDATION **2.12.13** Children who are undergoing surgery may be accompanied to the anaesthetic room by a parent or carer, or at least by a ward nurse who is familiar to the child. It is important, however, to respect the wishes of the parent or carer. Local policies should reflect a multi-disciplinary agreed protocol that supports this initiative.

RECOMMENDATION **2.12.14** Parents or carers should be considered a useful asset in the recovery area, and their presence should be encouraged.

RECOMMENDATION **2.12.15** Women taken to theatre for caesarean section may be accompanied in the theatre by their partners, if the woman so wishes. The partner should be appropriately prepared in the protocols to be observed during the perioperative phase.

RECOMMENDATION **2.12.16** Patients with language problems may be accompanied to theatre by a relative or friend who can interpret for them, or by an interpreter who is required to abide by policies and protocols.

RECOMMENDATION **2.12.17** Confused patients may be accompanied by someone they know.

RECOMMENDATION **2.12.18** Psychiatric patients may be accompanied by a registered mental nurse.

RECOMMENDATION **2.12.19** It is recommended that a designated waiting area is provided for relatives and friends that is situated away from the perioperative environment.

SECURITY OF PERSONS

RECOMMENDATION **2.12.20** There are certain instances when patients have to be accompanied by an officer (eg: royalty and patients under police custody). The attendance of these officers has to be given special consideration.

MEDICAL DEVICE REPRESENTATIVES

There are implications for the medical device representative, medical staff and the hospital, that must be addressed prior to admission being granted. These implications include patient consent, medical indemnity, confidentiality, health screening and the role of the representative within the perioperative environment.

RECOMMENDATION **2.12.21** The theatre manager or designated deputy must undertake a risk assessment of visitors such as a medical device representative in accordance with the Health and Safety at Work Act (HMSO 1974) and *Management of Health and Safety at Work Regulations* (HMSO 1992a). These regulations state: *'Every employer shall make a suitable and sufficient assessment of the risk to health and safety of persons not in his employment, arising out of or in connection with the conduct by him or his undertakings.'*

RECOMMENDATION **2.12.22** The risks involved with the visit should be assessed prior to the visit and the companies made aware of the potential risks involved.

The following guidelines should be followed:

- Medical device companies have a duty of care to provide the theatre manager with an appropriate risk assessment for the purpose and practicalities of the visit, including any medical devices or equipment to be brought in. This will include informing the theatre manager if the medical device representative is an expectant mother.
- Medical device representatives may act only as a resource regarding the representative's product, and may not scrub or actively participate in patient care.
- Medical device representatives should have attained a validated professional award in access to the operating theatre before being permitted access to the perioperative environment.
- Demonstrations of new technology should take place in a workshop or laboratory setting, and perioperative staff should be familiar with the technology prior to direct patient use.
- The operating surgeon must notify the theatre manager of the date, time and procedure where a medical device representative has been requested to attend.

WORK OBSERVATION STUDENTS

The management of underage visitors/external contractors to the perioperative environment raises health and safety, consent, confidentiality and risk management issues. A young person is *'any person who has not attained the age of 18'* (Health and Safety Executive 1997).

The *Health and Safety (Young Persons) Regulations* (Health and Safety Executive 1997) and Regulation 3 of the *Management of Health and Safety at Work Regulations* (Health and Safety Executive 1992) clearly state: *'An employer shall not employ a young person unless a risk assessment has been made or reviewed in relation to the risks to health and safety of young people'*.

Even though these regulations refer to employment of the individual, this will also include any visitors/external contractors to the organisation's premises, for example, under 18 year olds visiting the operating department. Within health and safety law, such students are deemed as employees of the hospital organisation.

RECOMMENDATION **2.12.23** The employer has responsibility to:

- assess all risks to young people before they start work
- ensure the risk assessment takes into account their psychological or physical immaturity, inexperience and lack of awareness of existing or potential risks
- introduce control measures, or minimise the risks so far as is reasonably practicable.

RECOMMENDATION **2.12.24** The student should undergo a comprehensive risk assessment to determine their level of inexperience, immaturity and lack of awareness to risks. This should be carried out by the human resources department or theatre manager.

The risk assessment needs to include:

- the nature, degree and duration of potential exposure to physical, chemical and biological agents, including exposure to radiological procedures or potentially harmful disinfection solutions
- organisation of processes and activities, including the layout of the operating theatre in relation to sterile areas so as not to compromise patient care.

RECOMMENDATION **2.12.25** It is recommended that:

- all potential work observation students receive a formal trust induction programme and are made aware of medico-legal issues in relation to their presence within the perioperative setting
- the occupational health department ensures that the students complete a health questionnaire.

RECOMMENDATION **2.12.26** It is essential that:

- the patient is made aware that the student is still of school age but is hoping to pursue a medical career – if the patient refuses to give consent this decision must be respected
- in situations where a patient is unable to give valid consent due to incapacity, work observation students should not be allowed access into the theatre
- all members of staff must be informed that the students are on work observation, are supernumerary and therefore are not permitted to be directly involved in any aspect of patient care.

REFERENCES

British Standards Institute 1993 *Medical Electrical Equipment Part 2 : particular requirements for the safety of diagnostic therapeutic laser equipment* BS EN 60601-2-22 (IEC 601-2-22: 1922; BS724 : Section 2.122:1993) London, BSI

British Standards Institute 1994a *Radiation Safety of Laser Products: equipment classification, requirements and user's guide* EN 60825-1 London, BSI

British Standards Institute 1994b *Specification for Filters and Equipment used for Personal Eye Protection Against Laser Systems* BS EN 207 London, BSI

British Standards Institute 1995 *Fire Detection and Alarm Systems for Buildings: code of practice* BS 5839-6 London, BSI

Faulkner A 1999 All Pierced Up: managing body piercing in perioperative practice *British Journal of Theatre Nursing* 9 (10) 468–471

Harrington J 1987 The Health of Anaesthetists *Anaesthesia* 42 131–132

Health and Safety Commission 1999 *General COSHH ACOP Approved Codes of Practice* London, HSE Books

Health and Safety Commission 2002 *Code of Practice: control of substances hazardous to health regulations* London, HSE Books

Health and Safety Executive 1992 *Management of Health and Safety at Work Regulations: approved code of practice* London, HSE Books

Health and Safety Executive 1997 *The Health and Safety (Young Persons) Regulations* London, HSE Books

Health and Safety Executive 1998a *Lifting Operations and Lifting Equipment Regulations* London, HSE Books

Health and Safety Executive 1998b *Guidance on Manual Handling Operations Regulations* London, HSE Books

HMSO 1971 *The Fire Precautions Act* Norwich, The Stationery Office

HMSO 1974 *Health and Safety at Work Act* Norwich, The Stationery Office

HMSO 1987 *Consumer Protection Act* Norwich, The Stationery Office

HMSO 1990a *Food Safety Act* Norwich, The Stationery Office

HMSO 1990b *Environment Protection Act* Norwich, The Stationery Office

HMSO 1992a *Management of Health and Safety at Work Regulations* Norwich, The Stationery Office

HMSO 1992b *The Controlled Waste Regulations* S1 1992/588 Norwich, The Stationery Office

HMSO 1992c *Personal Protective Equipment Regulations* (EC Directive No 3139) Norwich, The Stationery Office

HMSO 1992d *Manual Handling Operations Regulations* Norwich, The Stationery Office

HMSO 1994 *Management of Health and Safety at Work (Amendment) Regulations* Norwich, The Stationery Office

HMSO 1996 *Reporting of Injuries, Diseases and Dangerous Occurences Regulations (RIDDOR)* Norwich, The Stationery Office

HMSO 1997 *Fire Precautions (Workplace) Regulations Act* Norwich, The Stationery Office

HMSO 1998a *Working Time Regulations* Norwich, The Stationery Office

HMSO 1998b *The Provision and Use of Work Equipment Regulations* Norwich, The Stationery Office

HMSO 1998c *Human Rights Act* London, The Stationery Office. www.hmso.gov.uk/acts/acts1998

HMSO 1999a *Approved Code of Practice: management of health and safety at work regulations* Norwich, The Stationery Office

HMSO 1999b *Food Standards Act* Norwich, The Stationery Office

HMSO 1999c *Ionising Radiation Regulations: equipment used for medical exposure* Norwich, The Stationery Office www.legislation.hmso.gov.uk/si/si1999/19993232.htm

HMSO 2002a *The Control of Substances Hazardous to Health Regulations* Norwich, The Stationery Office

HMSO 2002b *Dangerous Substances and Explosive Atmosphere Regulations (DSEAR)* Norwich, The Stationery Office

Hoerauf K, Funk W, Harth M, Hobbhahn J 1997 Occupational exposure to servoflurane, halothane and nitrous oxide during paediatric anaesthesia *Anaesthesia* 52 (3) 215–219

Hoerauf K, Wiesner G, Schroegendorfer KF et al 1999 Waste anaesthetic gases induce sister chromatid exchanges in lymphocytes of operating theatre personnel *British Journal of Anaesthesia* 82 (5) 764–766

Medical Devices Agency 1996 *Guidance of the Safe Use of Lasers in Medical and Dental Practice* DB9602 London, MDA

Medical Devices Agency 1997a *Mobile Communications: interference with medical devices* SN9706 London, MDA

Medical Devices Agency 1997b *Electromagnetic Compatability of Medical Devices with Mobile Communications* DB9702 London, MDA

Medical Devices Agency 2000 *Use of Spirit-Based Solutions During Surgical Procedures Requiring the Use of Electrosurgical Equipment* London, MDA

Monson R 1990 *Occupational Epidemiology* Broca Raton, CRC Press

National Association of Theatre Nurses 2002 *Risk and Quality Management System* Harrogate, NATN

NHS Estates 1994 *Sterilisation* Health Technical Memorandum 2010 London, HMSO

NHS Estates 2000 *Ventilation in Healthcare Premises: validation and verification* Health Technical Memorandum 2025 London, HMSO

NHS Estates 2001 *Decontamination Programme Technical Manual* London, Engineering and Science Group, DH

NHS Executive 1996 *Advice on the implementation of the health and safety commission's occupational exposure standards for anaesthetic agents* London, DH

Royal College of Nursing 1993 *Code of Practice for Handling of Patients* London, RCN

Spence A 1987 Environmental Pollution by Inhalation Anaesthetics *British Journal of Anaesthesia* 59 93–103

Tri JL, Hayes DL, Smith TT, Severson RP 2001 Cellular Phone Interference with External Cardiopulmonary Monitoring Devices *Mayo Clinic Proceedings* 76 11–15

FURTHER READING

Adomat R 1999 Filming in Hospitals: ethical and methodological issues *Nursing Standard* 14 (2) 37–39

American Operating Room Nurses 2004 *Standards, Recommended Practices and Guidelines* Denver, AORN Inc

American Operating Room Nurses 2004 *Fire Safety Study Guide* Denver, AORN Inc

Austin PR, Austin PJ 1996 Measurement of Nitrous oxide concentrations in a simulated post anaesthesia care unit environment *Journal of Perianaesthesia Nursing* 11 (4) 259–266

Australian College of Operating Room Nurses 2002 *Standards, Guidelines and Policy Statements* Adelaide, ACORN

Australian College of Operating Room Nurses 2004 *Standards for Perioperative Nursing* Adelaide, ACORN

Badgwell JM 1997 A Clinical Evaluation of an Operational Post-Anaesthesia Care Unit Source Control System *Journal of Perianaesthesia Nursing* 12 (2) 73–81

Barnett J 2003 Health Implications of Body Piercing and Tattooing: a literature review *Nursing Times* 99 (37) 62–65

Beesley J 2002 Answers Supplied *British Journal of Perioperative Nursing* 12 (3) 84–85

Beesley J 2003 Did You Know You Can Minimise the Risk to Patients? *Target* 3 (8) 19

Beesley J 2004 Answers supplied *British Journal of Perioperative Nursing* 14 (7) 286–288

British Standards Institute 1995 *Guidance on Airway Management During Laser Surgery of Upper Airway* ISO TR11991 London, BSI

British Standards Institute 1998 *Tracheal Tubes Designed for Laser Surgery: requirements for marking and accompanying information* ISO 14408 London, BSI

Champion J 2000 Laser Safety Management *British Journal of Perioperative Nursing* 10 (8) 428–432

Chivers L 2002 Body Adornment: piercings and tattoos *Nursing Standard* 16 (34) 41–45

Coleman S 1999 Manual Handling in the Operating Theatre *Professional Nurse* 14 (10) 682–686

Collins F 2003 Writing a Manual Handling Policy *Nurse2Nurse* 3 (2) 11–13

Craig K 2003 Prone Positioning Made Easy *British Journal of Perioperative Nursing* 13 (12) 522–527

Croners 1999 *Health Service Risks Management and Practice* London, Croner Publications Ltd

Department of Health 1987 *Directory of Fire Document* Norwich, The Stationery Office

Department of Health 2000 *Mobile Phones and Health* Norwich, The Stationery Office. www.dh.gov.uk

Department of Health 2001 *Reference Guide to Consent for Examination or Treatment* Norwich, The Stationery Office. www.dh.gov.uk

Department of Health 2001 *Building a Safer NHS for Patients* Norwich, The Stationery Office

Department of Health 2001 *An Organisation with a Memory: report of an expert group on learning from adverse events in the NHS, chaired by the chief medical officer* Norwich, The Stationery Office

Department of Health 2003 *Confidentiality: NHS code of practice* Norwich, The Stationery Office. www.dh.gov.uk

Department of Health 2003 *Essence of Care: patient focused benchmarks for clinical governance* Norwich, The Stationery Office

Department of Trade and Industry Maternity Rights (PL958) – www.dti.gov.uk/er/maternity.htm

Dimond B 2002 Risk Assessment and Management to Ensure Health and Safety at Work *British Journal of Nursing* 11 (6) 396–397

Dimond B 2002 Statutory Provisions of the Health and Safety at Work Act *British Journal of Nursing* 11 (11) 1372–1374

Dimond B 2002 Responsibilities in Relation to Controlling Hazardous Substances *British Journal of Nursing* 11 (14) 941–943

European Community Directive 1992 *Consumer Protection, Personal Protective Equipment Statutory Instruction* 1992/3139 Norwich, The Stationery Office

European Community Directive 1992 *Personal Protective Equipment Statutory Instruction* 1992/2966 Norwich, The Stationery Office

Farquhar-Thomson DR, Goddard JM 1996 The Hazards of Anaesthetic Gas Scavenging Systems *Anaesthesia* 51 860–862

Green S 1996 Positioning of Patient for Surgery *British Journal of Theatre Nursing* 6 (5) 35–38

Gilmour D 2000 Risks for the New or Expectant Mother Working in the Perioperative Environment *British Journal of Perioperative Nursing* 10 (6) 306–310

Grundeman B, Magnum S 2001 *Infection Prevention in Surgical Settings* London, WB Saunders

Hassan S, Kay S 2003 Brachial Plexus Injury *Surgery* 21 (10) 262–264

Health and Safety Agency 1985 *The ionising radiation regulations (Northern Ireland) protection of persons against ionising radiation arising from any work activity: approved code of practice* Belfast, HMSO

Health and Safety Executive 1998 *Essentials of Health and Safety at Work* London, HSE Books

Health and Safety Executive 1998 *The Reporting of Diseases and Dangerous Occurences Regulations 1995: guidance for employers in the healthcare sector* London, HSE Books

Health and Safety Executive 1999 *A Guide to Risk Assessment Requirements* London, HSE Books

Health and Safety Executive 1999 *Fire Safety: an employer's guide* London, HSE Books

Health and Safety Executive 1999 *Managing Health and Safety: five steps to success* London, HSE Books

Health and Safety Executive 2000 *Occupational Exposure Limits* EH40/2000 London, HSE Books

Health and Safety Executive 2000 *The Ionising Radiation (Medical Exposure) Regulations* London, HSE Books

Health Services Advisory Committee 1999 *Safe Disposal of Clinical Waste* 2nd ed, Norwich, The Stationery Office

Hind M, Wicker P 2000 *Principles of Perioperative Practice* London, Harcourt

HMSO 1978 *Health and Safety at Work Order (Northern Ireland)* Norwich, The Stationery Office

HMSO 1985 *The Ionising Radiation Regulations (Northern Ireland)* Belfast, HMSO

HMSO 1993 *Management of Health and Safety at Work Regulations (Northern Ireland)* Norwich, The Stationery Office

HMSO 1998 *Data Protection Act* Norwich, The Stationery Office

HMSO 1998 *Collection and Disposal of Waste Regulations* Norwich, The Stationery Office

HMSO 1999 *Ionising Radiations Regulations* Norwich, The Stationery Office

Hoerauf K, Harth M, Wild K, Hobbhahn J 1997 Occupational exposure to desflurane and isoflurane during cardiopulmonary bypass: is the gas outlet of the membrane oxygenator an operating theatre pollution hazard? *British Journal of Anaesthesia* 78 378–380

Hoerauf K, Koller C, Jakob W, Taeger K, Hobbhahn J 1996 Isoflurane Waste Gas Exposure During General Anaesthesia: the laryngeal mask compared with tracheal intubation *British Journal of Anaesthesia* 77 189–193

Institute of Sterile Services Management 2000 *Standards and Practice* Truro, ISSM. www.issm.org.uk

Larkin B 2004 The Ins and Outs of Body Piercing *AORN Journal* 79 (2) 333–342

Layzell M 2000 The Air We Breathe *British Journal of Perioperative Nursing* 10 (5) 272–275

Mackenzie M, Richardson B, Kidd R, Tracy M 1997 A Novel Limb-Support System to Reduce Postural Load in Theatres *British Journal of Theatre Nursing* 6 (10) 28–30

Malan T, Mcindoe A 2003 Positioning the Surgical Patient *Anaesthesia and Intensive Care Medicine* 4 (11) 360–365

Marenzi B 2001 Body Piercing *The Dissector* 29 (2) 12–15

Mather S, Sellek G 2004 Hidden Danger of Inhalational Anaesthesia *The Clinical Services Journal* 3 (2) 37–39

McEwen D 1996 Intraoperative Positioning of Surgical Patients *AORN Journal* 63 (6) 1059–1079

Medical Devices Agency 1999 *Mobile Communications: interference with medical devices during the millennium period* MDA SN 1999/39 London, MDA

Medical Devices Agency 2001 *Update on Electromagnetic Compatibility of Medical Devices with Mobile Communications: TETRA (terestrial trunked radio system) and outside media broadcasts from hospital premises* MDA SN 2001/06 London, MDA

Myerson S, Mitchell A 2003 Mobile Phones in Hospitals *British Medical Journal* 326 (1) 460–461

National Association of Theatre Nurses 1998 *Safeguards for Invasive Procedures: the management of risks* Harrogate, NATN

National Association of Theatre Nurses 1998 *Principles of Safe Practice in the Perioperative Environment* Harrogate, NATN

National Association of Theatre Nurses 2000 *Back to Basics: perioperative practice principles* Harrogate, NATN

National Association of Theatre Nurses 2001 *Universal/Standard Precautions* Harrogate, NATN

National Association of Theatre Nurses 2001 *Control and Scavenging of Waste Anaesthetic Gases* Harrogate, NATN

National Association of Theatre Nurses 2002 *Risk and Quality Management System* Harrogate, NATN

National Confidential Enquiry into Perioperative Deaths 1997 *Who Operates When?* London, NCEPOD

NHS Estates 1996 *Firecode Alarm and Detection Systems* HTM 82 Norwich, The Stationery Office

NHS Estates 1997 *Medical Gases* HTM 2022 Norwich, The Stationery Office

NHS Estates 2004 *Facilities for Surgical Procedures* Health Building Notes HBN26 Norwich, The Stationery Office

NHS Scotland 2003 *NHS Code of Practice on Protecting Patient Confidentiality* Edinburgh, Scottish Executive

NHS Scotland 2003 *Waste Incineration (Scotland): regulations and practical guidance* Edinburgh, Scottish Executive

Nursing and Midwifery Council 2002 *Code of Professional Conduct* London, NMC

Peate I 2000 Body Piercing: could you answer your patient's queries? *British Journal of Nursing* 9 (20) 2163–2168

Peate I, Lancaster J 2000 Safe Use of Medical Gases in the Clinical Setting: practical tips *British Journal of Nursing* 9 (4) 231–236

Pirie S 2004 Answers Supplied *British Journal of Theatre Nursing* 14 (6) 246–247

Pressly V 2000 Waste Anaesthetic Gases *British Journal of Perioperative Nursing* 10 (6) 299–304

Rogers R, Salvage J, Cowell R 1999 *Nurses at Risk: a guide to health and safety at work* 2nd ed, London, Macmillan

Royal College of Nursing, Institute of Physics and Engineering in Medicine 2003 *Ionising Radiation Safety: a handbook for nurses* York, Institute of Physics and Engineering in Medicine

Royal Marsden Hospital 2000 *Manual of Clinical Nursing Procedures* 5th ed, Oxford, Blackwell Publishing

Servant C, Purkiss S 2002 *Positioning Patients for Surgery* Oxford, Greenwich Medical Media

Scott E, Summerbell L 2004 Managing the Risk in the Perioperative Environment *Nursing Standard* 18 (30) 47–52

Smith B 1997 Attendance of Company Representatives in the Operating Theatre *British Journal of Theatre Nursing* 7 (1) 40–43

Sprague J 2000 A Risky Business *British Journal of Perioperative Nursing* 10 (12) 612–617

Stevens V, Walker L 2001 Accidents Don't Just Happen *British Journal of Perioperative Nursing* 11 (8) 342–345

Taylor M, Campbell C 1998 Lasers. In Clarke P, Jones J (eds) *Brigdens Operating Department Practice* Edinburgh, Churchill Livingstone

Tunner P 1997 Establishing a Protocol for Parental Presence in Recovery *British Journal of Nursing* 6 (14) 794–799

Wicker P 2000 Manual Handling in the Perioperative Environment *British Journal of Perioperative Nursing* 10 (5) 255–259

Wilson J 1995 Clinical Risk Management: building provider awareness in the administration of anaesthesia *British Journal of Perioperative Nursing* 4 (12) 8–11

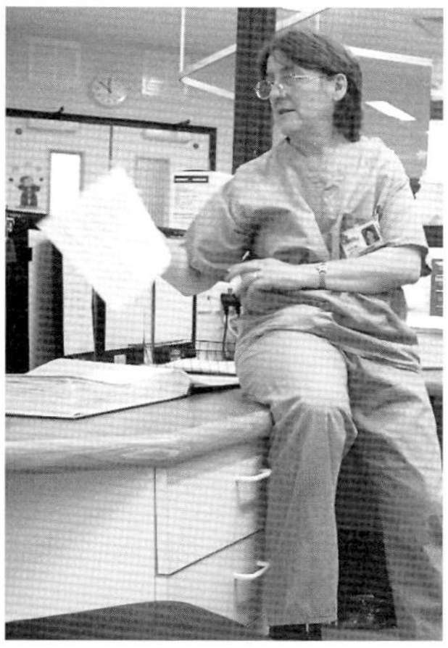

3 MANAGEMENT/HUMAN RESOURCES

3.1 DEPARTMENTAL MANAGEMENT

STANDARD There is a system in place that supports effective management of the perioperative environment. All activities support the best interests and safety of patients and staff.

The effective management of an operating theatre suite, either small or large, depends on a number of key elements: good communication and administration, trained competent staff, appropriate facilities, equipment and resources.

The day to day running of the theatre department should be in the hands of a designated theatre manager who is responsible for co-ordinating effective communication systems within the department. Staff should be allocated efficiently to respond to the planned theatre activity. Staff rotas should be managed to ensure high standards of competent patient care and staff should be informed of their duty requirements at least one calendar month in advance.

Efficiency of the theatre suite is influenced by many outside factors, namely, effective pre-operative planning and assessment, bed status, decontamination services and adequate staffing levels. Clear planning and scheduling will enable the theatre department to be used to its maximum capacity. This allows more work to be carried out at a reasonable time, whilst improving patient and carer experience, and employee satisfaction and morale.

The theatre manager should support the development of clinical governance within the department and assist in the setting of standards of care. The theatre manager should implement and monitor theatre information systems to capture theatre utilisation, cancelled operations and theatre activity information. This is necessary to identify trends and take remedial action where required in order to improve clinical effectiveness.

A culture of good timekeeping within the theatre department should be encouraged and enforced by the theatre manager. This should curtail overruns and cancellations and should ensure that all patients requiring surgery are treated within the allocated time-frame.

RECOMMENDATIONS FOR LOCAL POLICY

Management considerations

There are three major aspects of organisational management which need to be applied to all areas of the operating department.

STRATEGIC

Effective organisations develop a three to five year strategic plan which gives direction to the core and secondary roles of the organisation and which clarifies ongoing and new business developments.

RECOMMENDATION **3.1.1** Operating departments should reflect the overall strategy and identify specific developments by producing their own strategic direction statement and ensuring that this is published widely to all staff. When constructing a strategic planning document, the following areas require attention:

- A philosophy statement identifies the key role of the department and establishes the quality of care which can be expected for all patients and describes the working environment for staff.
- Key objectives (such as financial, improvements against major performance indicators, effective staffing establishments, developments in clinical practice, team management, education and training/continual professional development, clinical supervision, research and evidence-based practice, risk management, recruitment and retention strategy) must be written down, so that outcomes are clearly defined, measurable and have dates for achievement.

TACTICAL

RECOMMENDATION **3.1.2** Tactical organisation involves setting and agreeing standards for the department as a whole. It should be linked to the departmental strategic direction statement. These standards will relate to the quality of:

- patient care delivery
- information in order to assist the decision-making
- process (including that about patients, staff, equipment theatre users)
- education and training.

RECOMMENDATION **3.1.3** Use of existing facilities (capacity planning), budgetary control and overall organisation of elective and emergency workload (demand scheduling) are all aspects which fall under the remit of tactical management.

RECOMMENDATION **3.1.4** All objectives must be written down, so that the outcomes are clearly defined, measurable and have dates for achievement. Formal systems are essential for monitoring, evaluating and reviewing these standards.

OPERATIONAL

RECOMMENDATION **3.1.5** Each operating department should have an up-to-date operational policy. This involves setting and agreeing standards which relate to the day to day function of perioperative clinical services in order to ensure a high quality service and safe practices. These standards should reflect the tactical outcomes and be written down, so that the outcomes are clearly defined and measurable with dates for achievement. These policies should be reviewed annually. They will relate to:

- the cost of effective service delivery
- resource scheduling and allocation level of cancelled procedures
- demand scheduling and throughput use of emergency theatre during normal working hours, maintaining agreed standards of theatre use
- procedures and policies for the collection of information, the development of individuals and teams.

Topics for development

RECOMMENDATION **3.1.6**

- **Patient care** A quality assurance system will establish the effect of departmental procedures on the overall surgical patient process, the standards for ensuring a safe environment and the maintenance of records and documentation.
- **Staff** The operating department is a stressful and complex environment. The continuous recruitment and development of new staff is very costly, and it is therefore incumbent upon the operating department manager to ensure that effective support systems are in place in order to encourage the retention of staff.

RECOMMENDATION **3.1.7** It will be necessary to include:

- the observance of local policies, employment legislation and the *Agenda for Change* conditions of service
- job descriptions and person specifications for each grade/band of staff
- systems for monitoring, reviewing and evaluating workforce and utilisation
- personnel and occupational health procedures to ensure good employment practice
- an education and training programme which is non-discriminatory and can be applied with equity for all staff – this will be based on the outcome of individual personal development plans
- a system of individual performance review with associated individual development planning.

ACTIVITY

RECOMMENDATION **3.1.8** It will be necessary to include:

- provision of suitable operating facilities for patients who are undergoing anaesthetic and/or surgery as inpatients or outpatients
- information describing the length of elective and emergency procedures which allows operating sessions to be planned and negotiated effectively
- communication pathways to ensure that prepared patients receive the expected procedure and arrive in the operating department in an optimum condition
- defined procedures for booking cases into scheduled and emergency systems with clear direction about the staff who must be involved
- support for the decision-making process, by clarifying the type of information required about operating department activity, for example patient cancellations, over-runs, under-runs, staff sickness levels, high cost procedures
- patient information systems that can support the collection of data in the operating department and ensure the continuity of care and information for patients
- a major incident plan.

MAINTENANCE

RECOMMENDATION **3.1.9** Healthcare organisations have agreed programmes for maintaining the building, and mechanical standards of the building, with programmes for planned major plant repair and replacement. There must be systems to ensure that the fabric of the building and mechanical and electrical plant are maintained in good order. Policies to ensure safe functioning of the mechanical and electrical installations in the operating department must be in place.

EQUIPMENT

RECOMMENDATION **3.1.10** Systems should be in place for the planned replacement of expensive items, for monitoring the purchase and maintenance of all equipment and for reporting ineffective or broken equipment. Standards must be set at an operational level for safe usage of equipment which must relate to the manufacturer's guidelines.

CONSUMABLES

RECOMMENDATION **3.1.11** Systems should be in place for enabling the purchase of an adequate and effective supply of consumables, for monitoring, evaluating and reviewing consumable supplies to ensure the maintenance of adequate and relevant stock levels and for ordering, receiving and storing supplies to maintain agreed stock levels.

HEALTH, SAFETY AND WELFARE

RECOMMENDATION **3.1.12** Health, safety and welfare issues relating to the environment, staff and patients must be considered at all times. Managers should ensure that staff comply with the Health and Safety at Work Act (HMSO 1974) and the *Management of Health and Safety at Work Regulations* (HMSO 1992).

Benchmarking

A benchmark is defined as a standard or point of reference.

Perioperative patient care has been delivered using many different standards over the years, and can vary from organisation to organisation and sometimes within an operating department itself. The NATN *Risk and Quality Management System* (NATN 2002a) provides a benchmark for auditing standards of patient care provided in the perioperative setting.

Best practice versus accepted practice can experience a huge gap, and benchmarking is an essential tool. Structuring the approach to sharing and comparing practice enables the practitioner to identify best practice and to take appropriate actions to correct poor practice in a non-threatening situation.

RECOMMENDATION **3.1.13** The Department of Health (DH 2003a) has published *The Essence of Care* which is a process of comparing, sharing and developing practice in order to achieve and sustain best practice. Nursing care in the perioperative setting should be benchmarked against the standards stipulated in this publication.

RECOMMENDATION **3.1.14** Benchmarking is a positive activity for perioperative practice and can be used for a variety of reasons. Managers can use it for:

- local monitoring of standards and to reduce complacency
- target setting to ensure efficiency targets are met
- resource allocation
- key performance indicators.

RECOMMENDATION **3.1.15** Perioperative practitioners can use benchmarking for:

- comparing standards and learning from others
- reducing misconceptions from those outside the operating department
- ensuring that patients receive the best possible perioperative care.

Clinical leadership

Good leadership is essential to motivate staff and improve the quality of services. The need for quality leadership as a skill has not been overlooked by government in recent years. The NHS *Leadership Qualities Framework* was launched in October 2002. The framework was originally commissioned by the NHS Leadership Centre to provide a set of competencies but the new framework is designed to be a user-friendly tool for all team leaders and managers in the NHS to help them understand what defines good leadership in the NHS. The introduction of the modern matron post and the creation of leadership courses such as the National Nursing Leadership Projects, Leading an Empowered Organisation (LEO) courses have redefined the qualities needed to lead a team. Robust leadership is at the forefront of health reforms and is the key to assisting perioperative personnel to face the challenges of the modernisation agenda.

RECOMMENDATION **3.1.16** It is the role of managers and team leaders to facilitate a working environment that is conducive to learning. There is evidence of a relationship between a good learning environment and a good leader, as there is a relationship between a friendly, positive environment and better patient outcomes. Such environments increase the professional confidence and self esteem of practitioners, and improve recruitment and retention of staff.

RECOMMENDATION **3.1.17** Clinical leaders must maintain and grow their personal credibility by ensuring their knowledge, skills and competencies are kept up to date. One way of supporting team members, and a key quality of a good leader, is to be a good role model.

RECOMMENDATION **3.1.18** HOW TO LEAD A TEAM EFFECTIVELY

- **Know yourself** Use structured reflections to increase awareness of your strengths and weaknesses. Invite open feedback from your colleagues.
- **Know your team** A team needs a range of skills and competencies. Allow them opportunities to do things they are good at and support them in developing those areas in which they are not so strong.
- **Be a good role model** Use your position as an opportunity to demonstrate good practice.
- **Adopt a flexible leadership style**.

RECOMMENDATION **3.1.19** The qualities and activities of good leadership should include the following:

- **Vision** A fluid concept and open to change, vision is described as having the ability to see a way forward to a desired outcome, and selling that vision with enthusiasm, realism and commitment.
- **Empowerment** Facilitating the potential in all team members by sharing knowledge and information, giving constructive feedback, investing in others' development, and setting boundaries of acceptable standards and behaviours which provide stability and security for the team members.

- **Team building** Uniting all the members of a group into a team who share purpose, who collaborate together in achieving goals, and who respect each other's strengths and weaknesses.
- **Communicating** Effective communication skills are essential.

RECOMMENDATION **3.1.20** Staff within an operating theatre that have leadership qualities need to be identified, nurtured and facilitated in reaching their maximum potential. Staff in senior positions who lack leadership qualities should be identified and should engage in continual professional development activities to enhance their abilities. Staff in senior positions who fail to develop effective leadership skills and cannot fulfil the management responsibilities adequately should be redeployed in a position that maximises their strengths within the theatre team.

Clinical governance

The NHS Executive (1999) introduced a framework known as clinical governance to improve the quality of care throughout the NHS. Clinical governance was also introduced into Scotland with the document *Designed to Care* (DH 1997).

Clinical governance is defined as *'the means by which organisations ensure the provision of quality clinical care by making individuals accountable for setting, maintaining and monitoring performance standards'* (NHS Executive 1999).

Clinical governance is an initiative which recommends local actions to ensure that national standards are reflected in the delivery of patient care within the NHS.

The elements of clinical governance are:

- **Corporate accountability for clinical performance** Under this section, NHS Trust chief executives and boards, and private sector managers, are accountable for the performance of their practitioners and the quality of care they deliver.
- **Internal mechanisms for clinical performance** This focuses on individual accountability and self/professional regulation. Health professionals are empowered to set their own standards of practice, conduct and discipline. There is an emphasis on lifelong learning and continuous professional development, evidence-based practice and risk management. These will ensure that improvements in patient care are in place.

RECOMMENDATION **3.1.21** A non-blame culture must be adopted, with staff being encouraged to report adverse events or near miss situations. These mistakes can be identified early and learnt from in this environment.

RECOMMENDATION **3.1.22** Clinical governance is everyone's business and must be brought to life within the culture of all healthcare organisations. Good practice and innovation should be recognised and shared.

RECOMMENDATION **3.1.23** Senior practitioners possessing clinical leadership, team building and change management skills, should take the lead in clinical governance and ensure that their juniors are empowered to be confident and proactive in assuring a collaborative approach to high quality patient-centred care.

RECOMMENDATION **3.1.24** The following aspects should be implemented to ensure quality care:

- Clinical effectiveness programmes to identify and build on good practice. They should include protocols, care pathways and evidence-based practice.
- Dissemination of good practice.
- Clinical risk assessment programmes to facilitate risk reduction.

- Adverse events and near miss incidents detected, documented and investigated in a no-blame culture to promote improvement.
- Complaints dealt with promptly and positively and information used to improve organisation and delivery of care.
- Self regulation and clinical leadership development.
- High quality and performance audits to monitor clinical care and to support practitioners who deliver that care.
- Poor performance dealt with in an appropriate manner which ensures staff and patient safety.
- Staff supported in 'whistle-blowing' situations.
- Continuous professional development encouraged for all staff.

Clinical governance has had a significant influence on the future of patient care and has therefore given all practitioners the opportunity to shape the service to meet the needs of patients.

Formulating policies and protocols

Managers and team leaders require written standards giving specifics on principles and procedures, in order to be able to lead and direct their staff effectively. Policies and protocols can become a meaningful part of practice if they are used appropriately and successfully.

RECOMMENDATION **3.1.25** When formulating policies or protocols, the following should be considered:

- The need for the policy or protocol has been raised and needs to be explored either by an individual, steering group or working party.
- Relevant information should be collected and existing policies examined.
- The departmental staff should be involved in the process, so that they can take ownership of the finished product. It is a good idea to talk to other departments and colleagues to find out if anyone else has looked at this particular area of practice before.
- Decide what is to be accomplished from this policy, set clear guidelines and define expectations.
- If the protocol encompasses national policy or direction, this should be made clear and referenced.
- Once agreement has been reached on the technical aspects of the policy, details should be built in.
- The document needs to be approved – with the team who worked on it, and then the departmental manager and the clinical effectiveness team or designated manager.
- When approval occurs, the policy can be implemented.
- A review date should be set.

Audit and inspection for principles of safe practice

Clinical audit has long been suggested as a means of assessing developments in practice within a department, ensuring that standards are met and identifying areas for improvement. Benchmarking constituted a similar exercise but outcomes were generally used as a starting position or as a comparison with others using the same criteria.

NATN has long advocated the use of such tools to measure practice and management outcomes. The *Risk and Quality Management System* (NATN 2002a) is the most comprehensive audit tool for perioperative practice in the United Kingdom.

With the advent of clinical governance and a more thorough understanding of risk management, audit has been increasingly used in the acute sector. Organisations such as the Commission for Health, Audit and Inspection (CHAI), Welsh Risk Pool, and Quality Improvement, Scotland (NHSQIS) are using a variety of audit tools to measure and define standards, as a mechanism for comparison across NHS trusts and the independent healthcare sector. The Health Care Commission is responsible for measuring standards within the private sector and has provided an extensive set of standards by which all units are measured (SH 2002). The organisations send a team of inspectors to the hospitals and report to the chief executive and board.

PREPARATION FOR AUDIT

RECOMMENDATION **3.1.26** Perioperative areas preparing for inspections and audit should review their policies and protocols to ensure that they are accessible, up-to-date, and most importantly, in use. Undertaking some patient follow-throughs will identify that all aspects of patient safety are being managed properly, and ensure that staff are well informed about health and safety procedures. The NATN *Risk and Quality Management System* (NATN 2002a) provides an excellent framework for internal mock audits.

RECOMMENDATION **3.1.27** Auditors should be experienced practitioners with a perioperative background and be well versed in up-to-date safety notices and hazard warnings. Whilst most auditors are realistic about working conditions and do not expect everything to be absolutely perfect, they are also present to ensure that patient safety is paramount in all perioperative activity. A constructive feedback at the end of the inspection will ensure that findings are acted upon without delay. Written reports containing an action plan should be made to the hospital or department within weeks, to have the best effect on safe patient care.

3.2 MANAGEMENT OF OPERATING SESSIONS

STANDARD Human and physical resources are used effectively through proactive co-ordination, in order to facilitate the delivery of high quality patient care to patients admitted for elective and scheduled surgery.

INTRODUCTION

Effective organisation by all members of the perioperative caring team is essential for the efficient management of elective and scheduled operating sessions. Managers responsible for calculating staffing establishments should comply with the recommendations set out in the NATN publication *Staffing for Patients in the Perioperative Setting* (NATN 2003).

The aim is to reduce and prevent the cancellation of elective and scheduled surgery by ensuring that allocated theatre time is planned effectively and that perioperative personnel are deployed appropriately to meet the identified service demand.

A policy is essential to ensure that all theatre users are aware of the optimal means of utilising allocated theatre time, and its associated resources, for the delivery of an elective/scheduled operating session. The criteria should be viewed annually.

DEFINITIONS USED

Theatre co-ordinator/team leader

The most senior nurse/operating department practitioner. The theatre co-ordinator/team leader is in charge of the theatre team on a particular shift.

Elective

An operative list organised and delivered at a time that is planned within the operating schedule/contract as agreed by the Theatre Users' Committee or relevant forum.

Emergency

The requirement for an operative procedure or collection of procedures as a result of a condition that is judged to be life-threatening, or requires prioritising over and above the needs of patients scheduled for an elective list.

RECOMMENDATIONS FOR LOCAL POLICY

Times of operating sessions

The start of the theatre session is defined as '*when the anaesthetist takes charge of the first patient in preparation for anaesthesia*'. The end of the session is defined as '*when the anaesthetist has finished handing over the last patient to the recovery staff and is free to start another task*' (RCA 2000).

RECOMMENDATION **3.2.1** The operating session should allow for three and a half hours of operating time, and half an hour for the postoperative recovery of a patient and the effective decontamination of the operating theatre.

- The morning session may be defined as 0900–1230 operating time and 1230–1300 recovery and cleaning time.
- The afternoon session may be defined as 1330–1700 operating time and 1700–1730 recovery and cleaning time.
- In the case of a planned all day operating list, the allocated sessions should be from 0900–1600.

RECOMMENDATION **3.2.2** It is the responsibility of the consultant operating surgeon or nominated theatre scheduler when planning elective and scheduled operating lists that, as far as is reasonably practicable, allocated operating session times are not exceeded. Theatre resources can then be utilised appropriately and staff can be assured meal and rest breaks. There is also a reduced need for overtime.

Cancellation of elective/scheduled patients

RECOMMENDATION 3.2.3 In situations where the operating surgeon is about to, or has actually run out of allocated session time, the co-ordinator or designated team leader of the theatre concerned, in collaboration with the consultant anaesthetist, should cancel any further cases to prevent the operating list from over running.

RECOMMENDATION 3.2.4 The surgical team responsible for the operative list should ensure that all patients affected by the decision to curtail the list receive an explanation as to why it was deemed necessary to postpone or cancel their planned surgery.

RECOMMENDATION 3.2.5 The appropriate clinical incident form, must be completed by the co-ordinator or designated team leader, stating the reason for cancellation and who was involved in making this decision.

RECOMMENDATION 3.2.6 In the absence of a co-ordinator or designated team leader, the anaesthetic assistant should seek advice from the most senior member of staff on duty within the operating department.

RECOMMENDATION 3.2.7 To ensure effective management of perioperative resources it must be accepted by all staff that only the co-ordinator or designated team leader have the authority to authorise the collection of or sending for patients.

RECOMMENDATION 3.2.8 All cancellations should be audited monthly to determine whether theatre scheduling has been effective. This process should include Anaesthetic and Surgical Directorates, the main co-ordinator/scheduler and medical secretaries as recommended by NCEPOD (2001).

Planned over-running of sessions

RECOMMENDATION 3.2.9 In situations where it is anticipated that the complexity of a procedure or the nature of the operative case will result in a longer than scheduled operating time, it is the responsibility of both the consultant surgeon and the anaesthetist to liaise with the co-ordinator/designated team leader. The priority is to ensure that the appropriate physical and staff resources can be organised and secured.

RECOMMENDATION 3.2.10 In circumstances where a consultant surgeon or anaesthetist may wish to commence the scheduled operating list at an earlier time than that allocated or published, they must liaise with the co-ordinator or designated team leader to ensure that appropriate human and physical resources are available. If the necessary resources are not available then the co-ordinator/designated team leader should inform both the consultant surgeon and the anaesthetist as soon as is reasonably practicable.

Ensuring an effective response to emergency situations

RECOMMENDATION 3.2.11 If the organisation wishes to provide a responsive emergency service then a designated 24-hour operating theatre, managed by trained and competent staff, must be resourced (NCEPOD 1997).

RECOMMENDATION 3.2.12 The staff rostered/designated to provide emergency cover must not be used to supplement the staffing establishment for elective or scheduled cases; they must be available to provide an immediate response to emergency incidents.

RECOMMENDATION **3.2.13** In situations where emergency teams comprise a minimum of three trained personnel, and a risk assessment regarding prioritisation of service and patient dependency has been conducted at the discretion of the co-ordinator or designated team leader, one individual may be directed to assist where a significant staffing problem has occurred. This is acceptable only on the understanding that the individual will be recalled in the advent of an emergency situation.

RECOMMENDATION **3.2.14** Emergency lists should be organised and staffed by senior anaesthetists and surgeons working to a fixed sessional pattern (AAGBI 2003). Anaesthetists and surgeons rostered for emergency work should be free from other commitments to routine work or outpatient clinics (NCEPOD 1997).

Cancellation/changes to the operating list

RECOMMENDATION **3.2.15** All operating lists should arrive in theatre 16–24 hours in advance of a scheduled session, in order to ensure patient safety and the effective utilisation of resources (NATN 1998). The theatre manager is responsible for facilitating the formulation of a policy to ensure that planned surgical activity in printed or electronic form is clearly posted, well in advance and in all appropriate locations (AAGBI 2003).

RECOMMENDATION **3.2.16** Any changes to the list or cancellations must be relayed immediately to the person in charge of the operating list.

- All copies of the operating list or send-for slips must be amended as appropriate by the person making the changes. All appropriate members of staff must be notified (AAGBI 1995).
- The persons making the amendments must sign and add a note to the side of the list which says 'note change to order'. The appropriate untoward incident form should be completed detailing the reasons why the change in order was indicated.
- All relevant staff should be informed, including the wards, radiological departments and support services as appropriate.

RECOMMENDATION **3.2.17** It must be acknowledged by all staff that to change the order of an operating list creates the potential for error, and that changes to a published schedule should only occur in extreme circumstances and only when absolutely necessary. The importance of documenting the circumstances of any change, via the appropriate untoward incident form, should be viewed as fundamental to securing improvements in future scheduling practice.

Staffing of elective/scheduled operating lists

RECOMMENDATION **3.2.18** It is the responsibility of the co-ordinator or designated team leader to ensure that every elective and emergency operating list is staffed by a team of appropriately trained and competent personnel who are equipped with the skills and abilities to administer high quality patient care, and who are able to identify and minimise any risks to the patient as they journey through the perioperative environment. It is recommended that the formulae for calculating staffing establishment advocated by NATN (2003) are utilised.

These include:

- one qualified anaesthetic assistant practitioner for each session involving an anaesthetic
- two qualified scrub practitioners as a basic requirement for each session, unless there is only one planned case on the operating list
- one trained circulating practitioner for each session
- two trained circulating practitioners where the operative procedure involves two cavities being opened simultaneously and has two operating teams at the operating table
- one qualified post-anaesthetic recovery practitioner for the immediate postoperative period. There may be occasions where two qualified staff are required if there is a quick throughput of patients requiring minor procedures, such as in a surgical day unit.

RECOMMENDATION **3.2.19** If the patient is not returning to a special care area such as a high dependency unit immediately after surgery, they need to be cared for by practitioners who are trained and experienced in post-anaesthetic care.

Theatre efficiency

RECOMMENDATION **3.2.20** The document *Step Guide to Improving Operating Theatre Performance* (Modernisation Agency 2002) recognised that a major non-clinical reason for cancellation of elective surgery is the lack of availability of beds. The Association of Anaesthetists of Great Britain and Ireland (2003) recommended that efficiency could be improved by admitting all patients to a preoperative preparation area on the day of surgery. The area could be integrated with preoperative assessment and day case areas adjacent to theatres, and would provide an efficient use of space and competent staff. It would also facilitate transport to and from theatre.

RECOMMENDATION **3.2.21** If a bed is not available, patients must be contacted by telephone in good time and the patient must be offered another date for admission within the next 28 days (DH 2000).

RECOMMENDATION **3.2.22** A holding area for patients, staffed by registered practitioners, is recommended in the operating department to assist with the efficient running of operating lists. Patients that are not sedated and are medically fit should be encouraged to walk to theatre with a suitably trained escort.

RECOMMENDATION **3.2.23** Patients must be ready for theatre when they are sent for and theatres should liaise closely with ward areas and the bed manager at all times, especially if the order of the operating lists has changed (AAGBI 2003).

RECOMMENDATION **3.2.24** The incidence and reason for all cancellations, delays and overruns should be documented and audited by the theatre management team. Electronic computerised systems for collecting data are recommended, as such systems make it easy for managers to predict probable overruns and therefore take the necessary action to review theatre scheduling.

3.3 HUMAN RESOURCE MANAGEMENT

STANDARD Perioperative personnel responsible for human resource management are knowledgeable and competent in employment law, including codes of practice and European laws relevant to the perioperative setting.

INTRODUCTION

Good employment practice is governed by legislation which is aimed at protecting both staff and employers in the workplace. Local policies should be in place which reflect current legislation, local agreements and management guidelines that have been implemented to govern the conduct of employers in relation to employees.

Staff wages consume a vast portion of a hospital's total expenditure. Effective human resource management is therefore essential in order to achieve the aims and objectives of the organisation.

The success of a hospital or department depends on having the right number of staff with the required skills and abilities. Large organisations have dedicated human resource departments whose function is to oversee the recruitment process, whilst a smaller organisation may devolve the responsibility to line managers.

EMPLOYMENT LAW

Employment law comes from a variety of sources, not only common law and statute but also codes of practice and European Commission law.

This area is constantly changing. Governments legislate to amend the rights of the employer and employee, discrimination law and trade unions. Membership of the European Community requires changes that strengthen the protection provided for employees and those subject to discrimination. The employer has a legal responsibility to ensure that no unlawful sex, race or disability discrimination occurs in the recruitment and selection process.

Local agreements pertaining to pay and conditions of service must be readily available to managers and staff alike. These will have been agreed by the employer and represented union officials jointly. Managers should also be up to date with the NHS pay and conditions of service which are integral to *Agenda for Change* (DH 2003b).

Employment legislation

Initial employment processes will be governed by various employment legislation. The main areas are:

- Asylum and Immigration Act 1996
- Contracts (Rights of Third Parties) Act 1999
- Directive 97/81/EC Part-time Work Directive as extended to the UK by Directive 98/23/EC
- Disability Discrimination Act 1995
- Dispute Resolution Regulations 2004
- Employment Act 2002
- Employment Rights Act 1999
- Employment Relations Act 1996
- Employment Relations Act 1999
- Employment Equality (Religion or Belief) Regulations 2003
- Employment Equality (Sexual Orientation) Regulations 2003
- Equal Pay Act 1970
- Fixed Term Employees (Prevention of Less Favourable Treatment) Regulations 2002
- Human Rights Act 1998
- List 99 Department of Education and Employment
- Management of Health and Safety at Work Regulations 1992
- Police Act 1997
- Protection of Children Act 1999
- Race Relations Act 1976
- Race Relations Act 2003
- Rehabilitation of Offenders Act 1974 (Exemptions) Order 1975
- Sex Discrimination Act 1975
- Sexual Offenders Act 1997
- Trade Union and Labour Relations (Consolidation) Act 1992
- Trade Union Reforms and Employment Rights Act 1993
- Working Time Regulations 1998

RECOMMENDATIONS FOR LOCAL POLICY

The various aspects of staff management that should be adhered to by both the employer and employee are included below.

Initial employment process

In organisations such as the NHS or other healthcare providers, the line manager, with contributions and advice from the human resource department, usually undertakes the selection and employment of staff. The role of the human resource manager is to ensure that procedures in selection and recruitment are followed, to provide support and advice on all aspects of equal opportunities, and to ensure that all documentation related to the selection and recruitment process is completed in a timely fashion.

Employment statutes are beyond the remit of this publication, but the basic principles of the initial employment process are outlined, and cover the contract and statutory rights of the employee.

Good employment practice will encompass and provide protocols and standards for the following:

WORKFORCE PLANNING AND JOB ANALYSIS

RECOMMENDATION **3.3.1** Managers should review the demands of the service every year, or more frequently if service changes are anticipated. This entails identifying the skills required in the department to undertake the caseload in a safe and competent manner. They must ensure staff are in place with the necessary skills and training to carry out the work expected of them.

RECOMMENDATION **3.3.2** Human resource planning should include:

- assessing the future requirement needs
- formulating a training programme
- developing a promotion and career development policy
- developing a flexible workforce
- controlling staff costs
- assessing the future requirements for capital equipment and technological training needs.

JOB ANALYSIS AND EVALUATION

Job analysis and evaluation is a key function of management and is essential for all processes leading to effective performance in the workplace. It is inextricably linked to workforce planning (ie: ensuring that job descriptions and specifications match the skill required for the job).

RECOMMENDATION **3.3.3** A job should be reviewed regularly and changed when appropriate. Several components should be examined when undertaking this task:

- **Job specification** This specifies the skills, knowledge and attitudes required to perform the job. It should clearly specify any out of hours commitments.
- **Job description** This specifies the component tasks, duties and standards required, and the environmental circumstances of a job. It should reflect the level of skill required to carry out the job. A job description is seen as a guide to the skills required and is not definitive. A job description is not regarded in law as setting out the terms of a contract.
- **Person specification** This is an interpretation of the job specification in terms of the kind of person needed to perform the job effectively. Its main use is in the selection process, where it can be used to assess/score against suitability for the post.

Recruitment of staff

It is recommended that personnel involved in human resource management adhere to the following guidance, in conjunction with the publication *Recruitment and Retention Strategies for Perioperative Staff* (NATN 2000).

RECOMMENDATION **3.3.4** The public image projected by an organisation can determine the quality of staff it is able to recruit. A positive image is crucial in attracting suitable applicants. The wording and placement of advertisements must be carefully considered. Employers must comply with legal requirements, especially discrimination laws, when recruiting staff. It is unlawful for employers to advertise vacancies, select interview candidates or offer employment in a way that discriminates on the grounds of sex, race or marital status. An employee or job applicant who feels that they have been discriminated against can raise a complaint with the Equal Opportunities Commission, the Commission for Racial Equality or an employment tribunal.

RECOMMENDATION **3.3.5** Recruitment and selection should be an efficient systematic process which enables optimum choice, otherwise the process will not be cost-effective or an efficient use of resources.

The process should consider:

- the extent of vacancies following job analysis
- the preparation and publication of information including an explicit job summary, description and personal specification
- marketing of the employing organisation – projecting a good image to attract applicants
- a closing date which allows adequate time for distribution and return of application forms
- a schedule which allows applicants sufficient time for preparation (eg: eight working days' notice of an interview)
- inclusion of all documents necessary for the applicant to bring to interview, including a map showing the location of the hospital and directions to the place of interview.

JOB ADVERTISEMENT

RECOMMENDATION **3.3.6** It is good employment practice to prepare a written job description and job specification with the job title. From this written description an employer can specify the most important duties of the vacant post as follows:

- Qualifications and experience required
- Specific skills and competencies required
- Experience with specific equipment
- Salary and benefits offered
- The person to contact
- Required references.

It is recommended that the human resource department is always consulted.

SELECTION OF CANDIDATES

RECOMMENDATION **3.3.7** The following checklist outlines what the employer should do during the selection process:

- Process all applications in the same way.
- Formulate standard questions which are consistent for each interviewee.
- Ask questions at interview which relate to the requirements of the vacant post.
- Keep records of interviews showing why applicants were or were not appointed.
- Use a scoring system to benchmark candidates.

All interviews, whether informal or formal, need careful preparation if they are to be successful.

RECOMMENDATION **3.3.8** Good interview practice should include the following:

- Potential staff should be afforded privacy and uniformity during the interview.
- Interviews should be structured to discover all relevant information and to assess the competencies of the applicant.
- The interview should have a consistent format – which is particularly important if there is more than one applicant.
- Interview should be undertaken in a quiet environment, guaranteed free from interruption. Interviewers' bleepers should be switched off and telephones diverted for the duration of the interview.
- A clear statement of terms and conditions of employment should be made at the beginning of the interview.
- Two references must be obtained before the initial employment process is finalised.
- Security clearance with the Criminal Records Bureau and health clearance from occupational health must be attained before an offer of employment is made.
- Once the preferred candidate accepts the offer of employment, rejection letters should be sent to the unsuccessful candidates. The letter should indicate that they can contact a designated person to obtain constructive feedback on why they were unsuccessful.
- Verbal promises at interview and when the job offer is made constitute implied contracts. Employers cannot change terms and conditions offered at interview.

REFERENCES

RECOMMENDATION **3.3.9** It is illegal for an employer or employee to write an untrue reference. A reference should offer an accurate view of the candidate and his or her ability to do the job in question. Opinions expressed in a reference should be supported by facts. Negative comments should be justified so that the reader can make an informed decision.

RECOMMENDATION **3.3.10** The Data Protection Act (HMSO 1998a) allows all employees to access their personal file including references. It is recommended that there is a policy that supports showing an employee a copy of any references.

RECOMMENDATION **3.3.11** References should be obtained before interview, to avoid having to make an offer of a job subject to references.

Retention of staff

Staff need to feel valued, particularly in today's ever-changing healthcare environment. Staff shortages affect many of us, and can have a stressful and damaging affect on the team as a whole, putting relentless pressure on performance, sometimes at almost unsustainable levels.

RECOMMENDATION **3.3.12** Effective leadership is an essential element of staff retention. Support and guidance is required at all levels to maintain a happy and safe working environment. Managers require financial support to enable them to provide training development to staff. Statutory training alone requires much organisation and time, and staff also have other developmental needs. Adequate resources are an essential requirement to support training and development, which in turn is crucial in aiding recruitment and retention.

RECOMMENDATION **3.3.13** An initial induction period will have a lasting effect on new staff, and it is vital that they are introduced into the workplace by an efficient employment process and a well-supported induction period.

CONTRACT OF EMPLOYMENT

RECOMMENDATION **3.3.14** There is no legal requirement for the contract of employment to be in writing. It can be written, oral or a mixture of both. However Section 1 of the Employment Relations Act (HMSO 1996) states that employers are required to give a written statement of particulars of employment within two months of commencement of a post. The statement should set out minimum details about the terms governing the employment relationship and should contain:

- name of employer and employee
- date when employment began
- period of employment, if a fixed term contract
- scale or rate of remuneration and intervals of pay
- any terms relating to holidays, holiday pay and pensions
- job title, job description and job specification
- place of work
- hours of work
- leave entitlement
- notice entitlement
- sickness entitlement
- disciplinary rules
- grievance procedure
- details of local collective agreements affecting employment.

RECOMMENDATION **3.3.15** The employee is under a contractual duty to exercise reasonable care and skill in the performance of his or her duties. An employee would therefore be in breach of this duty if his/her duties were performed negligently or incompetently.

RECOMMENDATION **3.3.16** During employment, an implied term of a contract is for the employee not to reveal any confidential information.

HOSPITAL INDUCTION

The human resource department is responsible for ensuring that new staff receive information on certain policies and procedures, such as pension schemes, equal opportunities, statutory sick pay, and working time directives.

RECOMMENDATION **3.3.17** A local induction should be undertaken within one month of initial employment for all staff new to the hospital. This should consist of an introduction to the hospital environment, and mandatory training including manual handling, COSHH, fire, basic life support, waste disposal and infection control.

DEPARTMENTAL INDUCTION AND MENTOR/PRECEPTORSHIP

RECOMMENDATION **3.3.18** All new staff, regardless of their grade, should be provided with a departmental staff induction pack to guide them in their initial few weeks. This should aid their orientation to the area, outline the working schedule of the department, the various roles performed by staff, and the objectives expected of them within time-scales.

RECOMMENDATION **3.3.19** New staff should be appointed to a preceptor or mentor for their period of departmental induction, who should be an experienced perioperative practitioner. The length of this induction will depend on their previous experience. It should be carefully planned by both parties, have clear objectives and time-scales. A review date should be set.

TRAINING AND DEVELOPMENT PROGRAMME

RECOMMENDATION **3.3.20** The perioperative environment must have a comprehensive training programme, to ensure that individuals are trained and supported within the multi-professional environment.

RECOMMENDATION **3.3.21** Policies and guidelines must be in place, and reviewed regularly to reflect current best practice. Flexible positive measures must be available to enable a person to reach their full potential and aid retention of staff. Appraisal, or individual performance review, is an integral part of this process and should be carried out each year.

Grievance procedures

In any organisation employees may have problems or concerns about their work, working environment or working relationships that they wish to have addressed. Grievance procedures enable an individual or group to raise issues with management about their work or about the actions of fellow employees which affect them. Examples may be issues around health and safety, terms and conditions of employment, new working practices, organisational change, equal opportunities or bullying at work.

RECOMMENDATION **3.3.22** Disciplinary and grievance procedures should comply with Section 1 of the Employment Relations Act (HMSO 1996), the Employment Act 2002 and the *Dispute Resolution Regulations* (HMSO 2004a). Failure to comply could lead to employment tribunals and heavy penalties for the transgressor, whether the employer or the employee.

RECOMMENDATION **3.3.23** Whilst employers are not required by statute to have a grievance procedure, it is seen as good practice in employment relations to provide workers with a reasonable and prompt opportunity to seek redress of any grievance. Employers are required by statute to specify, in the written statement of terms and conditions of employment, a means by which an employee can contact a person within the organisation if they have a grievance.

RECOMMENDATION **3.3.24** Management must be responsible for developing grievance procedures. A formal grievance procedure must be acceptable to those covered by the procedure and those who have to implement it. Policies should be written in accordance with the Advisory Conciliation and Arbitration Service guidelines (ACAS 2000) and in consultation with local trade union representation within the hospital. A formal procedure must follow stages, although it is to be hoped that most grievances are resolved at the first stage.

RECOMMENDATION **3.3.25** A grievance procedure provides a mechanism for issues to be dealt with fairly and speedily, with the aim of avoiding major difficulties by prolonged discussions and arbitration. It is important that grievances are dealt with quickly and at the lowest level possible within the hospital in order to obtain a speedy resolution. Most routine complaints or grievances are best resolved informally by discussion between the employee and their immediate manager. The formal grievance procedure should only be invoked where it has not been possible to deal with matters in this way. For example, there may be situations where the employee finds it difficult to raise the case with their manager because of its nature. In such a case the employee can choose to have a representative raise the case for them or can seek advice on the process to follow.

STAGE 1 – IMMEDIATE LINE MANAGER

RECOMMENDATION **3.3.26** The employee should raise their grievance, in writing, with their immediate line manager. If the grievance is against the manager, the next level of management should be the first point of contact. The manager should invite the employee to attend a hearing to discuss their complaint, and, depending on the nature of the grievance, inform them of their right to be accompanied by a union representative or work colleague. This hearing should be arranged as soon as possible after the grievance has been raised, preferably within 15 working days. The manager should respond to the grievance in writing within five working days after the hearing, although ideally the decision would be given verbally at the hearing. If this is not possible, the employee should be given an explanation for the delay and told when a response can be expected.

STAGE 2 – NEXT LEVEL OF MANAGEMENT

RECOMMENDATION **3.3.27** The employee can raise the matter to the next level of management if the problem is not resolved at Stage 1. They must do this in writing. The manager should arrange to hear the grievance within ten working days and should inform the worker of their right to be accompanied if appropriate.

STAGE 3 – HIGHER LEVEL OF MANAGEMENT (TRUST BOARD PANEL OR HOSPITAL MANAGEMENT COMMITTEE)

RECOMMENDATION **3.3.28** To evoke Stage 3 the employee or their representative must write to the director of human resources or whoever is responsible for these issues with the hospital. Within a trust hospital those involved at this level of appeal may include:

- director of human resources
- non-executive director of the trust
- executive director of the trust
- local representative of a trade union/professional association that has members employed by the trust
- human resource manager acting as secretary and advisor to the panel, but who will not have a vote.

RECOMMENDATION **3.3.29** This meeting should take place with the minimum of formality but should follow a basic framework, as recommended by ACAS. The panel must arrive at a decision, which may have to be a majority one. The panel should announce their decision at the meeting if possible and give written confirmation with a specified time (ie: 10–15 working days following the meeting).

RECOMMENDATION **3.3.30** If the matter is not resolved at Stage 3, the position is as follows:

- For an individual grievance there is no further right to appeal.
- For collective disputes (with the agreement of both management and trade union) the matter can be referred to ACAS.

Disciplinary procedures

Rules and procedures related to disciplinary matters are necessary in order to provide fair, constant and rational employment relations. The Employment Relations Act 1996 and the Employment Act 2002 require employers to provide written information for their employees regarding certain aspects of their disciplinary rules and procedures. All managers should be familiar with the process within their hospital.

RECOMMENDATION **3.3.31** Management is responsible for maintaining discipline and for ensuring that there are appropriate disciplinary rules and procedures covering issues of worker and capability (ACAS 2000).

RECOMMENDATION **3.3.32** Rules or policies should be readily available for staff, in booklets and intranet sites. Managers have a responsibility to ensure that staff are aware of the information and that it can be accessed. Ideally policy awareness should be part of a hospital induction programme.

RECOMMENDATION **3.3.33** Where a case calls for disciplinary procedures to be taken, a formal procedure should be followed:

- **First warning – oral** In response to minor infringements the employee should be given a formal oral warning. A note of the warning should be made but this should be disregarded for disciplinary purposes after a specified period of time (ie: six months).
- **First warning – written** If the infringement is deemed more serious, a formal written warning should be given, outlining the details of the complaint. The warning should also outline the changes or improvements required in behaviour, and the time-scale allowed for these. This warning should inform the employee that a final written warning may follow if there is no satisfactory change or improvement.
- **Final written warning** If there is no improvement or change during the period given, or if matters become worse, the employee should be given a final written warning. This again should explain the reasons for the warning and the improvements required, which if not achieved, will lead to dismissal or additional action such as transfer. It should refer to the right to appeal. A final written warning should be disregarded for disciplinary purposes after a specified time, but may be kept on file.
- **Dismissal or other authorisation** If the employee's conduct or performance fails to improve, the next step will depend on the organisation. Any action such as transfer, suspension without pay, loss of seniority or pay increment, demotion or dismissal will be made by an appropriate manager and human resource manager. Disciplinary outcome will depend on the seriousness of the event.

Whistle-blowing

There are two types of whistle-blowing – the first is where the employee reports another employee to the employer, and the other arises when an employee feels that there is no alternative but to go public because no one in the organisation will take a deficiency in the service seriously.

RECOMMENDATION **3.3.34** In the light of the Public Interest Disclosure Act (HMSO 1998b), healthcare organisations should have a whistle-blowing policy. The act protects staff from suffering employment detriment as a result of making disclosure about the acts or omissions of other members of the workforce, in the public interest. It therefore protects them against victimisation.

RECOMMENDATION **3.3.35** According to the NMC *Code of Professional Conduct* (NMC 2002) and the Health Professions Council *Code of Conduct* (HPC 2003), both nurses and operating department practitioners are required to bring hazards and dangers to the attention of management. Staff should initially voice their concerns and should support them in writing.

NURSES' RESPONSIBILITY

RECOMMENDATION 3.3.36 The nurse must comply with the following clauses of the NMC *Code of Professional Conduct* (2002):

- 8.2 *You must act quickly to protect patients and clients from risk if you have good reason to believe that you or a colleague, from your own or another profession, may not be fit to practise for reasons of conduct, health or competence. You should be aware of the terms of legislation that offer protection for people who raise concerns about health and safety issues.*
- 8.3 *Where you cannot remedy circumstances in the environment of care that could jeopardise standards of practice, you must report them to a senior person with sufficient authority to manage them and also, in the case of midwifery, to the supervisor of midwives. This must be supported by a written record.*

RECOMMENDATION 3.3.37 In situations which put patients and/or staff at risk, the nurse must communicate concerns to a manager. The manager should assess the report and communicate it to a senior person with sufficient authority, such as a risk manger where appropriate.

RECOMMENDATION 3.3.38 Protected disclosures are extensive and cover all concerns a registered practitioner is likely to have or be professionally bound by duty to disclose under their code of professional conduct. A hospital should have a range of policies which deal with standards of behaviour and conduct at work, and staff should use these procedures where necessary and appropriate. When situations occur where procedures do not apply, individuals may resort to the whistle-blowing guidelines for reporting justifiable concerns.

Justifiable concerns are:

- a criminal offence has been, is being or is likely to be committed
- a person has failed, is failing or is likely to fail to comply with any legal obligation to which he is subject
- a miscarriage of justice has occurred, is occurring or is likely to occur
- a health or safety of any individual has been, is being or is likely to be endangered
- the environment has been, is being or is likely to be damaged
- information tending to show any matter falling within any of the above paragraphs has been, is being or is likely to be deliberately concealed.

MANAGERIAL RESPONSIBILITIES

RECOMMENDATION 3.3.39 Hospital managers involved in a whistle-blowing issue have a responsibility to:

- take concerns seriously
- consider them carefully and undertake investigation if appropriate
- seek appropriate advice
- take prompt action to resolve the issue or refer it to a more appropriate person
- keep the individual who raised the issue informed of the process
- monitor and review the situation
- inform senior managers
- ensure as far as possible that individuals who genuinely raise concerns are not penalised.

RECOMMENDATION 3.3.40 A hospital should protect the confidentiality of those who raise concerns. It should not disclose the identity of an individual unless required to do so as part of an official investigation.

INFORMAL APPROACH

RECOMMENDATION **3.3.41** An informal approach for whistle-blowing would refer to:

- designated officers who are external to the formal line management structure
- staff/union representatives.

In all cases individuals have the right to discuss their concerns with the chief executive or equivalent and chair of the trust/hospital.

RECOMMENDATION **3.3.42** An informal procedure aims to resolve the concerns between the individual and an appropriate manager or professional head. A line manager is required to investigate the allegations thoroughly. The individual should receive an initial verbal response within a set number of days, followed by a written acknowledgement. In the event of an unsatisfactory outcome for the complainant the employee has the right to proceed to the formal stage.

THE FORMAL APPROACH

RECOMMENDATION **3.3.43** The formal procedure has two stages. Stage 1 involves:

- raising the concern with an executive director and chief executive
- arranging a strictly confidential meeting, and recording the concern
- agreeing action to investigate the concern.

RECOMMENDATION **3.3.44** If satisfaction is not obtained or the individual feels the above is inappropriate, Stage 2 involves a non-executive director to help resolve the issue. In exceptional circumstances, for example where there is a possible danger to life, individuals have the right to make a public disclosure without going through internal procedures.

Complaints

The legal framework for the NHS complaints procedure is set out in the directions made under powers conferred on the Secretary of State by Section 17 of the National Health Service Act (HMSO 1977), Section 1A of the Hospital Complaints Procedure Act 1985, and paragraph 6(2)(e) of Schedule 2 to the NHS and Community Care Act 1990.

The NHS *Complaints Procedure Regulations* (HMSO 2004b) were published to cover the arrangements for making a complaint in different parts of the NHS.

The directions require NHS trusts (and health authorities prior to their abolition in October 2002) to have written procedures for dealing with complaints within their organisation (local resolution) and to operate the second element of the complaints procedure (independent review).

RECOMMENDATION **3.3.45** Health, social care legislation and other public protection laws govern how patients and the public are protected. When things go wrong and lead to a complaint, managers and practitioners will need to know what these laws are, how they affect complaints casework and how to access the right information. Advice should always be sought from the organisational complaints manager as it is important to understand fully patients' rights for complaints to be managed effectively.

RECOMMENDATION **3.3.46** Most NHS hospitals have a procedure in place with which to handle complaints; private hospitals will have their own systems in place. Staff should be guided through the complaints procedure and should be able to demonstrate a reasonable knowledge of the system in their place of work. Staff should be able to handle a minor complaint when it arises, and have knowledge of the appropriate channels if the complainant wishes to pursue their grievance.

RECOMMENDATION **3.3.47** The system should reflect the foundation principles outlined in The NHS Training Division (1995) which came from the report of a review chaired by Professor Wilson (DH 1994):

- Responsiveness
- Quality enhancement
- Cost-effectiveness
- Accessibility
- Impartiality
- Simplicity
- Speed
- Confidentiality
- Accountability.

RECOMMENDATION **3.3.48** Formal proceedings and legal action would often not occur if the complainant was given an understandable explanation of what happened, and the steps being taken to resolve matters.

RECOMMENDATION **3.3.49** Any staff involved in an actual or potential complaint should notify their line manager immediately. If the complaint is of a serious nature and statements are required, the employee should take advice from their senior departmental manager or the solicitor to the employer. The employer must allow a member of staff time to consult their union representative if requested. The purpose of the statement must be clear as it will affect the style and content of the information supplied. In some situations it is recommended that brief details of an event are written down for later reference whilst the event is clear in the mind of the staff member, before any official statement is written. A statement should contain the following essential elements:

- Date and time of the incident
- Name, position, grade and location of author
- Full name of person involved
- Date and time the statement was written
- Signature
- A supporting statement which should exhibit accuracy, be factual, avoid hearsay, and be concise, relevant and legible.

A copy should always be retained.

RECOMMENDATION **3.3.50** Trusts and health authorities must have a complaints manager whose job it is to oversee the complaints procedure. The manager will receive the complaints and investigate them. The aim is to resolve complaints at the informal local resolution stage. If this is not to the complainant's satisfaction they can request an independent review.

RECOMMENDATION **3.3.51** A convenor, a non-executive director of the trust or health authority, will have to decide whether the complaint should be passed on to an independent review panel. If no review is recommended the complainant must be informed of their right to complain to the Ombudsman.

RECOMMENDATION **3.3.52** Complaints where no independent review is carried out include:

- where legal proceedings have commenced or are about to be initiated
- where the trust or health authority has investigated all practical action and established that no further action would be beneficial
- where further local action aimed at conciliation is deemed preferable – referring the action back to the local resolution process.

RECOMMENDATION **3.3.53** The final route for unresolved complaints is to the Health Service Commissioner (Ombudsman). Complaints channelled to this route will include those related to local authority services, matters involving clinical judgement of healthcare professionals and those services provided by GPs, dentists, pharmacists and opticians. The commissioner is not able to investigate personnel matters such as staff appointments, pay or discipline.

Harassment and bullying

RECOMMENDATION **3.3.54** It is recommended that managers and practitioners consult the publication *Challenging Behaviours in the Perioperative Environment* (NATN 2002b) when formulating guidance.

It is likely that a theatre practitioner will be involved in a complaint during their career, which could be related to their own or another person's conduct. The NHS Litigation Authority has a risk management standard which states that '*a hospital must ensure that an agreed system of managing complaints is in place*' (Clinical Negligence Scheme for Trusts 2002).

REFERENCES

Advisory Conciliation and Arbitration Service 2000 *Code of Practice on Disciplinary and Grievance Procedures* London, ACAS

Association of Anaesthetists of Great Britain and Ireland 1995 *Risk Management* London, AAGBI. www.aagbi.org

Association of Anaesthetists of Great Britain and Ireland 2003 *Theatre Efficiency* London, AAGBI. www.aagbi.org

Clinical Negligence Scheme for Trusts 2002 *Clinical Risk Management Standards* London, NHS Litigation Authority

Department of Health 1994 *Being Heard: the report of a review committee chaired by Professor Wilson on NHS complaints procedures* London, DH

Department of Health 1997 *Designed to Care (Scotland)* Edinburgh, The Scottish Office

Department of Health 2000 *NHS Plan: a plan for investment, a plan for reform in England* London, DH

Department of Health 2002 *Indepedent Healthcare: national minimum standards regulations* London, The Stationery Office

Department of Health 2003a *The Essence of Care: patient-focused benchmarking for healthcare practitioners* London, DH

Department of Health 2003b *Agenda for Change: a proposed agreement* London, DH

HMSO 1974 *Health and Safety at Work Act* Norwich, The Stationery Office

HMSO 1977 *The National Health Service Act* Norwich, The Stationery Office

HMSO 1985 *Hospital Complaints Procedure Act* Norwich, The Stationery Office

HMSO 1990 *NHS and Community Care Act* Norwich, The Stationery Office

HMSO 1992 *Management of Health and Safety at Work Regulations* Norwich, The Stationery Office

HMSO 1996 *Employment Relations Act* Norwich, The Stationery Office

HMSO 1998a *Data Protection Act* Norwich, The Stationery Office

HMSO 1998b *The Public Interest Disclosure Act: whistle-blowing in the NHS* Norwich, The Stationery Office

HMSO 2002 *Employment Act* Norwich, The Stationery Office

HMSO 2004a *Dispute Resolution Regulations* Norwich, The Stationery Office

HMSO 2004b *NHS Complaints Procedure Regulations* Norwich, The Stationery Office

HPC 2003 *Health Professions Council (Conduct and Competence Committee) (Procedure) Rules Order of Council.* www.hpc-uk.org/publications/rules_conduct_and_competence_committee.htm

Modernisation Agency 2002 *Step Guide to Improving Operating Theatre Performance* London, DH

National Association of Theatre Nurses 1998 *Safeguards for Invasive Procedures: the management of risks* Harrogate, NATN

National Association of Theatre Nurses 2000 *Recruitment and Retention Strategies for Perioperative Staff* Harrogate, NATN

National Association of Theatre Nurses 2002a *Risk and Quality Management System* Harrogate, NATN

National Association of Theatre Nurses 2002b *Challenging Behaviours in the Perioperative Environment* Harrogate, NATN

National Association of Theatre Nurses 2003 *Staffing for Patients in the Perioperative Setting* Harrogate, NATN

National Confidential Enquiry into Perioperative Deaths 1997 *Who Operates When? 1 April 1995 – 31 March 1996* London, NCEPOD. www.ncepod.org.uk

National Confidential Enquiry into Perioperative Deaths 2001 *Changing the Way We Operate* London, NCEPOD. www.ncepod.org.uk

NHS Leadership Centre 2002 *Leadership Qualities Framework* www.nhsleadershipqualities.nhs.uk

NHS Executive 1999 *Clinical Governance: quality in the new NHS* London, DH

NHS Training Division 1995 *Local Resolution Training Resources Pack* Leeds, NHS Executive

Nursing and Midwifery Council 2002 *Code of Professional Conduct* London, NMC

Royal College of Anaesthetists 2000 *Raising the Standard* London, RCA

FURTHER READING

Advisory Conciliation and Arbitration Service 2002 *Recruitment and Selection* London, ACAS. www.acas.org.uk

Association of Anaesthetists of Great Britain and Ireland 2002 *Immediate Post Anaesthetic Recovery* London, AAGBI. www.aagbi.org

Audit Commission 2000 *Getting Better all the Time: making benchmarking work* London, Audit Commission

Audit Commission 2001 *A Spoonful of Sugar* London, Audit Commission

Audit Scotland 1999 *Full House: theatre utilisation in Scottish hospitals* www.audit-scotland.gov.uk

Audit Scotland 2000 *Planning Ward Nursing – legacy or design?* www.audit-scotland.gov.uk

Benson L, Boyd A, Walshe K 2004 *Interim Report Learning from CHI: the impact of healthcare regulation* Manchester, Manchester Centre for Healthcare Management

Bynom S 1999 When is Blowing the Whistle not Whistle-blowing? *British Journal of Theatre Nursing* 9 (6) 265–267

Campbell L 1999 Never Say Never ... *British Journal of Perioperative Nursing* 9 (9) 396–402

Cook M 2001 The Attributes of Effective Clinical Nurse Leaders *Nursing Standard* 15 (35) 33–36

Department of Health 1989 *Working for Patients* London, DH

Department of Health 1993 *Guidance for Staff on Relations with the Public and the Media* London, DH

Department of Health 1997 *The New NHS: modern dependable* London, DH

Department of Health 1998 *A First Class Service: quality in the new NHS* London, DH

Department of Health 1998 *European Working Time Regulations* London, DH

Department of Health 1998 *Clinical Governance: quality in the New NHS* London, DH

Department of Health 1999 *Making a Difference: strengthening the nursing, midwifery and health visiting contribution to health and healthcare* London, DH

Department of Health 2000 *NHS Plan: a plan for investment, a plan for reform in England* London, DH

Department of Health 2000 *An Organisation with a Memory: report of an expert group on learning from adverse incidents in the NHS* London, DH

Department of Health 2000 *Improving Working Lives* London, DH. www.dh.gov.uk/PolicyAndGuidance/HumanResourcesAndTraining/ModelEmployer/ImprovingWorkingLives/fs/en

Department of Health 2001 *Building a Safer NHS for Patients* London, DH

Department of Health/Cabinet Office 2003 *Making a Difference – reducing burdens in healthcare inspection and monitoring* London, DH. www.cabinet-office.gov.uk

Department of Health 2003 *Agenda for Change: proposed agreement* London, DH. www.dh.gov.uk

Department of Health 2003 *A Health Service for all Talents* London, DH

Department of Health 2003 *The NHS Knowledge and Skills Framework* London, DH. www.dh.gov.uk

Department of Health 2003 *Making Amends: a consultation paper setting out proposals for reforming the approach to clinical negligence in the NHS – a report by the chief medical officer* London, DH

Department of Health 2003 *Making a Difference: a first class service* London, DH. www.dh.gov.uk

Department of Health 2003 *Choice, Responsiveness and Equity in the NHS and Social Care* London, DH

Department of Health, Social Services and Public Safety 2002 *Developing Better Services: modernising hospitals and reforming structures in Northern Ireland* London, DH

Dimond B 2002 Clinical Governance and Assessing and Managing Clinical Risk *British Journal of Nursing* 11 (22) 1438–1440

Dimond B 2004 *Legal Aspects of Nursing* 4th ed, Harlow, Longman

Ellis JM 1999 Our Stamp and its Effects *Journal of Child Health Care* 2 6–8

Ellis JM 2000 Sharing the Evidence: clinical practice benchmarking to improve continuously the quality of care *Journal of Advanced Nursing* 32 215–225

Gemperlain J 2003 *Suggestions for Formulating Standards and Workable Policies* Virginia, American Press Institute

General Medical Council 1998 *Good Medical Practice* London, GMC

Guelbert C 2003 Leadership Qualities Framework Provides a Useful Tool for Nurses *Professional Nurse* 19 (3) 178–179

Harvey J, Kitson A 1996 Achieving Improvements Through Quality: an evaluation of key factors in the implementation process *Journal of Advanced Nursing* 24 185–195

Healthcare Commission 2004 *Corporate Plan 2004/2008: inspecting, informing, improving* London, Fishburn Hedges. www.healthcarecommission.org.uk/assetRoot

Health Education Authority 1995 *Organisational Stress in the National Health Service: an intervention to enable staff to address organisational sources of work-related stress* London, Health Education Authority

Health Service Ombudsman 2002 *Investigations Completed August–November 2001 – part 1: summaries of investigations completed* HC 679-1 London, The Stationery Office

HMSO 1970 *Equal Pay Act* Norwich, The Stationery Office

HMSO 1975 *Employment Protection Act* Norwich, The Stationery Office

HMSO 1975 *Sex Discrimination Act* Norwich, The Stationery Office

HMSO 1984 *Data Protection Act* Norwich, The Stationery Office

HMSO 1993 *Standards of Business Conduct* Norwich, The Stationery Office

HMSO 1993 *Trade Union Reform and Employment Rights Act* Norwich, The Stationery Office

HMSO 1995 *Disability Discrimination Act* Norwich, The Stationery Office

HMSO 1998 *Human Rights Act* Norwich, The Stationery Office

HMSO 2000 *Race Relations (Amendment) Act* Norwich, The Stationery Office

Klein R, Day P 2004 *The NHS Improvers* London, The King's Fund

Lee D 2002 Benchmarking *British Journal of Perioperative Nursing* 12 (7) 234–236

Mayatt V 2002 *Managing Risk in Healthcare Law and Practice* Croydon, Butterworths

McHale J, Tingle J 2001 *Law and Nursing* Oxford, Butterworth Heinemann

McNeil B 1999 Clinical Governance: the whys, whats and hows for theatre practitioners *British Journal of Perioperative Nursing* 9 (5) 209–216

McSherry R 2002 Clinical Supervision and Clinical Governance *Nursing Times* 98 (23) 30–32

Meadows S, Levenson R, Baeza J 2000 *The Last Straw: explaining the NHS nursing shortage* London, King's Fund. www.kingsfund.org.uk

Medical Defence Union 1993 *Talking to Patients* London, MDU

Modernisation Agency 2001 *Tackling Cancelled Operations* London, DH

Modernisation Agency 2002 *Theatre Programme: step guide to improving operating theatre performance* London, DH

National Assembly for Wales 2001 *Improving Health: the NHS plan for Wales* Cardiff, NAfW

National Association of Theatre Nurses 2000 *Recruitment and Retention Strategies for Perioperative Staff* Harrogate, NATN

National Association of Theatre Nurses 2002 *Supporting Students in the Perioperative Setting* Harrogate, NATN

National Association of Theatre Nurses 2002 *Risk and Quality Management System* Harrogate, NATN

National Association of Theatre Nurses 2002 *Challenging Behaviours in the Perioperative Environment: dealing with bullying, violence and harassment* Harrogate, NATN

National Audit Office 2001 *Handling Clinical Negligence Claims in England* London, The Stationery Office

National Audit Office 2003 *Achieving Improvements Through Clinical Governance* HC1055 London, The Stationery Office

National Nursing Leadership Project – www.nursingleadership.co.uk

NHS Confederation 2003 *Re-reviewing the Reviewers: the NHS Confederation's second review of NHS trust experience of CHI clinical governance reviews* London, NHS Confederation

NHS Executive 2001 *Improving Working Lives Standard* Leeds, DH

NHS Litigation Authority 2000 *Clinical Negligence Scheme for Trusts (CNST) Risk Management Standards and Procedures, Manual of Guidance* London, NHSLA

NHS Reviews Co-ordination Group 2003 *Improving the Efficiency of Scrutiny of Risk Management: progress report* London, NHSRCG. www.chi.nhs.uk/nhsrcg

NHS Scotland 2000 *Our National Health: a new agenda in Scotland* Edinburgh, Scottish Executive

Nursing and Midwifery Council 1994 *The Future of Professional Practice: the council's standards for education and practice following registration* London, NMC

Nursing and Midwifery Council 1996 *Guidelines for Professional Practice* London, NMC

Nursing and Midwifery Council 1996 *Reporting Unfitness to Practice: information for employers and managers* London, NMC

Nursing and Midwifery Council 2002 *Employers and Prep* London, NMC. www.nmc-uk.org/nmc/main/publications/employersprep.pdf

Reilly J 2001 Clinical Governance in the Real World *Nursing Times* 97 (50) 36–37

Royal College of Nursing 1999 *Guidance on Good Management Practice* London, RCN

Royal College of Nursing 2000 *Guidance for Nurse Expert Witnesses* London, RCN

Royal College of Nursing 2003 *Guidance for Nurse Staffing in Critical Care* RCN Direct. www.rcn.org.uk/direct

Shaw A 2002 Lessons in Empowerment *Nursing Times* 98 (26) 36–37

Simons F 2003 Clinical Leadership Part 1: key components of the programme *Professional Nurse* 18 (11) 656–657

Simons F 2003 Clinical Leadership Part 2: transforming leadership *Professional Nurse* 18 (12) 716–717

Simons F 2003 Clinical Leadership Part 3: how to foster a leading role for everyone *Professional Nurse* 19 (1) 56–58

Stauch M, Wheat K, Tingle J 2002 *Source Book on Medical Law* 2nd ed, London, Cavendish Publishing

Wallace H, Mulcahy L 1999 *The Public Law Project, Cause for Complaint? An evaluation of the effectiveness of the NHS complaints procedure* London, University of London

Walshe K, Dineen M 1999 *Clinical Risk Management in the NHS: making a difference?* London, NHS Confederation and Healthcare Risk Resources International

Westwood F 2001 Leadership and Communication *British Journal of Perioperative Nursing* 11 (4) 190–194

Wilson J 1999 Healthcare Risk Management *British Journal of Nursing* 8 (12) 821–822

Woodhead K 2004 Clinical Leadership Examined *The Clinical Services Journal* 3 (1) 35–37

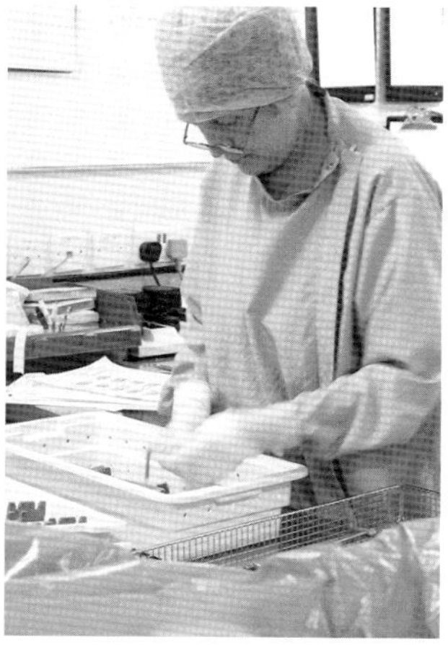

4 INFECTION CONTROL

4.1 STANDARD PRECAUTIONS

STANDARD A standard set of precautions is in place for every invasive procedure. An additional risk assessment of each patient is undertaken to determine whether extra precautions may be appropriate.

The emergence of the human immunodeficiency virus (HIV), hepatitis B (HBV) and C (HCV), tuberculosis (TB) and multi-resistant staphylococcus aureus (MRSA) have prompted the requirement for strict infection control procedures and the introduction of standard precautions for the protection of staff, patients and all present in clinical areas. An increase in the incidence of hospital acquired infection has emphasised the need to review regularly all infection control procedures within the perioperative setting to ensure that standard precautions are standard practice.

Infection control policies focus on minimising the risk of cross-infection in all healthcare settings. With increasing numbers of patients being treated, best practice recommends that all patients are treated as potentially infected. In the Centres for Disease Control recommendations for isolation precautions (CDC 1998) *'universal precautions'* have been replaced by *'standard precautions'*. Additional precautions can be taken when judged appropriate.

Standard precautions assess the activity to be completed and not the individual who is to receive the care. All patients have the right to be treated with dignity and respect, and the use of standard precautions eliminates the risk of random inappropriate practice, and permits staff to deliver high standards of care to all patients at all times. Standard precautions apply to the exposure to blood and body fluids. The management of these includes hand decontamination, decontamination of equipment and the environment, the safe disposal of clinical waste and the safe disposal of sharps.

Healthcare workers within the perioperative setting have a high risk of exposure to blood and body fluids. The activity assessment and use of standard precautions should therefore be strictly adhered to for all patients, in order to minimise the risk to healthcare workers, the patient and other members of the caring team. The healthcare worker must assess the risk factors inherent within each activity/procedure, must wear the appropriate protective equipment, and must take additional precautions dependent on the identified risk of contamination with blood and body fluids.

RECOMMENDATIONS FOR LOCAL POLICY

Management considerations

RECOMMENDATION **4.1.1** Infection control is an issue of health and safety and comes within the remit of various pieces of legislation: Health and Safety at Work Act (HMSO 1974), *Control of Substances Hazardous to Health Regulations* (HMSO 2002) and *Personal Protective Equipment Regulations* (HMSO 1992). The basic objective is to ensure that all staff are protected and that supplies of personal protective equipment are readily available.

RECOMMENDATION **4.1.2** All healthcare workers must take every precaution to minimise occupational exposure to potential pathogens.

RECOMMENDATION **4.1.3** An occupational health programme of hepatitis B vaccination is essential and must be available to all staff that work within the perioperative environment.

RECOMMENDATION **4.1.4** Any concerns which staff may have regarding occupational exposure, should be addressed to the local occupational health department in accordance with local policy.

RECOMMENDATION **4.1.5** In England and Wales perioperative departments must comply with the environmental standards issued by the DH, as well as controls assurance. It is the responsibility of all perioperative staff to ensure that the standards are monitored and maintained.

Patient considerations

RECOMMENDATION **4.1.6** All patients must be provided with clean bed/trolley linen and a theatre gown as preparation for going to theatre.

RECOMMENDATION **4.1.7** All patients must be treated with respect for their privacy and dignity throughout their perioperative phase. Only the number of personnel required to manage the case safely should be present in theatre.

RECOMMENDATION **4.1.8** There should be a restriction on movement and talking within the operating theatre.

RECOMMENDATION **4.1.9** An effective air changing ventilation system should be in operation.

RECOMMENDATION **4.1.10** The doors to the operating theatre should remain closed to ensure the effective ventilation of the area.

RECOMMENDATION **4.1.11** Disposable anaesthetic breathing circuits should be changed in accordance with local policy and filters changed after each patient.

RECOMMENDATION **4.1.12** All reusable equipment must be decontaminated in accordance with controls assurance and NATN decontamination guidelines (see Section 5).

RECOMMENDATION **4.1.13** Effective communication within the clinical area must always be practised to ensure a thorough knowledge of the patient and their condition. A patient known to be infectious is often scheduled at the end of a list where practicable.

Protection and precautions

The use of personal protective equipment such as eyewear or face protection, impervious gowns, aprons and gloves can minimise the risk of wound infection and can protect staff from occupational exposure to potential biohazards. Circulating staff should wear gloves, plastic aprons and eye protection whenever there is a risk of exposure to blood or body fluids, including the risk of splash and aerosol contamination.

SKIN

RECOMMENDATION **4.1.14** All cuts and skin abrasions must be covered with waterproof dressings which are identified as effective viral and bacterial barriers.

RECOMMENDATION **4.1.15** Personnel who have exudative lesions or weeping dermatitis should be reviewed by the occupational health department and should not be permitted to administer direct patient care or handle medical devices used in invasive procedures.

HAND WASHING

RECOMMENDATION **4.1.16** Effective hand washing techniques must always be used, as soon as patient safety permits, especially if contaminated with blood or body fluids. Frequent hand washing is the single most important measure in the prevention of nosocomial infection.

RECOMMENDATION **4.1.17** Hands must be washed before and after every patient contact and immediately after direct contact with body fluids even if wearing gloves.

The use of gloves does not preclude the need for hand washing before and after patient contact.

GLOVES

RECOMMENDATION **4.1.18** Gloves must comply with European Community Standards: being of an acceptable quality, free from pinholes and must not tear or split easily.

RECOMMENDATION **4.1.19** Gloves must be changed and discarded after each procedure or patient episode or if visibly contaminated.

RECOMMENDATION **4.1.20** Double gloving when scrubbed reduces the risk of microbial contamination from glove perforation, and further protects the member of staff.

EYES AND MOUTH

RECOMMENDATION **4.1.21** The risk of splash or aerosol contamination must be assessed. If necessary, either mask and goggles or full-face visor must be worn to prevent exposure from blood and body fluids to the skin and mucous membranes.

RECOMMENDATION **4.1.22** Masks must be removed and discarded immediately after each procedure and if visibly contaminated.

RECOMMENDATION **4.1.23** Hand to mouth contact should be avoided.

RECOMMENDATION **4.1.24** Eating, drinking and applying cosmetics, contact lenses or lip balm should be prohibited in clinical areas.

GOWNS AND APRONS

RECOMMENDATION **4.1.25** Disposable aprons must be worn if close contact with the patient may lead to contamination of clothing from body substances.

RECOMMENDATION **4.1.26** Disposable aprons must be worn by circulating staff whenever there is an assessed risk of contamination during a procedure.

RECOMMENDATION **4.1.27** Gowns and drapes, whether single use or reusable, must comply with European Standards on resistance to penetration by blood and other body fluids. They must be able to maintain their integrity and be durable.

RECOMMENDATION **4.1.28** Additional measures (ie: fluid collecting drapes) should be taken if there is a risk of excessive blood/body fluid loss during a procedure.

SHARPS

RECOMMENDATION **4.1.29** Awareness and adherence to the local policy when handling and disposing of sharps is essential by all staff.

RECOMMENDATION **4.1.30** Sharps bins must comply with national standards (UN 3291, BS 7320).

Bins should be:

- assembled according to the manufacturer's instructions
- free from protruding sharps
- stored off the floor.

The temporary closure mechanism should be utilised when the bin is not in use.

RECOMMENDATION **4.1.31** Sealed and locked bins should be stored in a locked holding area, cupboard or container away from public access.

RECOMMENDATION **4.1.32** Needles must never be re-sheathed.

RECOMMENDATION **4.1.33** Needles and syringes must not be disassembled prior to use or disposal and should be discarded as one unit.

RECOMMENDATION **4.1.34** An appropriate instrument/device for the careful application and removal of surgical blades to and from a handle must be used.

RECOMMENDATION **4.1.35** Sharps and needles should not be passed hand to hand by the surgical team and handling should be kept to a minimum. A neutral zone where sharps can be placed in a receiver for safe use and retrieval should be promoted.

RECOMMENDATION **4.1.36** A disposable device should be used to contain needles and sharps and this should be disposed of safely at the end of the procedure.

SPILLAGE

RECOMMENDATION **4.1.37** Staff must adhere to the local policy on dealing with spillages.

RECOMMENDATION **4.1.38** If there is a risk of excessive blood/body fluid loss, collecting drapes should be used to reduce the risk of spillage.

RECOMMENDATION **4.1.39** The operating table should be protected and covered with a non-permeable sheet.

RECOMMENDATION **4.1.40** Floor suction devices should be considered to reduce the risk of spillage.

RECOMMENDATION **4.1.41** All spillages must be dealt with as soon as is reasonably practicable. All spillages should be cleaned up before disinfecting the area.

RECOMMENDATION **4.1.42** All agents used to manage the spillage must be used in accordance with manufacturer's instructions.

RECOMMENDATION **4.1.43** The contaminated area should be cleaned with 1% sodium hypochlorite.

ACCIDENTAL EXPOSURE

RECOMMENDATION **4.1.44** In the event of an injury, encourage bleeding if the skin has been punctured, wash the area with running water and soap, or wash the eye with saline.

RECOMMENDATION **4.1.45** Report the incident to the occupational health department or other medical source as per hospital policy.

RECOMMENDATION **4.1.46** Advise the line manager of the incident and document the nature of event and outcome.

WASTE DISPOSAL

RECOMMENDATION **4.1.47** All clinical waste must be segregated and placed in the appropriate container – yellow sacks, sharps container or other receptacle.

RECOMMENDATION **4.1.48** All waste for incineration must be labelled at point of origin.

RECOMMENDATION **4.1.49** Containers must be no more than three-quarters full, closed and sealed.

RECOMMENDATION **4.1.50** Yellow sacks must be no more than three-quarters full, and tied at the neck to ensure an effective seal.

RECOMMENDATION **4.1.51** Disposal of fluid waste must be handled with care to prevent splashing of contents – ideally within closed suction containers, which are single use.

RECOMMENDATION **4.1.52** Body parts and tissue must be separated into another yellow sack or identified suitable receptacle for incineration.

RECOMMENDATION **4.1.53** Linen must be segregated in accordance with DH guidance (NHS Estates 1995), depending on use, to prevent contamination of laundry workers. Laundry bags are colour coded as per local policy.

4.2 ENVIRONMENTAL CLEANING

STANDARD A system is in place for the management of effective environmental cleaning in the perioperative setting. Patients are provided with a safe, clean environment.

Most infections in postoperative surgical wounds are acquired during surgery. They may be endogenous from the patient's own flora (ie: from the skin, mucous membranes or gastro-intestinal tract) or exogenous from the operating theatre personnel or, infrequently, from the environment.

The national standards of cleanliness issued by the NHS Estates (2002), enables trusts to have in place a robust programme through which *'technical standards'* of cleanliness can be routinely and accurately measured. This in turn provides information by which performance may be assessed in relation to standards achieved at other healthcare facilities.

Within the healthcare environment, cleaning procedures are determined by the extent of the risk posed by the area. A ward or department is assigned one of four risk categories namely: very high risk, high risk, significant risk and low risk. The criteria used to determine the categorisation are based on the following:

- The risk of infection
- The risk of poor public image
- Lack of confidence
- An occupational health and safety risk for staff and public
- The clinical governance agenda
- Risk of the service providing poor value for money
- Litigation.

The operating department is categorised as 'very high risk'. The service level required is for consistently high cleaning standards to be maintained throughout the day. Areas adjoining very high risk areas (ie: staff lounges, offices and bathrooms) must also receive intensive levels of cleaning.

The hospital environment must be visibly clean, free from dust and soil and must be acceptable to patients, visitors and staff. This is a category three recommendation (Pratt et al 2001).

RECOMMENDATIONS FOR LOCAL POLICY

RECOMMENDATION **4.2.1** A policy for environmental cleaning in the operating theatres should be developed in collaboration with the local infection control team (ICT) and housekeeping services. The policy should adhere to current microbiological recommendations. Personnel should wear personal protective equipment including gloves, eye protection, face mask or visor, and disposable apron when cleaning.

Between case cleaning procedures

RECOMMENDATION **4.2.2** Surfaces that do not have direct patient contact (eg: floor, wall and light) do not become contaminated more by 'dirty' than 'clean' operations. Surfaces such as operating tables, other furniture, and instruments that make contact with more than one patient have a greater potential for transmission of infection between dirty and subsequent cases.

RECOMMENDATION **4.2.3** Disposal of clinical waste, laundry and used instruments should be in accordance with national and local policies.

RECOMMENDATION **4.2.4** The operating table and related accessories that came into contact with the previous patient should be wiped down between cases in accordance with local policy.

RECOMMENDATION **4.2.5** Any mattress that is torn or damaged in any way should be repaired immediately (not taped) to prevent contamination with blood or other body fluids. If this is not practical the mattress should be decommissioned and removed from circulation.

Terminal daily cleaning procedures

RECOMMENDATION **4.2.6** All equipment should be cleaned and all portable equipment removed from the theatre.

RECOMMENDATION **4.2.7** Windowsills, overhead lights, cabinets, waste receptacles, equipment, and furniture should be cleaned with detergent solution and a disposable cloth.

RECOMMENDATION **4.2.8** Scrub sinks in scrub areas should be cleaned with detergent and water applied with a disposable sponge/cloth.

RECOMMENDATION **4.2.9** Shelves should be emptied, wiped with detergent and water, and dried before replacing supplies.

RECOMMENDATION **4.2.10** Suture storage boxes should be wiped with detergent and water and dried before being replaced on the shelves.

Management considerations

RECOMMENDATION **4.2.11** Surfaces should be kept free from visible dirt, and special attention should be given to areas that are likely to become heavily contaminated (ie: upward facing surfaces).

RECOMMENDATION **4.2.12** Walls with intact surfaces acquire very few bacteria even if left unwashed for long periods. However they must not be allowed to become visibly dirty, and washing at least every six months is recommended by the Hospital Infection Society (2002).

RECOMMENDATION **4.2.13** Areas of wall with peeling paint must be repainted or covered with a new wall finish.

RECOMMENDATION **4.2.14** For other surfaces, normal housekeeping methods are adequate (eg: daily damp cleaning of ledges and shelves).

RECOMMENDATION **4.2.15** Floors of the operating room should be disinfected at the end of each session and be scrubbed daily. Floors should be free of litter, dust, marks, water or spillages.

RECOMMENDATION **4.2.16** Floors should be free of floor polish build-up.

RECOMMENDATION **4.2.17** Specific spillages of blood or body fluids should be dealt with immediately.

RECOMMENDATION **4.2.18** Mop buckets for spillage should be emptied after each use and kept dry until the next occasion when they are required.

RECOMMENDATION **4.2.19** Disposable single use lint free cloth is recommended for all operating theatre cleaning.

RECOMMENDATION **4.2.20** The team leader should undertake a visual audit of the environment for cleanliness before the commencement of the operating list and take action where appropriate.

Cleaning equipment and materials

RECOMMENDATION **4.2.21** Before equipment is brought into the operating theatre it should be inspected for dust and cleaned.

SCRUBBING MACHINES

RECOMMENDATION **4.2.22** Cleaning machines should be cleaned and decontaminated according to local policy.

RECOMMENDATION **4.2.23** Floor-scrubbing machines should have detergent reservoirs that can be cleaned. The brushes and pads of scrubbing machines should be detachable and should be removed and thoroughly washed and dried after each use.

RECOMMENDATION **4.2.24** Brushes and pads used in operating theatres should be autoclaved at least weekly. Each theatre should preferably have its own brushes and pads.

SUCTION MACHINES

RECOMMENDATION **4.2.25** If suction machines are used in theatres they must be cleaned and dried thoroughly after use.

MOPS

RECOMMENDATION **4.2.26** A clean mop must be used in each theatre every day.

RECOMMENDATION **4.2.27** Mops should be washed in detergent after each use during the day.

RECOMMENDATION **4.2.28** Mop heads should be laundered daily.

RECOMMENDATION **4.2.29** The dual mop bucket system must be used.

RECOMMENDATION **4.2.30** The detergent solution must be made immediately before use in the theatre.

RECOMMENDATION **4.2.31** Mop buckets for spillage should be emptied after each use and kept dry until the next occasion when they are required.

DETERGENTS AND DISINFECTANTS

RECOMMENDATION **4.2.32** Detergents and disinfectants should be used according to the manufacturer's instructions and local infection control policies.

RECOMMENDATION **4.2.33** Disinfectants must be used at the correct concentration. Personnel handling disinfectants or using them must be adequately trained and supervised.

RECOMMENDATION **4.2.34** Disinfectants must be stored and labelled correctly according to COSHH regulations (HMSO 2002).

4.3 PREPARATION OF PERSONNEL

STANDARD All personnel entering semi-restricted and restricted areas of the operating department wear designated theatre attire, thus decreasing potential for wound infections in surgical patients.

Although surgery takes place in numerous types of settings, a patient's surgical outcome is greatly influenced by the creation and maintenance of an aseptic environment. The aim of all perioperative personnel must therefore be to minimise the introduction of microorganisms into the perioperative setting.

Personnel are able to influence the environment by maintaining personal hygiene, wearing theatre attire correctly, reporting potential health problems, monitoring visitors and maintaining a clean environment.

All departments must have written procedures stating the correct preparation for staff and visitors entering and leaving all areas of the perioperative environment. Staff must be made aware of these policies and procedures.

Personal protective equipment should be worn in accordance with standard precautions, and health and safety guidelines. Employees have a responsibility to co-operate with any measures that their employer may take to protect their health in the workplace.

The purpose of theatre attire is to provide a barrier that protects the patient from microorganisms which are shed into the environment from the skin and hair of theatre personnel and to protect the outside environment from theatre contaminants.

RECOMMENDATIONS FOR LOCAL POLICY

Theatre attire

It is essential that all staff receive instruction as to the correct manner of dress within the operating department, including information about the need for strict personal hygiene, good health and the implications of these to patient care. Theatre attire is also a means of identifying theatre personnel.

RECOMMENDATION **4.3.1** Theatre attire is designed to minimise the transfer of microorganisms from the mucous membranes, skin and hair of the surgical team to the patient. It also provides the surgical team with some protection from the patient. At present, there are few studies showing that special theatre attire actually decreases infection rates and it is believed that linen used for surgical suits should be no more than socially clean. Despite this, when selecting theatre clothing, it is important to consider the quality of material in relation to the dissemination of airborne bacteria and bacterial strike-through.

RECOMMENDATION **4.3.2** All personnel who enter the restricted/semi-restricted area of the theatre suite should don the attire intended for use within the surgical environment. Each perioperative environment has established traffic patterns. The design of the department often predetermines these patterns and each area should be clearly indicated:

- **Unrestricted areas** Traffic is not limited.
- **Semi-restricted areas** Traffic is limited to authorised, correctly attired personnel and patients.
- **Restricted areas** Traffic is very limited and personnel must be correctly attired. This includes the operating theatre.

RECOMMENDATION **4.3.3** Changing rooms should be situated in an area adjacent to the restricted/semi-restricted area of the theatre suite and reached through an outer corridor.

RECOMMENDATION **4.3.4** Changing areas should ensure privacy and have wash/shower facilities available. Changing areas should also have adequate provision for storing personal and theatre clothing. Storage areas should be clean and dry.

RECOMMENDATION **4.3.5** Sufficient supplies of theatre clothing should be provided daily and clean theatre clothing should be protected from possible contamination during transfer and storage.

RECOMMENDATION **4.3.6** Theatre attire should consist of a two-piece trouser suit. It should also be:

- made of a close-knit material with antistatic properties
- resistant to bacterial strike-through
- flame resistant
- lint-free, as lint can increase the number of airborne particulates
- coloured to reduce glare
- cool and comfortable with maximum skin covering
- professional.

RECOMMENDATION **4.3.7** Theatre attire should be provided freshly laundered and in good condition.

RECOMMENDATION **4.3.8** Non-scrubbed personnel should have fastening warm-up jackets available which have long sleeves cuffed at the wrists, for use when required.

RECOMMENDATION **4.3.9** Hands should be washed before and after donning theatre attire.

RECOMMENDATION **4.3.10** Theatre attire should be removed when it becomes wet or soiled, and placed into containers specially designed for contaminated laundry, to reduce the potential for cross-contamination.

RECOMMENDATION **4.3.11** Theatre attire should be changed following environmental cleaning of the operating theatre and before the commencement of a new operating list.

Cover gowns/lab coats

RECOMMENDATION **4.3.12** Ideally, all theatre personnel should change into outdoor clothing before leaving the theatre environment, however NATN recognises that this is not always feasible. If theatre personnel require to leave the theatre environment without changing, fully fastened and clean cover gowns or lab coats may be worn, as determined by the individual practice setting. There is currently little evidence showing that the wearing of cover gowns reduces the risk of surgical site infections (Hospital Infection Society 2002).

RECOMMENDATION **4.3.13** Theatre attire should be removed before leaving the theatre environment and placed into an appropriate container. When leaving the clinical area, personnel should change into their outdoor clothes.

- Fresh, clean attire should be donned on return to theatre.
- Used theatre attire should not be stored in lockers for further use.
- Theatre attire should not be worn outside the clinical area or in public places.

Laundering of theatre attire

RECOMMENDATION **4.3.14** The home laundering of theatre attire is not recommended, although there are no well-controlled studies showing a relationship between scrub suits and surgical wound infections. The rationale for laundering in an approved hospital facility is to prevent soiled clothing spreading contaminants into the home environment. Hospitals have approved laundry facilities in which laundry processes are monitored and assessed and laundry can be handled in conjunction with standard precautions.

RECOMMENDATION **4.3.15** Laundry should be contained during transfer to and from theatres.

Headwear

RECOMMENDATION **4.3.16** All head and facial hair should be covered completely by a head cover/cap. Surgical site infections have been traced to organisms isolated from the hair and scalp.

RECOMMENDATION **4.3.17** Headwear should be donned prior to donning the scrub suit. This eliminates the possibility of hair or dandruff being shed onto scrub clothing.

RECOMMENDATION **4.3.18** Disposable headwear is preferable, however cloth hats are permissible if laundered in an approved facility and not at home. Bouffant and hood style covers are preferred as they cover side hair, ears and hair at the nape of the neck.

RECOMMENDATION **4.3.19** Headwear should be changed daily, unless it becomes soiled, when it should be changed immediately.

RECOMMENDATION **4.3.20** Headwear should be discarded into an appropriate container for disposal or laundry after use.

RECOMMENDATION **4.3.21** Hands must be washed following the application and removal of headwear to avoid cross-infection occurring when in contact with patients or equipment.

RECOMMENDATION **4.3.22** Headwear should always be worn in laminar flow theatres during prosthetic implant operations (ICNA 2002).

Jewellery

RECOMMENDATION **4.3.23** It is recommended that jewellery is removed as it has been shown to increase surface bacterial counts when left in situ.

RECOMMENDATION **4.3.24** Removal or confinement of jewellery can prevent the risk of it falling onto the sterile area.

RECOMMENDATION **4.3.25** Neck chains create a risk because they may be broken or cause harm to the wearer if grasped by a patient.

RECOMMENDATION **4.3.26** Necklaces, earrings, watches and rings with stones should be removed; however, plain wedding bands may continue to be worn.

RECOMMENDATION **4.3.27** Surgeons working with metal prosthesis may be advised to remove wedding rings. This is because perforations have been found at the ring site on gloves worn during joint replacement surgery (Hospital Infection Society 2002).

Finger nails

RECOMMENDATION **4.3.28** Finger nails should be clean, short and free from nail varnish. Short nails are less likely to puncture gloves and therefore reduce the risk of harming the patient through transfer.

RECOMMENDATION **4.3.29** False finger nails should not be worn, as these have been shown to harbour microorganisms such as fungi and Gram-negative bacteria even after hand washing; they can also inhibit hand washing (Hedderwick et al 2000, McNeil 2000). Chipped nail varnish or varnish worn longer than four days has been shown to harbour more bacteria than natural or freshly polished nails.

Footwear

RECOMMENDATION **4.3.30** The Personal Protective Equipment at Work (HMSO 1992) Regulation 4 requires every employer to provide suitable PPE to each employee who may be exposed to any risk whilst at work. Footwear in theatres should provide adequate protection and a risk assessment should be done to determine whether the type of footwear is suitable for decontamination. The purpose of such footwear is to provide antistatic properties in accordance with EN 345 standard ('A', S1, S2 or S3).

RECOMMENDATION **4.3.31** Footwear should be well-fitting, supportive and protective. Shoes should provide protection from spillages and accidentally dropped equipment.

RECOMMENDATION **4.3.32** Shoes should have enclosed toes and heels.

RECOMMENDATION **4.3.33** Footwear worn in theatres should be for that use only and should be cleaned regularly (using appropriate PPE) to remove any contaminants. The use of washer-disinfectors or autoclaves is preferable for the decontamination of footwear (ICNA 2002). Autoclavable footwear should therefore be available to personnel. It is each individual health worker's responsibility to ensure that their footwear is decontaminated.

RECOMMENDATION **4.3.34** Footwear should not be left in a contaminated state or on changing room floors. Footwear should be clean and stored ready for use.

RECOMMENDATION **4.3.35** Studies of bacterial contamination of operating theatre corridor floors indicate that footwear should be removed as far from the operating theatre as is feasible (Hospital Infection Society 2002).

RECOMMENDATION **4.3.36** The use of overshoes is not recommended, except in anticipation of grossly contaminated cases, as these have been shown to increase floor bacterial counts (Humphreys et al 1991, Hospital Infection Society 2002), as well as the numbers of bacteria on the hands when applied or removed (Carter 1990, Hospital Infection Society 2002). The practice has also been highlighted in other studies to be a risk to patients (Carter 1990, Weightman & Banfield 1994).

Masks

RECOMMENDATION **4.3.37** The wearing of masks in theatre is recommended when sterile items are being opened or are already open, when surgery is about to commence or is already under way, and during surgical intervention. However their use is questionable, except during prosthetic implant operation (Hospital Infection Society 2002). At present the research regarding the wearing of masks is inconclusive, therefore, individual facilities should develop their own policies and guidelines in relation to the wearing of masks.

The rationale for wearing masks is to contain the microorganisms expelled from the mouth and nose. They also protect the wearer from body fluids and blood. Masks may offer some protection from inhalation of surgical smoke and laser plume. Filtration levels vary according to manufacturer's specification and masks should be selected according to the level of protection required.

RECOMMENDATION **4.3.38** Masks are classified as personal protective equipment (PPE) and as such should be disposable and have a high filtration to trap bacteria of all sizes.

RECOMMENDATION **4.3.39** Some masks have additional features, such as fluid shields. Protective face shields should be worn whenever activities could place personnel at risk of splashes or aerosol contamination.

RECOMMENDATION **4.3.40** Masks should cover the nose and mouth, fitting the contour of the face and should be tied securely.

RECOMMENDATION **4.3.41** The user should avoid touching the mask once it is applied. A used mask should be handled by the tapes only.

RECOMMENDATION **4.3.42** Used masks should be discarded into an appropriate container for disposal after each case or if soiled.

RECOMMENDATION **4.3.43** Masks should not be left around the neck or put into pockets for future use. Hands should be washed following mask removal.

Patient attire

RECOMMENDATION **4.3.44** It is common practice that patients entering the theatre environment remove all of their own clothing and change into clothing appropriate for surgery, for example, theatre gowns and caps. This reduces the risk of infection from the patient's own clothing which is a source of bacteria, especially staphylococcus aureus. More recently, many theatre facilities have allowed patients to enter the theatre area wearing their own clothes, particularly if it does not interfere with the surgical procedure, for example, cataract surgery. Most patients feel more comfortable in their own clothing, particularly if allowed to keep on their underwear. Recommendations for patient attire state only that clothing should be clean and that, if it is required to remove more clothing, then this should be done on an individual basis.

Personal hygiene

RECOMMENDATION **4.3.45** Personal hygiene should be of a high standard.

Visitors to the perioperative environment

Visitors to the theatre environment include:

- relatives (in particular parents)
- students (from various health professions)
- visiting professionals (visiting surgeons etc)
- allied health professionals (lab technicians, maintenance workers etc)
- medical device representatives.

RECOMMENDATION **4.3.46** Visitors under the age of 18 years should be discouraged.

RECOMMENDATION **4.3.47** People are the main source of infection, therefore the number of visitors to the theatre environment should be restricted. Patients in the perioperative environment have the right to confidentiality and to maintain their privacy and this should be reiterated to all visitors entering the theatre suite. It is therefore imperative that theatre facilities provide guidelines and policies for visitors entering the theatre environment. These guidelines and policies should take into account infection control standards and practices and restrictions on traffic in the theatre environment.

RECOMMENDATION **4.3.48** There is no evidence that visitors entering only the anaesthetic room increase the risk of infection. Cover gowns and overshoes therefore would not be required (Hospital Infection Society 2002). If visitors actually enter the operating theatre itself, then the clothing intended for use within that environment should be worn.

4.4 SCRUBBING, GOWNING AND GLOVING

STANDARD There is a standardised procedure for scrubbing, gowning and gloving based on current evidence, best practice and validated research. The patient's surgical outcome is enhanced by the promotion of an aseptic environment.

Effective hand decontamination results in significant reductions in the numbers of potential pathogens on the hands and decreases the incidence of preventable hospital acquired infection, and therefore patient morbidity and mortality (Pratt et al 2001).

The fundamental principles of aseptic technique must be adhered to when scrubbing, gowning and gloving prior to surgical intervention. Surgical scrubbing is an extension of hand washing. Scrubbing is undertaken immediately prior to donning sterile gowns and gloves before participating in surgical and invasive procedures, in order to reduce the risk of cross infection in event of glove perforations (Swarbrook et al 2003). It is necessary to have a standardised procedure and must be practised to a high level of competence.

RECOMMENDATIONS FOR LOCAL POLICY

General guidelines

RECOMMENDATION **4.4.1** Practice settings should establish guidelines and protocols in conjunction with infection control teams.

RECOMMENDATION **4.4.2** Regular education and training of staff, plus audit of practice should be undertaken.

RECOMMENDATION **4.4.3** Training and induction for all new personnel, both medical and perioperative staff should be undertaken to ensure compliance.

Facilities

RECOMMENDATION **4.4.4** It is recommended that the scrub area is separate from the operating theatre. There should be two entrances – one from the access corridor with a door barrier, and the other from the theatre itself with independent access.

- The size of the room should facilitate free movement of people with sufficient space for a minimum of three people.
- The scrub room should be large enough to enable staff to scrub up, gown and circulate concurrently without risk of contamination from each other or from the surrounding fittings.
- If an operating theatre has a recessed scrub area, this must be located away from the area containing laid-up instrument trolleys, in order to prevent water contamination.

RECOMMENDATION **4.4.5** The sink and furniture should be at a height to facilitate hand and arm washing. The design and drainage should ensure that the floor does not become wet during washing procedures.

- Foot pedals and/or elbow adjustments should be provided to operate taps and dispense scrub solution.
- Provision of hot and cold water is essential and water should flow at a steady rate.

The maintenance of these facilities should be included in a planned preventative maintenance programme.

RECOMMENDATION **4.4.6** Where sensor taps are in operation they must allow a sufficient run-on time for the scrub protocol to be completed. The run-on time should be a minimum of 20 seconds.

RECOMMENDATION **4.4.7** Wet floors are a potential hazard, with a risk of injury caused by slipping. It is important that floor surfaces should be anti-slip.

RECOMMENDATION **4.4.8** A shelf or other work surface should be provided on which to open gown packs. This should be at a height to facilitate gowning and gloving, and be wide enough to allow gown packs to be opened fully.

RECOMMENDATION **4.4.9** Storage facilities for all necessary sterile equipment should be available and located away from the sterile field. Where sterile equipment is stored in the scrub area, it should be situated away from the sink area, in order to prevent water contamination.

RECOMMENDATION **4.4.10** The shelf or work surface used to open gowns should not be directly below any storage.

RECOMMENDATION **4.4.11** Foot-operated disposal bins for used brushes and waster paper should be provided.

RECOMMENDATION **4.4.12** The scrub area should be kept adequately stocked with necessary equipment. Careful consideration should be paid to the number of sterile gowns required to be stored in the scrub area, ensuring adequate stock rotation.

RECOMMENDATION **4.4.13** Some individual perioperative staff have become allergic to some microbial scrub preparations. Alternative scrub solutions should be provided. Brushes must be provided for use on nails only.

RECOMMENDATION **4.4.14** It is not essential to have an opening door between the scrub room and theatre. If one is provided it must be an automatic self-closing door to prevent scrubbed staff from re-contaminating their hands.

Scrubbing procedures

The aim of the surgical scrub is to remove debris and transient microorganisms, to reduce resident microorganisms to a minimum and to inhibit rapid rebound growth on the hands, nails and forearms of surgical personnel (AORN 2004a).

RECOMMENDATION **4.4.15** All staff should be in the appropriate theatre attire before commencing a surgical scrub. The correct theatre attire includes top tucked into trousers with sleeves rolled up to above the elbow, all hair covered by a surgical hat, and clean hands and nails.

RECOMMENDATION **4.4.16** Finger nails must be short and free from polish or artificial nails. The risk of tearing gloves can increase if fingernails extend past the fingertips. Although there is no clear evidence that the wearing of nail polish increases microbial growth on the hands and leads to an increased infection rate, it is suggested that personnel wearing nail polish may be more concerned with the state of their nails than performing the surgical scrub to an appropriate standard. Artificial nails may harbour microorganisms that cannot be easily removed (NATN 1998).

RECOMMENDATION **4.4.17** Nails can be cleaned using a disposable nail pick under running water. There is no evidence that more than a two minute wash (decontamination) using aqueous disinfectants is required, before any procedure is regarded as 'sterile' (Hospital Infection Society 2002).

RECOMMENDATION **4.4.18** All jewellery must be removed and confined in a secure place before hand washing. Although there is no clear evidence that wearing finger rings increases the microbial growth on the hands and leads to an increased infection rate, microorganisms may be harboured beneath the jewellery and scrub solutions may accumulate and cause allergic reaction.

A SYSTEMATIC METHOD

Using a systematic method of hand washing ensures an effective way of cleansing all areas of the hands and arms (Gould 2000). Surgical hand antisepsis must be performed before donning sterile gloves for clinical invasive procedures.

RECOMMENDATION **4.4.19** Hands should be washed with plain antimicrobial solution and running water immediately before beginning the surgical scrub.

Hands and arms should be wet before applying scrub solution.

The first wash should encompass the hands and arms to the elbows, utilising a systematic method to cover all areas (Pratt et al 2001).

The six steps of hand washing should be used for scrubbing and social hand wash:

- Palm to palm
- Right palm over left dorsum and left palm over right dorsum
- Palm to palm, fingers interlaced
- Backs of fingers to opposing palms with fingers interlocked
- Rotational rubbing of right thumb clasped in left palm and vice versa
- Rotational rubbing backwards and forwards with clasped fingers of right hand in left palm and vice versa.

The use of a scrubbing brush is not necessary for reduction of bacterial counts and can lead to skin damage and an increase in skin cell shedding.

Subsequent washes should encompass two thirds of the forearms to avoid compromising the cleanliness of the hands.

Hands must be rinsed thoroughly from the fingertips to the elbows, allowing excess water to drain from the elbows into the sink.

Avoid splashing surgical attire, if surgical attire becomes excessively wet this can compromise the protection afforded by the gown. It may be necessary to change attire before beginning scrub procedure again.

Hands must be dried thoroughly – as wet surfaces transfer microorganisms more effectively than dry (Gould 2000). The skin should be blotted dry with the towels, as rubbing the skin in order to dry it will disturb skin cells. Adhering to the principle of working from the fingertips to the elbows and using one towel per hand is essential.

Hands are dried first by placing the opposite hand behind the towel and blotting the skin – then using a corkscrew movement to dry from the hand to the elbow. The towel must not be returned to the hand once the arm has been dried and must be discarded immediately.

The process is repeated for the opposite hand.

Hold hands higher than elbows and away from surgical attire.

RECOMMENDATION **4.4.20** Unless proceeding directly from one procedure to another, subsequent hand scrubs should be the same as for initial scrubs (AORN 2004a). Although evidence shows a reduction in microorganisms over time with a cumulative effect, this depends on the solution used and the technique. Advocating the same procedure for all scrubs reduces confusion and increases compliance. Alcohol hand rubs are an acceptable alternative to repeated washing (Hospital Infection Society 2002). Alcohol hand rubs are not appropriate for use when hands are visibly contaminated as these hand rubs do not remove soil or debris.

RECOMMENDATION **4.4.21** When proceeding directly from one procedure to another, cleaning the nails with a pick and scrubbing the nails can be omitted.

RECOMMENDATION **4.4.22** In order to minimise contamination during the scrubbing procedure, personnel should ensure:

- water is at a comfortable temperature with steady flow
- movements are steady
- the hands remain above the level of the elbows and away from theatre attire to avoid contamination from splashing (Pereira et al 1997, NATN 1998, AORN 2004a)

- rinsing is performed from the fingertips to the elbows using the water flow only
- vigorous shaking of the hands to dispel water is avoided.

RECOMMENDATION **4.4.23** The hands and forearms should be free from lesions or breaks in skin integrity. Minor lesions must be covered by a waterproof occlusive dressing. An individual with a major wound or infected wound must not scrub (AORN 2004a).

SURGICAL SCRUB SOLUTIONS

RECOMMENDATION **4.4.24** The scrub solution must be antiseptic or alcohol-based, fast acting and have a broad spectrum of action and a residual effect (AORN 2004a).

RECOMMENDATION **4.4.25** Alcohol-based solutions provide the most rapid and greatest reduction in microbial count, but are not effective at removing debris and soiling (Larson et al 1990, Hobson et al 1998, Pratt et al 2001).

RECOMMENDATION **4.4.26** Soap and water alone are not acceptable, as soap has no antimicrobial properties (Pereira et al 1990, Pratt et al 2001). Personnel who are allergic to scrub solutions should be allowed to use soap but must combine this with an alcohol solution/gel following consultation with the occupational health department.

RECOMMENDATION **4.4.27** Each scrub solution varies in the time needed for optimum effect and the manufacturer's instructions should be adhered to. Scrub solutions must be in adequate contact with the skin to achieve their optimal effect (Pereira et al 1990).

RECOMMENDATION **4.4.28** Approximately 5mls of solution should be used at each application. Using copious amounts of scrub solution with quick application and rinsing is neither efficient in technique nor cost-effective.

RECOMMENDATION **4.4.29** A scrub protocol with alcohol-based antiseptics is as effective as, and no more damaging to skin, than traditional methods (Pereira et al 1997).

Face and eye protection

RECOMMENDATION **4.4.30** Although surgical face masks were originally developed to protect the patient from micro-organisms expelled from the mouth and nasopharynx of surgical staff during procedures (Belkin 1996), they also provide a protective barrier for the surgical team. Given the anticipated risk of splash injuries from blood and body fluid, face and eye protection (that covers the side of the face) must be used by scrub personnel. Face masks should be positioned and secured prior to scrubbing to cover the nose and mouth. Masks should be handled only by the ties. Spectacles or microscopic glasses must also protect the sides of the face/eyes.

RECOMMENDATION **4.4.31** Perioperative personnel should also note the following:

- Specific face masks and/or eye protection are required when dealing with specific risks, for example, surgical smoke plume or lasers.
- Specific equipment must be donned for use within laminar flow enclosures, for example aspirators.
- Additional protective clothing may be indicated, for example lead gowns, plastic aprons.

Gowning procedures

RECOMMENDATION **4.4.32** Surgical gowns and clean air suits are medical devices whose essential requirements are to be controlled by the harmonised standard EN 13795: '*Surgical drapes, gowns and clean air suits, used as medical devices, for patients, clinical staff and equipment.*' (European Committee for Standardisation 2002)

RECOMMENDATION **4.4.33** The fabrics of gowns must be tested for the following characteristics:

- Resistance to microbial penetration (dry and wet)
- Cleanliness (from microbial and particulate matter)
- Linting
- Resistance to liquid penetration
- Bursting strength (dry and wet)
- Tensile strength (dry and wet).

RECOMMENDATION **4.4.34** The EN 13795 standard requires gowns to be able to withstand the user performing all that is required from the surgical procedure without compromising the sterile field, and to be resistant to liquid penetration and microbial penetration, with a minimal release of particles.

RECOMMENDATION **4.4.35** A variety of styles and specifications are available in both single use and reusable gowns. It is recommended gowns should be a wrap-around style to protect the sterile field.

RECOMMENDATION **4.4.36** Personnel must be aware of:

- the specification of the gown and its suitability for the procedure to be undertaken
- how it is packed and presented
- how it is donned
- once donned, what area of sterility it affords the wearer.

RECOMMENDATION **4.4.37** Gowns must be presented in a good state of repair. Any gown found not to have been processed to the standard should be discarded. The pack details should be noted and reported for quality control. A variety of sizes should be available to staff to avoid the use of too small or too large gowns which would compromise the safety of staff and patients.

RECOMMENDATION **4.4.38** When donning the gown, personnel must ensure they only touch the inside of the gown. The neck of the gown is located and held firmly. The rest of the gown is released with the inside facing towards the scrubbed individual. The armholes are located and both arms are inserted. The circulator assists the scrubbed personnel to secure the gown's fastenings and wrap-around.

Gloving procedures

Gloves act as a barrier to prevent transmission of infection between staff and patients, and as a personal protective barrier. Surgical gloves must fit appropriately for comfort, dexterity and sensitivity.

RECOMMENDATION **4.4.39** Surgical gloves must conform to the standard EN 455 – Parts 1, 2 and 3. The choice of surgical glove depends on the surgical procedure being undertaken.

RECOMMENDATION **4.4.40** Failure of surgical gloves from sutures, sharp instruments, bone fragments and natural 'wear and tear' is a common source of contamination of the hands of surgical personnel with blood and body fluids.

RECOMMENDATION **4.4.41** Double gloving provides an extra layer of protection and significantly reduces the number of perforations to inner gloves in all types of surgery (Tanner & Parkinson 2002). The decision to double glove should be based on the risk posed by the surgical procedure (eg: the exposure to sharps) and not the risk posed by the patient, or personal preference. Evidence supports the use of double gloving for all surgical procedures involving sharps and especially for orthopaedic surgery.

RECOMMENDATION **4.4.42** Wearing a coloured glove puncture indicator system has been shown to enable wearers to detect perforations in the outer gloves more easily than when wearing standard gloves (Tanner & Parkinson 2002).

RECOMMENDATION **4.4.43** Although double gloving reduces hand dexterity and sensation compared with single gloves, with sensory perception deficit greater than motor function, perforation rates do not alter significantly between single gloves and double outer gloves, indicating no significant problem with dexterity (Tanner & Parkinson 2002). A period of acclimatisation is needed to find a comfortable combination of gloves, especially in those who have not routinely used double gloving (Patterson et al 1998, Novak et al 1999).

RECOMMENDATION **4.4.44** Wearing gloves half a size larger underneath the outer glove can be more comfortable.

RECOMMENDATION **4.4.45** Aqueous fluids can affect the integrity of the glove (Doyle et al 1992). This indicates that the outer glove should be changed after preparation of the patient's skin for surgery.

RECOMMENDATION **4.4.46** Surgeons who are reluctant to double glove should consider double gloving on the non-dominant hand, which is more at risk of puncture (Avery 1999).

RECOMMENDATION **4.4.47** Alternative gloves must be available for individuals who are sensitised to natural latex proteins and/or other chemicals in gloves. Latex-free gloves must be available for use by all scrub personnel when dealing with latex sensitive patients or those in a high risk category.

RECOMMENDATION **4.4.48** The closed method of gloving is the preferred option for donning sterile gloves.

RECOMMENDATION **4.4.49** When gloves require changing intraoperatively due to a puncture or inadvertent contamination, the glove must be removed in a way that avoids further contamination. A new glove may be donned with assistance from a member of the surgical team. There is no evidence that perforated gloves increase the incidence of infection, and needle puncture of a glove is not an indication to change gloves. If any action is taken it is preferable to don a second pair of gloves to protect the operating surgeon or individual undertaking the procedure (Hospital Infection Society 2002).

Intraoperative and post procedure protocol

RECOMMENDATION **4.4.50** After personnel have scrubbed and gowned it is essential that they understand that the area of sterility includes:

- their gloved hands and forearms
- below nipple line to waist level. Hands must be kept at or above waist level and below shoulder level, and should be visible at all times in order to avoid inadvertent contamination.

RECOMMENDATION **4.4.51** Scrubbed personnel must only touch items or areas which are sterile. When not involved in a sterile procedure, scrubbed personnel should stand with their hands within the area of the sterile field.

RECOMMENDATION **4.4.52** At the completion of a sterile procedure, gowns and gloves are treated as clinically contaminated or clinical waste. When removing the gown, contaminated hands should not undo the gown. Once released it is pulled forward over the gloved hands, folding it onto itself. It is then discarded appropriately.

RECOMMENDATION **4.4.53** Gloves are removed by ensuring that glove surface comes into contact with glove, and skin with skin, to avoid contaminating the hands.

RECOMMENDATION **4.4.54** Face masks and single use eye protection must be discarded after each procedure.

RECOMMENDATION **4.4.55** Reusable eye protection must be cleaned between procedures according to manufacturer's instructions.

RECOMMENDATION **4.4.56** Personnel should inspect their hands post procedure for contamination.

RECOMMENDATION **4.4.57** Hands must be washed thoroughly once gown and gloves are removed.

Skin care

RECOMMENDATION **4.4.58** Personnel should ensure they care for their hands to ensure adequate hand decontamination and good practice.

RECOMMENDATION **4.4.59** When skin is damaged the microorganism count raises, leading to an increased risk of cross infection.

RECOMMENDATION **4.4.60** Scrub solutions and soap must only be applied to wet hands. Hands must be rinsed thoroughly (Gould 2000) to remove any soap residue and then dried properly.

RECOMMENDATION **4.4.61** Hand creams can be used but must be non-ionic to avoid their inhibiting actions on some scrub solutions and latex gloves. Hydrocarbon products are not compatible with latex; water-based hand creams are best. Products containing mineral oil, petroleum or lanolin should be avoided. The user should always check with the manufacturer of the skin care product to verify that it is compatible with the chosen hand antiseptic agent. Containers must not be communal as they can be contaminated (Gould 2000).

RECOMMENDATION **4.4.62** Abrasions and lesions must be covered with occlusive waterproof dressing. Infected lesions must be reported and personnel must not scrub (Gould 2000).

RECOMMENDATION **4.4.63** Occupational health guidance must be sought for any skin problems (Pratt et al 2001).

4.5 ASEPTIC TECHNIQUE

STANDARD There is a system in place for the effective management of surgical asepsis.

The outcome of a patient's surgical experience is influenced by the competence, knowledge and skill of application for aseptic technique by perioperative staff. All persons involved in the preparation and performance of surgical procedures are responsible for providing a safe environment for the patient. This is best achieved by maintaining asepsis and limiting the risk of contamination.

Measures to prevent surgical wound infection include provision of medical devices, supplies and equipment which are free of microbial contamination at the time of use. Sterilisation provides the highest level of assurance that an object is void of viable microbes.

The basic principles of aseptic technique prevent contamination of the open wound, isolate the operative site from the surrounding unsterile physical environment and create, maintain and promote a sterile field so that surgery can be performed safely.

RECOMMENDATIONS FOR LOCAL POLICY

General considerations

RECOMMENDATION **4.5.1** Perioperative staff with infected lesions of the skin or bacterial infections of the upper respiratory system should not participate in any aseptic technique.

RECOMMENDATION **4.5.2** Staff must be aware of differences between sterile items and non-sterile items and share the responsibility for monitoring aseptic practice.

RECOMMENDATION **4.5.3** The environment and all working surfaces must be cleaned in accordance with local infection control policies prior to the commencement of the procedure.

Equipment and medical devices safeguards

RECOMMENDATION **4.5.4** All pre-sterilised articles must be checked for damage, the integrity of packaging, and expiry date, prior to use. Any packs found to be in an unsatisfactory condition must be discarded.

RECOMMENDATION **4.5.5** Items used within a sterile field must be sterile. Any items that fall into an area of questionable cleanliness must be considered unsterile.

RECOMMENDATION **4.5.6** Sterile drapes should be used to establish a sterile field and conform to EN 13795 (European Committee for Standardisation 2002).

RECOMMENDATION **4.5.7** Sterile drapes should be handled as little as possible. The drapes should be applied from the surgical site to the periphery, avoiding reaching over non-sterile areas. Once placed, drapes should not be repositioned, to avoid contamination of the sterile field (AORN 2004b).

RECOMMENDATION **4.5.8** Scrubbed personnel should move draped sterile trolleys by placing hands on the horizontal surfaces only.

RECOMMENDATION **4.5.9** To maintain asepsis it is essential that all staff are aware of the correct method of opening different sterile packages to avoid the contamination of contents. Non-sterile persons should open wrapped sterile supplies by opening the wrapper flap furthest away from them first. The nearest wrapper should be opened last. Outer wrappers should be secured when presenting sterile items, to avoid contamination.

RECOMMENDATION **4.5.10** Sterile items should be presented to the scrubbed person or placed securely on a specific area of the sterile field identified and managed by the scrubbed person. Items should not be tossed onto a sterile field as they may roll off or cause other items to be displaced.

RECOMMENDATION **4.5.11** Sharps and heavy items must be presented to the scrubbed person to avoid penetration of the sterile field.

RECOMMENDATION **4.5.12** When dispensing solutions, the solution vessel should be placed near the trolley edge or held by the scrubbed person. The solution should be poured slowly to avoid splashing which could cause strike-through and compromise the sterile field.

RECOMMENDATION **4.5.13** The edge of a container is considered contaminated after the cap is removed and therefore the sterility of its contents cannot be guaranteed if the cap is replaced.

Scrubbed personnel

RECOMMENDATION **4.5.14** Staff participating in an aseptic technique should present themselves as recommended in Sections 4.3 and 4.4. If gown or gloves are contaminated they must be changed as soon as is reasonably practicable.

RECOMMENDATION **4.5.15** Scrubbed personnel should remain close to the sterile field and not leave the immediate area. If personnel leave the sterile field and exit the operating theatre they must rescrub before returning to the sterile field. Leaving the sterile field increases the risk for potential contamination.

RECOMMENDATION **4.5.16** Personnel participating within sterile procedures must stay within the sterile boundaries, and a wide margin of safety should be given between scrubbed and non-scrubbed persons.

RECOMMENDATION **4.5.17** When changing positions or moving between sterile areas, scrub personnel should turn back to back or face to face to avoid contamination.

RECOMMENDATION **4.5.18** Scrubbed personnel must keep their arms and hands within the sterile field at all times. Contamination may occur if hands are moved below the level of the sterile field.

RECOMMENDATION **4.5.19** Scrubbed personnel should only be seated when the operative procedure is to be performed at that level.

RECOMMENDATION **4.5.20** Circulating personnel should not walk between the two sterile fields and should be aware of keeping an adequate distance from the sterile field.

Special considerations

RECOMMENDATION **4.5.21** Dressings must be removed carefully from the wound to prevent scattering of microorganisms into the air. It is recommended that this is carried out by an assistant wearing gloves rather than a scrubbed member of the surgical team. Used and soiled dressings should be discarded immediately and in accordance with local infection control policy.

RECOMMENDATION **4.5.22** To reduce the risk of airborne cross infection, talking, movement, opening and closing doors, exposure of wounds, disturbance of clothing and linen, and number of personnel in the theatre should be kept to a minimum. Special consideration must be taken to maintain the integrity of the sterile field at all times.

RECOMMENDATION **4.5.23** The sterile field should be constantly monitored and maintained, as sterility cannot be assured without direct observation of the sterile field (AORN 2004b). Any break in sterility must be reported and acted on to ensure patient safety (Gruendemann & Fernsebner 1995).

RECOMMENDATION **4.5.24** Sterile fields should be prepared as close as possible to the time of use.

RECOMMENDATION **4.5.25** Preparation of sterile trolleys in advance, with the use of sterile sheets to cover them, is not recommended. The trolleys are subject to contamination over time and removal of sheets without contamination cannot be guaranteed.

RECOMMENDATION **4.5.26** If the operating theatre has ultra-clean ventilation the inclusion of a preparation room is not essential. The canopy of the ultra-clean ventilation system should be sized sufficiently to permit the laying up of instruments within its footprint.

4.6 TROLLEY PREPARATION FOR SURGICAL INTERVENTION

STANDARD The preparation of sterile instrument trolleys for surgical intervention is a skilled and precise procedure. Staff adhere to a strict aseptic technique throughout.

The type of instrument trolley used in a procedure may be influenced by the type of surgery being performed. All trolleys should adhere to the *Medical Devices Directive 93/42* (European Commission 1993) and be stable and robust enough for the intended job. The design choice of the instrument trolley will need to take into account ease of movement, height, and ease of cleaning in accordance with local infection control policies. Trolleys should be included in a planned prevention maintenance programme. Particular attention to wheel mechanism is required in order to allow free and smooth movement. Trolleys, mayo stands and bowl stands should be made of aluminium, stainless steel or mild steel covered in nylon. All trolleys should be free of abrasions and be in good working order.

RECOMMENDATIONS FOR LOCAL POLICY

General considerations

RECOMMENDATION **4.6.1** Medical devices such as surgical instruments must be prepared immediately prior to each individual surgical intervention, in accordance with the planned operative procedure and individual patient needs (Gruendemann and Fernsebner 1995).

RECOMMENDATION **4.6.2** A designated area, which affords sufficient space to open packs whilst maintaining a sterile field, should be identified for this procedure. There should be minimal movement of personnel within this area during preparation of the trolley.

RECOMMENDATION **4.6.3** All equipment for the surgical procedure must be gathered in advance and all packs must be checked for sterility, integrity of packaging and expiry date. Heavy items and instrument trays should be presented to the scrub person on separate trolleys.

RECOMMENDATION **4.6.4** Two members of staff are required for the preparation of sterile trolleys. It is essential that one of these members is scrubbed, gowned and gloved and follows the principles of aseptic technique.

RECOMMENDATION **4.6.5** All trolleys should be covered with at least two layers of sterile drapes which meet EU Standards. The drapes should be of a recommended material large enough to cover the horizontal plane of the trolley and enough vertical plane to avoid contamination. The trolley should be considered sterile on the horizontal plane only.

RECOMMENDATION **4.6.6** Sterile medical devices must be presented to the scrubbed person from the edge of the sterile field and received in such a way as to prevent glove contamination on the unsterile wraps (Gruendemann & Fernsebner 1995).

RECOMMENDATION **4.6.7** Items that extend over the edge of the trolley are at risk of contamination and should not be brought back into the sterile field.

RECOMMENDATION **4.6.8** When opening packs or trays on trolleys the circulator must open them away from their body first and then towards. The scrubbed person opens packs towards themselves first and then away to avoid contamination of the sterile item. Circulators should not reach over sterile fields.

RECOMMENDATION **4.6.9** When pouring solutions, containers should be placed at the edge of the trolley to avoid the circulator leaning over the sterile field and the danger of splashing or spillage.

RECOMMENDATION **4.6.10** Sharps should be opened into a container to avoid injuries or drapes penetration (Gruendemann & Fernsebner 1995).

RECOMMENDATION **4.6.11** Once prepared, the trolley must be attended at all times.

RECOMMENDATION **4.6.12** There should be a locally agreed method of laying out sterile instrument trolleys. All staff should adhere to this method in order to facilitate continuity of patient care and safety in the event of a sudden change of scrub person during the operative procedure.

RECOMMENDATION **4.6.13** Trolleys should be positioned close together to ensure there are no breaks in the sterile field.

RECOMMENDATION **4.6.14** Care must be taken to ensure that there is no undue pressure placed on any part of the patient's body or limbs which could cause injury, especially when positioning mayo tables.

RECOMMENDATION **4.6.15** All medical devices must be returned to the surface of the instrument trolley in order to prevent injury to the patient.

RECOMMENDATION **4.6.16** Any break in aseptic technique must be acted on immediately. Contaminated equipment must be removed from the sterile field using a suitable instrument to prevent compromising sterility of the procedure. Regloving and redraping should be carried out where appropriate.

RECOMMENDATION **4.6.17** The disposal of all equipment, drapes and sharps must be carried out in accordance with local and national guidelines. The scrub person should be considered the person of choice to dispose of all contaminated materials whilst still gowned and gloved.

4.7 SKIN PREPARATION

STANDARD The risk of postoperative surgical site infection is minimised through the effective management of skin preparation of the surgical site.

The skin is the largest organ in the body. It covers the body and protects the internal organs from the environment. The skin is made up of two layers called the epidermis and the dermis. The epidermis is the superficial or outer layer of skin and the dermis is the deeper layer, which is attached through subcutaneous tissue to the structures below – the hair follicles, sweat and sebaceous glands, blood and lymphatic vessels and the nerves. The skin is continually renewing itself with millions of new cells every day.

Skin preparation, skin prep or prepping is the process by which the skin is cleansed to reduce the number of transient (staphylococcus aureus) and resident (staphylococcus epidermis) skin bacteria before surgical incision. Transient bacteria do not normally colonise the skin and are easily removed, whereas resident bacteria grow on normal skin and are difficult to remove. Most wound infections are associated with the patient's own skin flora. The skin cannot be sterilised and therefore it must be prepared to reduce the risk of surgical site infection. Skin preparation removes dirt and debris from the patient's skin, reduces the number of microbes, inhibits the regrowth of further microorganisms and reduces the number of microorganisms entering the wound site. Skin preparation should not cause irritation to the skin.

In many areas, hair removal is a routine part of preoperative preparation. Staff and patients need to be aware of the evidence and rationale for this practice as research has shown that removal of hair is not always necessary, and should only be undertaken after assessment of the individual patient. For example, some patients undergoing removal of a lipoma from their back may not need the area to be shaved if there is minimal fine hair whereas another patient with thick hair would require the area to be prepared preoperatively to minimise the risk of postoperative infection.

The purpose of skin preparation is to reduce the number of microorganisms on the skin prior to surgical intervention thus reducing the potential of postoperative infection.

RECOMMENDATIONS FOR LOCAL POLICY

Types of solutions used in skin preparation

RECOMMENDATION **4.7.1** Antiseptics used for skin preparation should have a broad spectrum of activity with a fast and lasting effect against Gram negative and Gram positive bacteria, as well as viruses and fungi. They should be resistant to inactivation by organic matter, be non-toxic and acceptable cosmetically.

RECOMMENDATION **4.7.2** Antiseptics should be supplied in ready-to-use, single use containers or sachets, as there is an increased risk of contamination from using multiple use containers.

RECOMMENDATION **4.7.3** If multiple use containers are to be used, they should not be refilled and should be used within date.

RECOMMENDATION **4.7.4** If antiseptic needs to be reapplied, the same antiseptic should be used.

RECOMMENDATION **4.7.5** There are several types of skin preparation available and the type of solution used will depend on surgical preference, the condition of the skin, patient allergies, and the area which requires preparation. Types of skin preparations include:

- povidone-iodine alcoholic solution
- povidone-iodine aqueous solution
- chlorhexidine 0.5% in 70% industrial methylated spirits
- iodine 1% in industrial methylated spirits
- 70% iodine in spirit
- chlorhexidine gluconate 0.015% and cetrimide solution
- industrial methylated spirit 70%.

Alcohol solutions are deemed to be more efficient than aqueous solutions (Hospital Infection Society 2002).

RECOMMENDATION **4.7.6** When using an alcohol-based solution, it is imperative that the skin is allowed to dry completely after every application, and before applying electrocautery or laser treatment. Spontaneous combustion can occur when flammable solutions are exposed to an ignition source when oxygen is present (MDA 2000).

RECOMMENDATION **4.7.7** Skin preparation solutions should be kept in a locked cupboard and particular attention should be paid to storage of flammable solutions.

RECOMMENDATION **4.7.8** There are other solutions which may be used intraoperatively. Topical gels may be used for skin preparation. According to the manufacturers, gels reduce pooling under the patient and thus reduce the risk of chemical burns and skin irritation. Sodium chloride 0.9% can be used for wound irrigation and to clean the skin immediately after surgery. Sterile water is often used to clean instruments throughout the surgical procedure. Hydrogen peroxide 3% solution can be used to cleanse dirty and infected wounds and methylene blue 1% can be used to mark or stain the skin.

Preoperative skin preparation

RECOMMENDATION **4.7.9** Showering or bathing on the day of surgery is recommended (except in emergency situations). Transient skin bacteria are easily removed with soap and water. There is no evidence that chlorhexidine showers reduce the incidence of postoperative infection (Hospital Infection Society 2002). Removal of superficial soil, debris and transient microbes before applying anti-microbial agents reduces the risk of wound contamination by decreasing organic debris on the skin.

RECOMMENDATION **4.7.10** The skin should be assessed for any breaks, cuts, abrasions and sores as the effectiveness of the skin as a protective barrier is reduced if the skin is not intact. Any skin breaks should be documented. The presence of moles, warts, rashes or other skin conditions at the surgical site should also be documented.

RECOMMENDATION **4.7.11** Checks prior to surgery should be made to ensure that there are no allergies to antiseptic agents. If there are allergies to any cleansing agents, this should be documented and an alternative found. Attention should also be paid to any contraindications for surgical use, for example use of iodine during pregnancy.

Preoperative shaving

RECOMMENDATION **4.7.12** Research has shown that hair removal is best achieved with the use of a depilatory cream and not the use of a razor. The Hospital Infection Society (2002) make the following recommendation for preoperative skin preparation: *'Only the area to be incised needs to be shaved and if this cannot be done with depilatory cream the day before operation, it should be done in the anaesthetic room immediately preoperatively, using clippers rather than a razor.'*

RECOMMENDATION **4.7.13** The removal of hair is only necessary if it will directly interfere with access to the incision site, or if there is a risk it will contaminate the wound site. In cases where hair removal is necessary, the following is recommended:

- Patient consent must be obtained prior to hair removal, with a full explanation of the method to be used and why it is necessary.
- The method of hair removal should be decided between the patient and the surgical team with patient safety being the main priority. The person who performed the hair removal, the area from where the hair was removed and the method used should be documented.
- Hair removal should take place as close to the time of surgery as possible to minimise the risk of bacterial contamination to the skin surface.
- Hair removal should be carried out by an experienced practitioner in a clean area of the surgical suite, with good lighting, affording the patient privacy at all times.

RECOMMENDATION **4.7.14** The use of depilatory creams is an effective method of hair removal, causing the least risk of postoperative wound infection. The patients themselves can also carry it out effectively. However this method can be costly and care must be taken when used as it can cause skin irritation in some patients. A patch test is recommended prior to use, in accordance with the manufacturer's instructions.

RECOMMENDATION **4.7.15** The use of clipping for hair removal is a simple and less irritating method than shaving. It also has a reduced risk of postoperative wound infection than with shaving (Cruse & Foord 1990, Managram et al 1999). An electric or battery powered clipper with a disposable or reusable head that can be disinfected should be used. Clipping should take place immediately before surgery.

RECOMMENDATION **4.7.16** Wet shaving with a razor should only be used when the previously suggested methods are not suitable for use. This method causes the most trauma to the skin and carries the highest risk of postoperative wound infection (Cruse & Foord 1990). Shaving should take place as near to the time of surgery as possible.

RECOMMENDATION **4.7.17** When surgery is to be performed on an already contaminated wound, shaving prior to surgery is not recommended as this holds a high risk of postoperative wound infection (Mishriki et al 1990).

Intraoperative skin preparation

RECOMMENDATION **4.7.18** Skin solutions should be used in accordance with manufacturer's instructions and Control of Substances Hazardous to Health (COSHH) (HMSO 2002) guidelines. Special attention should be paid to guidelines concerning warming of solutions.

- Skin solutions should be checked by the scrub and circulating practitioner to ensure they are in date and sterile.
- Solutions should be poured into a container at the edge of the sterile field, from a height of approximately 10cm, to avoid contamination of the sterile area.
- Care should be taken to avoid spillage onto the sterile area.

RECOMMENDATION **4.7.19** Only personnel who are competent and skilled in skin preparation techniques should prepare the surgical site. This should be a member of the scrub team.

RECOMMENDATION **4.7.20** Skin preparation should be carried out using an aseptic and non-touch technique using holders. A non-touch technique will prevent contamination of sterile gloves. Sponges should be positioned on the holder in such a way that the end of the holder cannot traumatise the patient. Swabs which are used for prepping should be retained as part of the swab count.

RECOMMENDATION **4.7.21** To maintain dignity and needless heat loss, unnecessary exposure of the patient should be avoided. However, the area exposed should be sufficient to comply with recognised skin preparation guidelines and surgical preference.

RECOMMENDATION **4.7.22** Skin solutions should not be allowed to seep or pool under the patient. To prevent seepage or pooling absorbent or sterile towels can be placed under the patient. These should be removed if they become wet, as this may cause unnecessary skin irritation, even if the solution used is non-irritating.

RECOMMENDATION **4.7.23** Flammable solutions should be allowed to evaporate before placing the drapes to avoid fumes accumulating under them. This will reduce the risk of chemical burns (MDA 2000).

RECOMMENDATION **4.7.24** Great care should be taken to avoid solutions running onto diathermy electrode plates, electrocardiogram (ECG) leads and tourniquets. This will also reduce the risk of chemical burns (MDA 2000).

RECOMMENDATION **4.7.25** Only sufficient antiseptic solution should be applied.

RECOMMENDATION **4.7.26** Skin preparation should proceed from clean to dirty. Cleansing should begin at the incision site and continue outwards to the periphery in a circular motion. This prevents any micro-organisms being returned to the incision site. This process should be repeated several times with a clean sponge each time.

RECOMMENDATION **4.7.27** An adequate area of skin surface should be prepared in order to allow for safe extension of the incision, placement of drains and for any possible movement of the drapes.

RECOMMENDATION **4.7.28** Used sponges and holders should be discarded after each application. Once all applications are complete, the area should be blotted dry with a dry sponge or swab.

RECOMMENDATION **4.7.29** The type of skin preparation used, area prepped, condition of the skin, any visible hyper-sensitivity and the person who undertook the skin preparation should be documented.

Additional considerations

RECOMMENDATION **4.7.30** In cases where a contaminated area is within the area to be prepped, skin preparation should start at the surrounding skin.

RECOMMENDATION **4.7.31** Areas which are considered to be heavily contaminated such as the perineum, anus, vagina and axilla should be prepared last. The umbilicus should be prepared first to prevent dirty solution running onto clean skin. Special care should be taken to avoid pooling of skin preparation within the umbilicus.

RECOMMENDATION **4.7.32** Skin ulcers and draining sinuses are also considered heavily contaminated areas and should be prepped last.

RECOMMENDATION **4.7.33** Special consideration should be given to diabetic patients as they may be sensitive to microbial solutions.

RECOMMENDATION **4.7.34** Multiple incision sites should be prepped separately.

RECOMMENDATION **4.7.35** Additional care should be given to prepping malignant areas to prevent potential spread of cancer cells.

RECOMMENDATION **4.7.36** Traumatic wounds may require large amounts of irrigation in addition to skin preparation to remove larger amounts of dirt or debris.

RECOMMENDATION **4.7.37** Stomas should be sealed with adhesive drapes. If a stoma is within the area to be prepped, it can be covered with a sterile swab and the area around it should be prepared first. Once the surrounding area is cleansed, the swab can be removed, and the stoma cleaned.

RECOMMENDATION **4.7.38** Delicate areas, such as the eyes and ears may require special or diluted solutions. Chlorhexidine is not recommended for facial prep and iodine may cause corneal damage if introduced to the eye. Solutions should also not be allowed to pool on the patient's eyes. If solutions enter the inner ear they may cause sensorineural deafness. Chlorhexidine gluconate and alcohol or alcohol-based solutions should also be avoided on mucous membranes.

RECOMMENDATION **4.7.39** Skin preparation of wound sites following the removal of casts or dressings may require soaking with sterile solutions to remove skin squames or adherent dressings.

RECOMMENDATION **4.7.40** During preparation of limbs, additional personnel or equipment may be required to hold the limb securely thus allowing the whole circumference to be cleansed safely.

RECOMMENDATION **4.7.41** Graft and donor sites are prepared separately to prevent cross-contamination from one site to the other. The donor site is prepared first. Colourless antiseptic solutions allow the surgeon to evaluate the vascularity of the graft.

Documentation

RECOMMENDATION **4.7.42** In order to comply with the Consumer Protection Act 1987 the following should be documented (AORN 2004c):

- The condition of the skin at the surgical site
- Hair removal if performed, including method and time of removal
- Type of skin preparation used, including lot and batch number
- Personnel performing skin preparation
- Development of any patient hypersensitivity reactions
- Postoperative skin assessment.

4.8 DRAPING

STANDARD A sterile field is created by providing a barrier between sterile and non-sterile areas, thereby reducing the risk of surgical site infection.

INTRODUCTION

Draping is an essential aspect of aseptic technique. It is the process whereby sterile barrier materials are used to isolate the operative site and cover the non-sterile area immediately surrounding the operative site. The introduction of microorganisms into the wound site from the surgical team, the environment and the patient's own skin flora is reduced.

Draping occurs after the patient has been positioned on the operating table for surgery, and after the skin has been prepared by solutions which reduce the number of microorganisms present at the surgical site. As well as creating a sterile field, drapes are used to maintain the sterility of other equipment used during surgery, such as instruments. They can also be used to extend the sterile field and to cover equipment that cannot be sterilised. The extent to which drapes are used will depend on the condition of the patient, the type of surgery, the length of time the procedure will take, the amount of fluid contamination anticipated, the potential for infection and the type of surgical environment.

Surgical drapes are pieces of cloth or material, either disposable (single use) or reusable (multiple use). They must meet certain requirements.

THE STANDARD FOR SURGICAL DRAPES

In June 1998, the Medical Device Directive (MDD) 93/42/EEC (European Commission 1993) became mandatory. It has created a harmonised regulatory environment within the European Union (EU), and the European Fair Trade Association states and permits free trade of all medical devices that comply with it and therefore carry the CE mark. CE marking is a declaration by the manufacturer that the product meets all the appropriate provisions of the relevant legislation implementing certain European Directives. CE marking gives companies easier access into the European market to sell their products without adaptation or rechecking. The initials 'CE' do not stand for any specific words but are a declaration by the manufacturer that his product meets the requirements of the applicable European Directive(s). Only products that comply with the essential requirements in the MDD may be placed on the market and put into service.

The European Commission gave a mandate to the Comité Européen de Normalisation (CEN) to prepare a European standard to support essential requirements of the EU Directive 93/42/EEC (European Commission 1993) concerning surgical drapes, gowns and clean air suits, especially in relation to the prevention of infection and microbial transfer during surgical procedures.

Members of the CEN

CEN members are the national standards bodies of Austria, Belgium, Czech Republic, Denmark, Finland, France, Germany, Greece, Iceland, Ireland, Italy, Luxembourg, Malta, Netherlands, Norway, Portugal, Spain, Switzerland and the United Kingdom.

A new European standard, EN 13795, is currently being drafted by a European standards working group (CEN/TC205/WG14) entitled *Surgical drapes, gowns and clean air suits, used as medical devices, for patients, clinical staff and equipment*.

Surgical drapes, gowns and clean air suits are medical devices whose essential requirements are to be controlled by the harmonised standard EN 13795.

Within the frame of the standard EN 13795 will be three parts, part one of which has been published (European Committee for Standardisation 2002):

- **Part 1** General requirements for manufacturers, processors and products
- **Part 2** Tests methods
- **Part 3** Performance requirements and performance levels.

EN 13795 requires the following characteristics of fabrics to be tested:

- Resistance to microbial penetration (dry and wet)
- Cleanliness (microbial and particulate matter)
- Linting
- Resistance to liquid penetration
- Bursting strength (dry and wet)
- Tensile strength (dry and wet)
- Adhesive for fixation, for the purpose of wound isolation.

Surgical gowns are evaluated against the same criteria, but without the addition of adhesive for fixation.

There is no legal requirement to comply with European or international standards, although meeting harmonised European standards is the easiest way to demonstrate compliance with the requirements of the medical devices directive. Compliance with harmonised standards is voluntary, and manufacturers are free to choose any other technical solution that provides compliance with the essential requirements of the medical devices directive based on the intended purpose of the product (MHRA 2003).

CONSIDERATIONS FOR CHOOSING DRAPES

Sterile drapes including trolley covers should comply with the new harmonised European Standard EN 13795. Surgical drapes are classed as medical devices and therefore come under the Medical Devices Directive (European Commission 1993) which became mandatory in 1998. Drapes are required to:

- provide a barrier against fluids (be resistant to strike-through) and microorganisms including viruses even when wet
- be lint and particulate free – lint and other particulates can contaminate the wound and cause infection or delay the healing process
- not contain toxic substances, such as laundry residues and non-fast dyes
- assist in maintaining the patient's body temperature
- be resistant to tearing
- prevent glare from reflected light
- be easy to use and conform to the patient and equipment
- be fire retardant and anti-static. This is especially important during the use of electrocautery, lasers, fibreoptics and other electrical equipment. Manufacturers should adhere to fire regulation standards.

TYPES OF DRAPES

There are a huge variety of drapes available. Drapes are often designed for speciality-specific procedures and named accordingly. However, there are a number of other drapes, such as fenestrated drapes, split drapes, aperture drapes, major and minor drapes, medium drapes, split drapes, leggings, isolation drapes and sterile towels. Isolation drapes are transparent drapes used to isolate necessary equipment which cannot be sterilised, (eg: x-ray equipment). Sterile towels are used to frame the surgical site. Drapes can also be reinforced or treated to improve their performance. Some drapes also have pockets for holding equipment such as tubing or cabling or pouches for the collection of fluid.

As well as the varieties of drapes already mentioned, there are drapes available for microscopes, endoscopes, cameras, light handles and other surgical equipment.

Reusable drapes

Reusable (also known as linen or cotton) drapes are the traditional form of drapes used in hospitals. Reusable drapes are made from tightly woven textiles comprising of a blend of polyester and long-staple cotton which are treated with chemicals to provide a barrier against strike-through. The integrity and porosity of reusable drapes is determined by the thread counts and the finishes of the natural woven fibres.

Traditional drapes are comfortable, drapeable and strong when dry. However, without continual treatment to maintain their barrier effect, they can become porous. Densely woven treated cotton will allow moisture to penetrate after 75 washes and untreated cotton will allow penetration of moisture in as few as 30 washes. The efficiency of reusable drapes will also be affected by repeated drying and ironing and repeated steam sterilisation cycles. These processes all affect the structure of the fabric, therefore drying, ironing and sterilisation cycles of reusable drapes should be recorded, and when they are no longer effective, drapes should be discarded.

There have been technological advances in reusable drapes and they are now also available in a range of textile materials ranging from single layer micro-filament yarns to tri-laminates, which incorporate a micro-porous membrane. All these provide better barrier protection to the transfer of microorganisms than cotton.

Disposable drapes

Disposable or single use drapes are composed of a variety of materials, such as rayon, nylon and polyester, combined with cellulose (wood pulp) fibres and bonded together chemically or mechanically. The common factor with disposable drapes is that they are non-woven. Disposable drapes range from single-layered products, such as hydrophobic materials and impermeable plastic products, through to multi-layered products which combine a number of functions in one product, through reinforcement with materials such as polypropylene. Disposable drapes are available pre-sterilised by the manufacturer, or non-sterile for sterilisation within the hospital setting.

Adhesive drapes

Adhesive drapes (also known as incision, adhesive plastic or sticky drapes), originally introduced in the 1960s, may be used in addition to reusable or disposable drapes. These drapes are applied to the skin following skin preparation at the operation site. An incision is then made through the plastic. The purpose of adhesive drapes is to assist in creating a sterile area around the incision site by preventing bacteria migrating towards the wound. The success of these drapes is dependent on their adherence to the skin during surgery.

There are various sizes and designs of adhesive drapes available for use, including those impregnated with antimicrobial agents which slowly release iodine into the skin during surgery to assist further in reducing the number of organisms on the patient's skin. The ideal requirements for adhesive drapes are that they should:

- be easy to incise
- not allow bacteria to permeate through
- adhere well to the skin
- be non-irritating, elastic and transparent
- allow the skin to breathe.

Adhesive drapes can help keep the surgical drapes in position, define the surgical site, keep the skin clean and isolate areas considered heavily contaminated, such as stomas. However, there is no evidence to show that they actually reduce the rate of postoperative infection. Despite this, there is some evidence which shows that adhesive drapes, impregnated with iodine, reduce the rate of recolonisation on the surface of the skin.

STORAGE OF DRAPES

The storage arrangements for drapes will depend on the type of drapes being used. However, drapes must be easily accessible to staff and the storage areas, both within and outside the theatre, should be kept clean, dry and tidy.

RECENT CHANGES IN PRACTICE

In recent times, there has been increased awareness regarding hospital acquired infections (HAIs), including those HAIs acquired through surgery. This has led to a review of the materials used for drapes and gowns. At present, most hospitals use a combination of reusable and disposable drapes. However, recent research has shown that disposable drapes and gowns offer better protection from postoperative infection.

The European Standard for surgical drapes, gowns and clean air suits EN13795 (European Committee for Standardisation 2002) proposes uniform standards for disposable and reusable surgical drapes and gowns to minimise the spread of infection during surgery and assist in preventing postoperative surgical site infections.

The standard recommends that drapes and gowns are resistant to liquid and microbial penetration with a minimal release of particles, for example, lint. Comparisons of fabrics indicate that disposable, polypropylene, spun-bound laminate materials offer best protection, therefore, the further use of cotton and polyester-cotton blended drapes is not recommended.

The EN 13795 standard also ensures that the manufacturer and processor are able to demonstrate that single use and reusable devices are fit for practice. Reprocessing and testing requirements are the responsibility of each hospital department involved in the supply of drapes and gowns. NHS organisations purchasing drapes should be aware of the research evidence on this topic provided by the NHS Purchasing and Supply Agency (PASA 2003).

Policies and procedures devised for drape and gown selection should be reviewed and revised in accordance with evidence-based practice. Risk managers should be aware that failure to comply with EN 13795 has legal implications for the operating department. If a patient acquires an infection as a result of using a defective drape or gown the hospital authority and the user is legally liable for the consequences under contract and civil law.

RECOMMENDATIONS FOR LOCAL POLICY

Guidelines for draping

RECOMMENDATION **4.8.1** Prior to the start of surgery, it is recommended that the scrub team check the effectiveness of their draping procedures, paying particular attention to table fitments etc. Adequate time should be available for draping.

RECOMMENDATION **4.8.2** The scrub practitioner should also have good knowledge and understanding of the procedure being undertaken.

RECOMMENDATION **4.8.3** Sterilisation wrap products should not be considered to be sterile drapes and therefore should not be used for trolley covers.

RECOMMENDATION **4.8.4** The area surrounding the table and the patient should be as free as possible from equipment, to prevent contamination of the drapes whilst draping. Any equipment required for the procedure should be moved into place once draping has taken place.

RECOMMENDATION **4.8.5** The patient's skin should be dry prior to commencement of the draping procedure.

RECOMMENDATION **4.8.6** Drapes should be handled as little as possible and not fanned or waved in the air.

RECOMMENDATION **4.8.7** Drapes should be made of waterproof, disposable material (Hospital Infection Society 2002).

RECOMMENDATION **4.8.8** To protect sterile, gloved hands from the patient, the drapes are protected by folding the drape around the hand.

RECOMMENDATION **4.8.9** The scrub practitioner should stand away from the operating table to avoid contamination of their sterile gown and gloves. The drapes are carried to the operating table and the area closest to the scrub practitioner should be draped first.

RECOMMENDATION **4.8.10** The scrub practitioner should not reach across the operating table, or lean on the patient to place drapes.

RECOMMENDATION **4.8.11** Drapes should be held high enough to prevent contact with any non-sterile areas before placing them over the patient. The distal edges of the drapes should be allowed to fall naturally. The area below waist level is not considered sterile.

RECOMMENDATION **4.8.12** Once the drapes have been placed, they should remain in position until the end of the procedure, however if they become wet or soiled during surgery, they should be removed and replaced with new sterile drapes. Contaminated gloves should also be replaced.

RECOMMENDATION **4.8.13** If a hole is found in a drape, this must be covered with another drape or the drape discarded and replaced. If there is any doubt regarding the sterility of a drape, then it should also be discarded and replaced.

RECOMMENDATION **4.8.14** Hair or foreign bodies found on the sterile drapes should be removed and handed off the sterile field, along with any other item which has come into contact with the foreign body, such as gloves. The area should then be re-covered with another sterile drape. Alternatively, the whole sterile pack can be discarded and the process restarted using a new pack.

RECOMMENDATION **4.8.15** Layering of drapes, once a common practice, is now seldom required due to technological advances in draping materials.

RECOMMENDATION **4.8.16** Non-adhesive drapes should be held in place by an atraumatic towel clip to hold the drapes together. Where adhesive drapes are used, checks should be made of patient's sensitivity to adhesives.

RECOMMENDATION **4.8.17** The drapes should remain in place until the dressing has been applied.

RECOMMENDATION **4.8.18** The scrub practitioner should be considered the person of choice to dispose of all drapes into appropriate bags, for either launder or disposal, while still gowned and gloved. It is considered good practice to label any linen or waste leaving the theatre.

4.9 BLOOD-BORNE VIRUSES

STANDARD Personnel employed within the perioperative setting are aware of the risk of transmission of blood-borne viruses (BBVs) and adhere to immunisation protocols.

The emergence of the human immunodeficiency virus (HIV) and hepatitis B (HBV) and C (HCV) have prompted the development of much stricter infection control procedures and the introduction of standard precautions for the protection of staff and patients.

Blood-borne infections, namely HIV, HBV and HCV, pose an occupational risk to perioperative personnel. Risk of occupational transmission of blood-borne pathogens is very low if standard precautions are adhered to. However the risk of contracting HBV from needlestick exposure is much higher because of the greater infectivity of the virus (ICNA 2003). Just 0.00004ml of infected blood can transfer infection.

RECOMMENDATIONS FOR LOCAL POLICY

Health

RECOMMENDATION **4.9.1** Within an operating department environment it is important that all staff are in an optimum state of health and any incidents of ill health (eg: skin lesion or sore throats) must be reported to the team leader who will advise on appropriate action.

RECOMMENDATION **4.9.2** It is mandatory that all personnel receive the HBV vaccine. Department of Health guidelines for health clearance for blood-borne viruses (namely HIV, HBV and HBC) will be required for all healthcare workers moving into training or a post involving exposure prone procedures (EPPs) for the first time. New workers will require additional health clearance for serious communicable diseases, unless they already have a record of being tested for blood-borne viruses. This will include, for instance, junior doctors entering surgical specialities and post-registration nurses in operating theatres.

RECOMMENDATION **4.9.3** The standard health checks required for serious communicable diseases for healthcare workers new to the NHS are listed below:

- Immunisation for hepatitis B. Doses are given at 0, 1 and 6 month intervals. After a further 2–3 months, a blood sample is given to test for antibodies.
- Immunisation for hepatitis C.
- Healthcare workers are offered an HCV antibody test and, if positive, an HCV RNA test.
- Healthcare workers are offered an HIV antibody test.
- Additional health checks are required for healthcare workers new to the NHS who will perform EPPs.
- A test is undertaken for hepatitis B surface antigen (HBsAg).

- A negative result indicates the person should be immunised and the response to the vaccine checked for anti-HBs.
- A positive result (HbsAg) indicates current hepatitis B infection, and individuals should be tested for HVB e-antigen markers.
- If the e-antigen (HBeAg) is positive, the individual will not be allowed to perform EPPs.
- If the e-antigen is negative the hepatitis B viral load (HBV DNA) is tested.
- If the viral load is greater than 103 genome equivalents per ml, the individual will not be allowed to perform EPPs.
- Tests are repeated on an annual basis.

RECOMMENDATION **4.9.4** If individuals are positive for HCV antibodies they should be tested for HCV RNA to detect the presence of current infection.

RECOMMENDATION **4.9.5** HCV RNA positive individuals will not be allowed to perform EPPs. HCV infected healthcare workers who have been treated with antiviral therapy and who remain HCV RNA negative for at least six months after cessation of treatment, should be permitted to return to EPPs. Further checks to show that the worker is still HCV RNA negative are carried out six months later.

RECOMMENDATION **4.9.6** If an individual is HIV antibody positive they will not be allowed to perform EPPs, in accordance with HSC 1998/064 and HSC 2002/008 (NHS Executive 1998, 2002).

RECOMMENDATION **4.9.7** Healthcare workers who apply for a post or training which may involve EPPs and who decline to be tested for HIV, HBV and HCV should not be cleared to perform EPPs.

RECOMMENDATION **4.9.8** The *National Minimum Standards for Independent Care* (DH 2002) require all healthcare workers in the independent healthcare sector to comply with Department of Health guidelines about infections with blood-borne viruses, including Hepatitis C.

Sharps injury/conjunctiva/mucous membrane splash

RECOMMENDATION **4.9.9** All personal injuries or ill health occurring at work must be reported to the manager and statutory and local procedures followed (RIDDOR) (HMSO 1996). The theatre manager should liaise and take advice from the occupational health officer and infection control co-ordinator.

RECOMMENDATION **4.9.10** Under the Health and Safety at Work Act (HMSO 1974) all individuals should take responsibility for ensuring their own health and safety and should report/seek advice regarding concerns or hazardous practices to the local health and safety officer.

RECOMMENDATION **4.9.11** In the event of an injury, the following actions should be implemented immediately (ICNA 2003):

- Encourage bleeding of the wound by applying gentle pressure. Do not suck the wound.
- Wash the area well with running water.
- Dry and apply a waterproof dressing as necessary.
- If body fluids splash into the mouth do not swallow, rinse out several times with cold water.
- Irrigate eye splash with tap water or saline. It is recommended that eye bath stations should be positioned near sink areas and readily available.
- Report the incident to your line manager and complete an accident form.

RECOMMENDATION **4.9.12** If accidental inoculation of blood occurs from a patient known or suspected to have a blood-borne virus, consent must be obtained from the patient before a blood sample can be taken, stored and tested.

The patient should be offered counselling before the blood sample is taken.

RECOMMENDATION **4.9.13** The chief medical officers' expert advisory group on AIDS recommends that antiretroviral (EAGA 2000) post exposure prophylaxis (PEP) for HIV should be considered if there has been exposure to blood, body fluids or tissue known or suspected to be infected with HIV.

Access to anti-retroviral drugs should be available within an hour of injury, and treatment should last for four weeks.

If PEP is delayed and the risk of infection is high, PEP should still be considered up to two weeks after the incident.

4.10 MANAGEMENT OF PATIENTS WITH MRSA

STANDARD Evidence-based practices are promoted in order to minimise and prevent the spread of MRSA to patients and staff in the perioperative setting.

Methicillin resistant staphylococcus aureus (MRSA) poses a challenge to healthcare organisations and infection control teams. MRSA is a significant cause of hospital acquired infection (National Audit Office 2000). Perioperative practitioners can minimise the risk to themselves, other healthcare workers and patients by strictly adhering to and complying with standard precautions. Practices can be adapted to reduce the risk of cross-infection further.

Staphylococcus aureus is a common bacterium found in warm, moist areas of the body. It causes the host no harm, but can cause infections ranging from superficial abscesses and boils to the more serious infections such as pneumonia, osteomyelitis and septicaemia. In the 1960s certain strains of the bacterium became resistant to penicillin and methicillin, and as new antibiotics have been manufactured, so more resistance has been reported with epidemic strains (EMRSA) occurring in the mid 1980s. MRSA is now endemic in many hospitals.

Direct contact, usually with another person's hands, is the primary mode of transmission and various studies have isolated MRSA on door handles, light switches, other equipment and surfaces as well as hands (Fogg 2002).

MRSA has been isolated in postoperative wound infections (almost 25% of all wounds), intravenous tip catheters, chest drains and burn wounds (National Audit Office 2000). However it must be noted that the majority of these infections arise from transference of the patient's own skin flora to the site (endogenous), although some do come from the operating theatre and its staff.

RECOMMENDATIONS FOR LOCAL POLICY

General considerations

RECOMMENDATION **4.10.1** Screening of all patients with MRSA as part of a preoperative assessment process is not clinically effective. Screening is recommended for the patient undergoing prosthetic surgery, to prevent prolonged hospital stay, breakdown of the wound and prosthesis.

RECOMMENDATION **4.10.2** Clinicians should attempt to eradicate the infection prior to surgery by prescribing and administering teicoplanin or vancomycin (Working Party Report 1998).

RECOMMENDATION **4.10.3** Known MRSA patients may be operated on at the end of a list, as such patients are likely to disperse bacterium into the atmosphere and potentially pose a risk to subsequent patients and staff.

RECOMMENDATION **4.10.4** Standard precautions should be adhered to and theatre doors kept closed, with minimal numbers of staff entering the theatre, so that ventilation systems can function efficiently and effectively.

RECOMMENDATION **4.10.5** Personnel and movement in theatre should be kept to a minimum as MRSA may be released into the atmosphere on skin squames and fibres from clothing, or carried as dust particles.

RECOMMENDATION **4.10.6** Following adequate cleaning of the theatre at the end of the case further procedures can continue. All surfaces in contact with the patient should be disinfected according to manufacturer's instructions.

RECOMMENDATION **4.10.7** If standard precautions are followed there is no need to remove all non-essential equipment or further restrict personnel.

RECOMMENDATION **4.10.8** All equipment and inanimate objects in theatre should be kept clean and free from dust.

RECOMMENDATION **4.10.9** Known MRSA patients may be recovered in the theatre room itself. This is to reduce the risk of additional staff coming into contact with the patient and potentially infecting other patients and staff. Strict hand washing protocols must be in place.

RECOMMENDATION **4.10.10** If there is a risk of exposure to blood or body fluids then appropriate barrier protection must be used. Clothes need to be changed if contamination has occurred, depending on the contact with the patient as assessed by the individual healthcare worker.

RECOMMENDATION **4.10.11** Regular theatre cleaning, as well as cleaning following spillages, should be managed as per local policy.

RECOMMENDATION **4.10.12** The most effective method of preventing and controlling the spread of MRSA is by the effective decontamination of hands after every patient episode or contact (Storr 2000).

4.11 TRANSMISSIBLE SPONGIFORM ENCEPHALOPATHY (TSE) AGENTS: SAFETY AND INFECTION PREVENTION

STANDARD There is a system in place that minimises the risk of infection with transmissible spongiform encephalopathy agents for both patients and staff in the perioperative environment.

The identification of variant Creutzfeldt-Jakob disease (vCJD) in March 1996, and the suggested link with consuming bovine spongiform encephalopathy (BSE) infected beef led the Advisory Committee on Dangerous Pathogens (ACDP) to review its current guidance on the agents of transmissible spongiform encephalopathies (TSEs).

TSEs are unique infectious agents, currently thought to be proteins known as prions, which do not share the properties of viruses or bacteria. They also exhibit resistance to conventional decontamination processes.

The ACDP

The Advisory Committee on Dangerous Pathogens is a pan government advisory committee which advises the Health and Safety Commission, the Health and Safety Executive, Health and Agricultural Ministers and their counterparts in Scotland, Wales and Northern Ireland, as required, on all aspects of hazards and risks to workers and others from exposure to pathogens.

In recent years the scientific community have provided healthcare workers with more detailed information on TSEs. However many uncertainties remain, for example the routes of infection and the potential number of people who may be incubating vCJD. It is important that employers responsible for the welfare of employees ensure that they are kept up to date with new research and guidance.

The following guidance by the Independent Spongiform Encephalopathy Advisory Committee (SEAC) is recommended to be included in local policy. The guidance advises on the management of TSEs in the perioperative setting.

RECOMMENDATIONS FOR LOCAL POLICY

Risk management

RECOMMENDATION **4.11.1** A risk assessment model which examined the risk of transmission of vCJD via surgical instruments was undertaken by the Department of Health and published in March 2001 (DH 2001). It concludes that effective decontamination is the key to reducing the risk of transmission via surgery. The Health Service Circular HSC 2000/032 (DH 2000) sets out the action necessary to ensure that decontamination of medical devices is carried out to the highest standard. The measures to be taken when performing invasive surgery will depend on:

- how likely the patient is to be carrying the infectious agent
- how likely it is that infection could be transmitted by the procedure being carried out.

RECOMMENDATION **4.11.2** All staff caring for patients with potential CJD or vCJD must have received training in the control of infection in accordance with the Controls Assurance Standard (Infection Control criterion 12) (NHS Estates 2001).

RECOMMENDATION **4.11.3** All medical devices, decontamination equipment and surfaces should be appropriately dealt with after use on patients who are definite, probable or possible CJD cases, and where the patient falls into a risk category for developing CJD or vCJD:

- Where surgical instruments have been used in procedures involving tissues designated as having high or medium infectivity, or on possible CJD or vCJD patients, instruments must be quarantined pending a confirmed diagnosis.
- All instruments used on definite or probable CJD patients, and those used on at-risk patients where there has been exposure to brain, spinal cord or eye tissue, must be disposed of by incineration.
- Manual handling of contaminated instruments should be kept to a minimum and automated decontamination processes should be used wherever possible.
- The manual handling of instruments intended for quarantine should be kept to a minimum, therefore instruments should only be rinsed to remove gross soil. Where instruments have been used on the low risk tissues of a definite, probable or possible CJD/vCJD case, or where the patient falls into an at-risk category for developing CJD/vCJD, then no special precautions are necessary.

RECOMMENDATION **4.11.4** Instruments should be reprocessed according to best practice, therefore automated decontamination processes should be used wherever possible:

- Neutral or enzymatic detergent suitable for use with this reprocessing equipment should be used.
- Contaminated instruments should be processed through an automated washer/disinfector in which no other instruments are being cleaned.
- Items should be cleaned as soon as possible after use to minimise drying of blood and body fluids onto the item which may be then be more difficult to remove. Items should not be soaked in disinfectant prior to cleaning.
- Following processing of instruments, the automated washer/disinfector should be run through an empty cycle.
- Any solid waste/tissue should be disposed of by incineration and liquid waste disposed of safely.
- Any cleaning aids such as brushes should be incinerated.

Manual cleaning

RECOMMENDATION **4.11.5** Care should be taken to avoid splashing and generating aerosols. Instruments should be held below the surface of the water in a sink into which water is running and draining out continuously.

Instruments should not be held directly under a flowing tap as this is likely to generate splashes.

RECOMMENDATION **4.11.6** Operators should wear personal protective equipment (PPE) when cleaning instruments and must take care to avoid penetrating injuries.

RECOMMENDATION **4.11.7** Instruments intended for quarantine after washing should be rinsed and placed on a disposable instrument tray and allowed to air dry.

Autoclaving

RECOMMENDATION **4.11.8** After cleaning contaminated items they should be processed in a porous load (high vacuum) steam steriliser using either:

- a single cycle of 134–137°C for a minimum holding time of 18 minutes
- six successive cycles of 134–137°C for a minimum holding time of 3 minutes for each cycle.

Other cycles are not recommended. Downward or upward displacement autoclaves must not be used.

Chemical disinfectants

RECOMMENDATION **4.11.9** If the item is unable to tolerate the moist heat porous load cycles specified, then liquid chemical treatment may be considered.

RECOMMENDATION **4.11.10** Chemical agents and contact times that are effective include:

- 20,000ppm available chlorine of sodium hypochlorite for one hour
- 2M sodium hydroxide (caustic soda – 8% w/v) for one hour.

10,000ppm hypochlorite must not be used as it is ineffective against the agents of TSE at this concentration. Sodium dichloroisocyanurate (presept) has also been shown to be ineffective.

Chemical agents used at these concentrations and contact times may have a corrosive effect on clinical instruments and equipment and should only be used after seeking advice from the manufacturer. Special care is required with electrical cables. Providing they have not been contaminated by the procedure, cables may be wiped down with 2M sodium hydroxide.

Quarantine of instruments

RECOMMENDATION **4.11.11** Suspected contaminated instruments should be placed in an impervious rigid plastic container with a close fitting lid, or a dedicated TSE bin.

RECOMMENDATION **4.11.12** The lid should be sealed with heavy duty tape such as autoclave tape and labelled with the patient's identification details including name, date of birth and hospital number. The label should also state the surgical procedure in which the instruments were used and the name of the responsible person such as the theatre manager or sterile services manager.

RECOMMENDATION **4.11.13** A responsible member of the theatre team should accompany the instruments to the incineration unit.

RECOMMENDATION **4.11.14** The instruments should be stored in a sealed box indefinitely in a suitable designated place until the outcome of any further investigations is known. If the patient is confirmed as suffering from CJD or vCJD, the box and its contents should be incinerated without any further examination. If an alternative diagnosis is confirmed, the instruments may be removed from the box by the responsible person (the theatre manager or named deputy), reprocessed according to best practice and returned to use. Additional decontamination procedures are not required.

Precautions

RECOMMENDATION **4.11.15** Where it is believed that the patient will fall into one of the various categories of CJD, then single use surgical instruments should be used as far as is reasonably practicable.

RECOMMENDATION **4.11.16** After completion of a surgical procedure on a possible CJD or vCJD patient, single use instruments should be separated and disposed of by incineration.

RECOMMENDATION **4.11.17** Some expensive items of equipment such as drills may be prevented from being contaminated by using shields, guards or coverings so that the entire device does not need to be incinerated. The drill bit or other parts in contact with high risk tissue and the protective covering would need to be incinerated. Advice should be sought from the manufacturer to ascertain if this is feasible.

RECOMMENDATION **4.11.18** Where possible, procedures should be performed at the end of the operating list to allow effective decontamination of the theatre.

RECOMMENDATION **4.11.19** Records must be kept of all decisions and the sterile service department must be informed about the decision before the instruments are sent for routine reprocessing.

Decontamination of endoscopes

Decontamination of endoscopes should be in accordance with the general procedures set out in MDA Device Bulletin MDA DB2002 (05) (MDA 2002) available at www.medical-devices.gov.uk

RECOMMENDATION **4.11.20** Aldehyde disinfectants with fixative qualities tend to stabilise, rather than inactivate prions. The use of non-fixative disinfectants, if this is in accordance with manufacturer's instructions, is therefore preferable.

RECOMMENDATION **4.11.21** Disinfectants with fixative properties should not be used on flexible endoscopes for any procedure on patients with a diagnosis of definite, probable or possible CJD, where the diagnosis of CJD is unclear, or the patient is at risk of developing CJD.

RECOMMENDATION **4.11.22** If it is necessary for an endoscopic procedure to be performed on a confirmed CJD or vCJD patient, a single use endoscope should be used and incinerated after use. For suspect CJD or vCJD patients the endoscope should be quarantined pending a confirmed definite diagnosis.

Blood

RECOMMENDATION **4.11.23** Careful attention must be given to standard infection control precautions to minimise any risks from blood.

RECOMMENDATION **4.11.24** Drug administration by injection should involve the same precautions and special care is required to avoid sharp injuries and other forms of parenteral exposure.

RECOMMENDATION **4.11.25** Compliance with standard infection control precautions are required in accordance with *Guidance for Clinical Health Workers: protection against infection with blood-borne viruses* (DH 1998).

Specimens

RECOMMENDATION **4.11.26** Specimen samples should be marked with a bio-hazard label and it is recommended to inform the laboratory in advance that a specimen sample is being sent. Consideration should be given to maintaining the patient's confidentiality.

Spillages

RECOMMENDATION **4.11.27** Infectious agents associated with TSEs are resistant to inactivation techniques, so special care is required at all times to avoid unnecessary spillages.

RECOMMENDATION **4.11.28** Dilution is the most important element in cleaning up the spillage and minimising the risk.

Exposure to high concentration (20,000ppm available chlorine) sodium hypochlorite for one hour is known to be effective.

RECOMMENDATION **4.11.29** Potentially infectious materials should be removed using absorbent material and any waste disposed of as clinical waste.

Intraoperative death

RECOMMENDATION **4.11.30** On the intraoperative death of a patient with a definite/probable or possible case of CJD/ vCJD, or where the patient falls into a risk category for developing CJD, the removal of the body from the theatre to the mortuary should be carried out using normal infection control procedures.

RECOMMENDATION **4.11.31** It is recommended that the deceased patient is placed in a cadaver bag prior to transportation to the mortuary, in line with normal procedures for where there is a known infection risk.

RECOMMENDATION **4.11.32** An infection control notification sheet should be completed and given to the undertakers concerned with the deceased.

REFERENCES

American Operating Room Nurses 2004a *Standards, Recommended Practices and Guidelines: recommended practices for surgical hand antisepsis/hands scrubs* Denver, AORN Inc

American Operating Room Nurses 2004b *Standards, Recommended Practices and Guidelines: recommended practices for maintaining a sterile field* Denver, AORN Inc

American Operating Room Nurses 2004c *Standards, Recommended Practices and Guidelines: recommended practices for skin preparation of patients* Denver, AORN Inc

Avery CM, Gallagher P, Birnbaum W 1999 Double gloving and a glove perforation indication system during the dental treatment of HIV positive patients: are they necessary? *British Dental Journal* 186 (1) 27–30

Belkin NL 1996 A Century after their Introduction: are surgical face masks necessary? *AORN Journal* 64 (4) 602–607

Carter R 1990 Plastic Overshoes – an unacceptable risk? *Nursing Times* 86 (13) 63–64

Centres for Disease Control and Prevention 1998 Perspectives in Disease Prevention and Health Promotion Update: universal precautions for prevention of transmission of human immunodeficiency virus, hepatitis B virus, and other blood-borne pathogens in healthcare settings *Morbidity and Mortality Weekly Report* 37 (24) 377–388

Cruse PJ, Foord R 1980 The Epidemiology of Wound Infection: a 10-year study of 62,939 wounds *Surgical Clinics of North America* 60 27–40

Department of Health 1998 *Guidance for Clinical Health Workers: protection against infection with blood-borne viruses* HSC 1998/063 London, DH. www.dh.gov.uk/PublicationsAndStatistics/fs/en

Department of Health 2000 *Decontamination of Medical Devices* HSC 2000/032 London, DH. www.dh.gov.uk/PublicationsAndStatistics/fs/en

Department of Health 2001 *Risk Assessment for the Transmission of vCJD via Surgical Instruments: a modelling approach and numerical scenarios* London, DH. www.dh.gov.uk

Department of Health 2002 *Independent Healthcare: national minimum standards* London, DH

Doyle PM, Alvis S, Johanson R 1992 The Effectiveness of Double Gloving in Obstetrics and Gynaecology *British Journal of Gynaecology* 99 83–84

EAGA 2000 *Chief Medical Officers' Expert Advisory Group on AIDS: HIV post-exposure prophylaxis* London, DH

European Commission 1993 *Medical Devices Directive 93/42* EEC European Communities, Luxembourg. http://europa.eu.int/comm/enterprise/medical_devices/index.htm

European Committee for Standardisation 2002 *Part 1: surgical drapes, gowns and clean air suits used as medical devices for patients, clinical staff and equipment* EN13795 European Committee for Standardisation CEN

Fogg D 2002 Clinical Issues *AORN* 76 (1) 175

Gould D 2000 Hand Decontamination *Nursing Standard* 15 (6) 45–50

Gruendemann BJ, Fernsebner B 1995 Principles of Aseptic Technique. In *Comprehensive Perioperative Nursing* Boston, Jones & Barlett

Hedderwick SA, McNeill SA, Lyons MJ, Kauffman CA 2000 Pathogenic Organisms Associated with Artificial Fingernails Worn by Healthcare Workers *Infection Control and Hospital Epidemiology* 21 (8) 505–509

HMSO 1974 *Health and Safety at Work Act* Norwich, The Stationery Office

HMSO 1987 *Consumer Protection Act* Norwich, The Stationery Office

HMSO 1992 *Personal Protective Equipment* (EC Directive Regulations) No 3139 Norwich, The Stationery Office

HMSO 1996 *Reporting of Injuries, Diseases and Dangerous Occurences Regulations (RIDDOR)* Norwich, The Stationery Office

HMSO 2002 *The Control of Substances Hazardous to Health Regulations (COSHH)* Norwich, The Stationery Office

Hobson DW, Woller W, Anderson L, Guthery E 1998 Development and evaluation of a new alcohol-based surgical hand scrub formulation with persistent antimicrobial characteristics and brushless application *American Journal of Infection Control* 26 (5) 507–512

Hospital Infection Society 2002 *Behaviours and Rituals in the Operating Theatre* Dublin, HIS Working Party

Humphreys H, Marshall RJ, Ricketts VE, Russell AJ, Reeves DS 1991 Theatre Overshoes do not Reduce Operating Theatre Floor Bacterial Counts *Journal of Hospital Infection* 17 (2) 117–123

Infection Control Nurses Association 2002 *Protective Clothing: principles and guidance* Edinburgh, ICNA

Infection Control Nurses Association 2003 *Infection Control Guidance for General Practice* Edinburgh, ICNA

Larson EL, Butz AM, Gullette DL, Laughon BA 1990 Alcohol for Surgical Scrubbing? *Infection Control and Hospital Epidemiology* 11 (3) 139–143

Managram AJ, Horan C, Pearson M, Silver L, Jarvis W 1999 Guidelines for Prevention of Surgical Site Infection *Infection Control and Hospital Epidemiology* 20 (4) 256–258

Maunder JA, Sargent RJ, Taylor R 2003 *Removal of Nail Polish and Finger Rings to Prevent Surgical Infection* (Cochrane Review). In The Cochrane Library, Issue 4, Chichester, John Wiley & Sons Ltd

McNeil SA, Foster CL, Hedderwick SA, Kaufman CA 2000 Effect of hand cleansing with antimicrobial soap or alcohol-based gel on microbial colonisation of artificial fingernails by healthcare workers *Clinical Infectious Diseases* 32 (3) 367–372

Medical Devices Agency 2000 *Use of Spirit-based Solutions During Surgical Procedures Requiring the Use of Electrosurgical Equipment* SN 2000(17) London, MDA

Medical Devices Agency 2002 *Decontamination of Endoscopes* MDA DB 2002 (05) London, MDA

MHRA 2003 *Surgical Gowns, Drapes and Coverings* London, Medicines and Healthcare Products Regulatory Agency. www.medical-devices.gov.uk/mda/mdawebsitev2.nsf

Mishriki SF, Law DJ, Jeffrey PJ 1990 Factors Affecting the Incidence of Postoperative Wound Infection *Journal of Hospital Infection* 16 223–230

National Association of Theatre Nurses 1998 *Safeguards for Invasive Procedures: management of risks* Harrogate, NATN

National Audit Office 2000 *Management and Control of Hospital Acquired Infection in Acute NHS Trusts in England* Norwich, The Stationery Office

NHS Estates 1995 *Hospital Laundry Arrangements for Used and Infected Linen* HSG (95) 18 London, DH

NHS Estates 2001 *A Review of the Decontamination of Surgical Instruments in the NHS in England* London, The Stationery Office

NHS Estates 2002 *Infection Control in the Built Environment* London, DH

NHS Executive 1998 *Pre and Post Appointment Checks for all Persons Working in the NHS in England* HSC 1998/064 Leeds, DH

NHS Executive 2002 *Management of Health and Safety and Welfare Issues for NHS Staff* HSC 2002/008 Leeds, DH

Novak CB, Patterson JM, Mackinnon SE 1999 Evaluation of Hand Sensibility with Single and Double Latex Gloves *Plastic Reconstruction Surgery* 103 (1) 128–131

PASA 2003 *Annual Report and Accounts 02/03* NHS Purchasing and Supply Agency. www.pasa.nhs.uk/annrpt

Patterson JM, Novak CB, Mackinnon SE, Patterson CA 1998 Surgeons' Concern and Practices of Protection Against Blood-borne Pathogens *American Surgery* 228 266–272

Pereira LJ, Lee GM, Wade KJ 1990 The effect of surgical hand washing routines on the microbial counts of operating room nurses *American Journal of Infection Control* 18 354–364

Pereira LJ, Lee GM, Wade KJ 1997 An evaluation of five protocols for surgical hand washing in relation to skin condition and microbial counts *Journal of Hospital Infection* 36 49–65

Pratt RJ, Pellowe C, Loveday HP, Robinson N, Smith G et al 2001 The Epic Project: developing national evidence-based guidelines for preventing healthcare associated infections *Journal of Hospital Infection* 47 (Supplement) S1–S82

Storr J 2000 MRSA *Nursing Times* 96 (10) 3–4

Swarbrook S, Stuart J, Tanner J 2003 *Surgical Scrubbing to Reduce Surgical Site Infection* (Protocol for a Cochrane Review). In The Cochrane Library, Issue 4, Chichester, John Wiley & Sons Ltd

Tanner J, Parkinson H 2002 Double Gloving to Reduce Surgical Cross-infection. In *Cochrane Database Systematic Reviews 2002(3): CD003087*

Weightman NC, Banfield KR 1994 Protective Overshoes are Unnecessary in a Day Surgery Unit *Journal of Hospital Infection* 28 (1) 1–3

Working Party Report 1998 Revised Guidelines for the Control of Methicillin-resistant Staphylococcus Aureus Infection in Hospitals Ayliffe Prof GA *Journal of Hospital Infection* 39 253–290

FURTHER READING

Agarwal M, Hamilton-Stewart P, Dixon RA 2002 Contaminated Operating Room Boots: the potential for infection *American Journal of Infection Control* 30 (3) 179–183

Alexander JW, Fischer JE, Boyajian M, Palmquist J 1983 The Influence of Hair Removal Methods on Wound Infections *Archives of Surgery* 118 347–352

American Operating Room Nurses Association 2004 *Standards, Practices and Guidelines* Denver, AORN Inc

American Operating Room Nurses Association 2004 *Recommended Practices for Standard and Transmission-based Precautions in the Perioperative Practice Setting* Denver, AORN Inc

Association of Anaesthetists of Great Britain and Ireland 2002 *Infection Control in Anaesthesia* London, AAGBI

Atkinson LJ, Fortunato NM 1996 *Berry & Kohn's Operating Room Technique* 8th ed, USA, Mosby

Australian Council of Operating Room Nurses 2004 *Environmental Management Standards for Perioperative Nursing* Adelaide, ACORN

Australian Council of Operating Room Nurses 2004 *Standards for Perioperative Nursing* Adelaide, ACORN

Ayliffe GA, Fraise AP, Geddes AM, Mitchell K 2000 *Control of Hospital Infection: a practical handbook* 4th ed, London, Arnold

Ayliffe GA, English MP 2003 *Hospital Infection from Miasmas to MRSA* 1st ed, Cambridge, University Press

Bartlett GE, Pollarol TC, Bowker KE, Bannister GC 2002 Effects of Jewellery on Surface Bacterial Counts of Operating Theatres *Journal of Hospital Infection* 52 (1) 68–70

Beesley J 2001 Answers Supplied *British Journal of Perioperative Nursing* 11 (8) 336

Beesley J 2002 Open Forum: as a professional registered nurse, you have a duty of care to the patient *British Journal of Perioperative Nursing* 12 (3) 84–85

Belkin NL 1997 Use of Scrubs and Related Apparel in Healthcare Facilities *American Journal of Infection Control* 25 401–404

Belkin NL 2001 Home Laundering of Soiled Surgical Scrubs: surgical site infections and the home environment *American Journal of Infection Control* 29 (1) 58–64

Bernthal L 2000 Two Gloves or not Two Gloves? That is the question *British Journal of Perioperative Nursing* 10 (2) 102–107

Brown M, Cumberland N 2000 Is it Time to Change? – theatre protocols for methicillin resistant staphylococcus aureus (MRSA) positive patients *British Journal of Infection Control* 1 (4) 13–14

Caunt H 1991 The Evolution of Theatre Dress *Nursing* 4 (42) 23–24

Clark L 2003 Hospital Acquired Infection *Nurse 2 Nurse* 3 (1) 46–48

Davidson K, Dobb M 2003 Surgical Draping Practices – a national survey *British Journal of Perioperative Nursing* 13 (3) 109–114

Department of Health 1998 *Scottish Infection Control Manual – guidance on core standards for the control of infection in hospitals, healthcare premises and at the community interface* Edinburgh, The Scottish Office

Department of Health 1998 *AIDS/HIV Infected Healthcare Workers: guidance on the management of infected healthcare workers and patient notification* London, DH

Department of Health 1999 *Hospital Acquired Infection: a framework for a national system of surveillance for the NHS in Scotland* Edinburgh, The Scottish Office

Department of Health 2003 *Health Clearance for Serious Communicable Diseases: new healthcare workers. Draft guide for consultation* London, DH. www.dh.gov.uk/healthclear

Department of Health 2003 *Winning Ways: working together to reduce healthcare associated infection in England* London, DH

East J 1998 Risk Management. In Clarke P, Jones J (eds) *Brigden's Operating Department Practice* Edinburgh, Churchill Livingstone

Edwards P 2001 Contamination of the Surgical Field – what does the published research say about face masks *British Journal of Perioperative Nursing* 11 (12) 543–546

Fairchild SS 1996 *Perioperative Nursing – principles and practice* 2nd ed, USA, Little, Brown and Company (Inc)

Fogg DM 1999 Clinical Issues: body piercing, perineal preps, insects in the operating room, wound classification systems, recommended practices *AORN Journal* 70 (1) 120–124

Garcia R 2000 To Attire or Not to Attire – the question of what to wear in surgery *Surgical Services Management* 6 (3) 30–35

Garner BD 1995 Infection Control. In Meeker MH, Rothrock JC (eds) *Alexander's Care of the Patient in Surgery* St Louis, Mosby

Gilmour D 2003 MRSA – here to stay? *Changing Practice* 9 5–8

Glasgow D, Sommers J 2003 Lint Shedding Cannot be Overlooked *Clinical Services Journal* 2 (3) 28–31

Gruedemann BJ, Mangum SS 2001 *Infection Prevention in Surgical Settings* 1st ed, USA, WB Saunders Company

Hambraeus A, Bengtsson S, Laurell G 1978 Bacterial Contamination in a Modern Operating Theatre: importance of floor contamination as a source of airborne bacteria *Journal of Hygiene* 80 57–67

Hedderwick S, McNeil SA, Lyons MJ, Kauffman CA 2000 Pathogenic Organisms Associated with Artificial Fingernails Worn by Healthcare Workers *Infection Control and Hospital Epidemiology* 21 (8) 505–509

HMSO 1990 *Environmental Protection Act* Norwich, The Stationery Office

Hoffmann KK, Clontz EP, Rutlala WA, Weber DJ 2001 Patient Attire in Ambulatory Surgery *American Journal of Infection Control* 29 (5) 345–346

Hospital Infection Control Practices Advisory Committee 1996 Guidelines for Isolation Procedures in Hospitals. Part II: recommendations for isolation precautions in hospitals *American Journal of Infection Control* 124 32–45

Independent Multi-Disciplinary Working Group 2001 *Surgical Drapes and Gowns in Today's NHS: moving forward from traditional textiles* Hertfordshire, HSD Communications

Independent Multi-Disciplinary Working Group 2003 *Considering the Consequences: an evaluation of infection risk when choosing surgical gowns and drapes in today's NHS* Rickmansworth, HSD Communications

Independent Multi-Disciplinary Working Group 2003 *Under Scrutiny – are you at risk? Making Sense of New EU regulations in Medical Devices: a case study* EN13795 Rickmansworth, HSD Communications

Infection Control Nurses Association 2002 *Guidelines for Hand Hygiene* Edinburgh, ICNA

Joint Scottish Executive Health Department and NHS Scotland Working Group 2001 *Managing the Risk of Healthcare Associated Infection in NHS Scotland* NHS Health Department Letters 53

Jurkovich P 1999 Rationale for Home Laundering of Scrub Attire *AORN Journal* 69 (5) 1024–1025

Kent S 2000 Antiseptic Skin Preparation Revisited *British Journal of Perioperative Nursing* 10 (7) 364–372

Kjonniksen I, Anderson BM, Sondenaa VG, Segadal L 2002 Preoperative Hair Removal – a systematic literature review *AORN Journal* 75 (5) 928–938

Larson EL, Aiello AE, Heilman JM, Lyle CT, Cronquist A, Stahl JB, Della-Latta P 2001 Comparison of Different Regimens for Surgical Hand Preparation *AORN* 73 (2) 412–432

Line S 2003 Decontamination and Control of Infection in Theatre *British Journal of Perioperative Nursing* 13 (2) 70–75

Lipp A 2003 An Assessment of the Clinical Effectiveness of Surgical Drapes *Nursing Times* 99 (49) 28–31

Lipp A, Edwards P 2002 Disposable Surgical Face Masks: a systematic review *Journal of Advanced Perioperative Care* 1 (2) 41–46

Loeb MB, Wilcox L, Smaill F, Walter S, Duff Z 1997 A Randomised Trial of Surgical Scrubbing with a Brush Compared to Antiseptic Soap Alone *American Journal of Infection Control* 25 11–15

Makoni T 2002 MRSA: risk assessment and flexible management *Nursing Standard* 16 (28) 39–41

Mallet J, Dougherty L 2000 *The Royal Marsden Hospital Manual of Clinical Nursing Procedures* 5th ed, Oxford, Blackwell Science

Meeker MH, Rothrock JC 1999 *Alexander's Care of the Patient in Surgery* 11th ed, USA, Mosby

Meyers GM 2001 Recommendation for Surgical Skin Preparation: an integrative review of literature *Journal of Knowledge Synthesis for Nursing* 2 (10) (online)

Moolenaar RL, Crutcher JM, San Joaquin VH et al 2000 A prolonged outbreak if pseudomonas aeruginosa in a neonatal intensive care unit: did staff fingernails play a role in disease transmission? *Infection Control Hospital and Epidemiology* 21 (2) 80–85

National Association of Theatre Nurses 1997 *Universal Precautions and Infection Control in the Perioperative Setting* Harrogate, NATN

National Association of Theatre Nurses 2000 *Back to Basics: perioperative practice principles* Harrogate, NATN

NHS Executive 2000 *Hepatitis B Infected Healthcare Workers: guidance on implementation of HSC 2000/020* Health Service Circular 1000/020 Leeds, DH

OR Manager Inc 1996 Should Scrub Suits be Laundered at Home? *OR Manager* 12 (8) 21–22

Rohrlach G 2001 Open Forum: a literature review demonstrated little to support the use of shoe covers *British Journal of Perioperative Nursing* 11 (4) 150

Royal College of Nursing 2000 *Universal Precautions* London, RCN

Royal Marsden Hospital 2000 *Manual of Clinical Nursing Procedures* 5th ed, Mallett J, Dougherty L (eds) London, Blackwell Publishing

Salisbury DM, Hutfilz P, Treen LM, Bollin GE, Gautam S 1997 The Effect of Rings on Microbial Load of Healthcare Workers' Hands *American Journal of Infection Control* 25 (1) 24–27

Scottish Executive Health Department Working Group 2001 *The Decontamination of Surgical Instrument and other Medical Devices* NHS Health Department Letters 10

Small SP 1996 Preoperative Hair Removal: a case report with implications for nursing *Journal of Clinical Nursing* 5 (2) 79–84

Sommers J 2003 The Impact of European Norms on the Selection of Drape and Gown Materials *Institute of Sterile Services Management Journal* 9 (2) 7–8

Spry C 1997 *Essentials of Perioperative Nursing* 2nd ed, USA, Aspen

Wilson J 2001 *Infection Control in Clinical Practice* 2nd ed, Edinburgh, Balliere Tindall

Working Party Report 2001 *Surgical Drapes and Gowns in Today's NHS: moving forward from traditional textiles.* Report from an independent multi-disciplinary working group Rickmansworth, HSD Communications

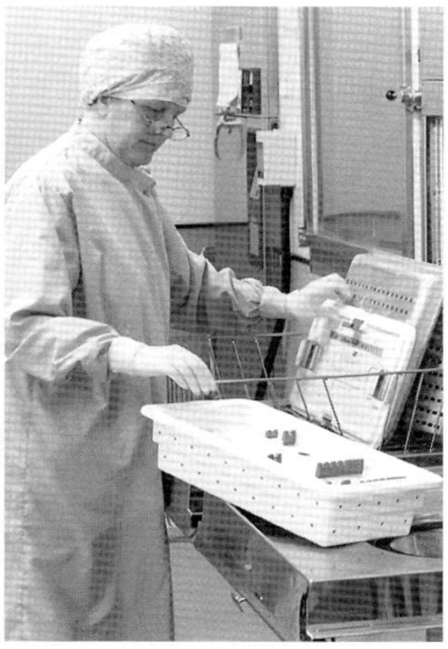

5 DECONTAMINATION

5.1 INTRODUCTION

STANDARD There is a system in place that ensures, as far as is reasonably practicable, that all reusable medical devices are properly decontaminated and that the risks associated with decontamination facilities and processes are adequately managed (Health Care Standards Unit 2002).

Decontamination is the combination of processes including cleaning, disinfection and sterilisation, which are used to render a reusable device safe for further use on patients and for handling by staff.

If decontamination processes are not correctly undertaken, either individually or collectively, the likelihood of infectious agents being transferred to individuals or the environment may be increased.

The decontamination process is required to make medical devices:

- safe for users to handle
- safe for use on the patient.

In 2001 a decontamination life cycle was published (NHS Estates 2001). This highlighted the extent to which decontamination can affect the whole organisation as well as any perioperative setting or areas which process medical devices. Effective decontamination requires the attainment of acceptable standards at all stages of the life cycle.

Decontamination life cycle

Diagram reproduced by kind permission of NHS Estates

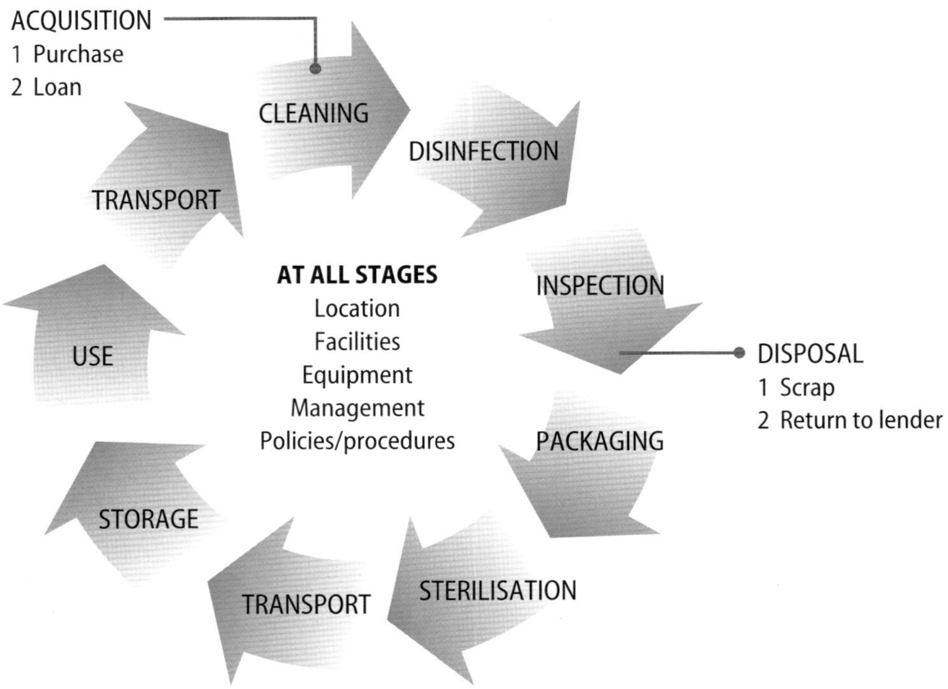

The reusable medical device life cycle comprises the processes of acquisition, cleaning, disinfection, inspection, disposal, packaging, sterilisation, transportation, and storage before use. The cycle is used to render a reusable item safe for further use.

RECOMMENDATIONS FOR LOCAL POLICY

RECOMMENDATION **5.1.1**

At all stages of reprocessing, the following issues need to be taken into account:

- The location and activities where decontamination takes place
- Facilities and equipment at each location
- Validation, maintenance and testing of equipment, in accordance with manufacturer's guidelines and legislation
- Effective management arrangements
- Policies and procedures for all aspects of decontamination work
- Understanding of risk reduction by all users.

5.2 RISK MANAGEMENT

STANDARD There is a system in place for the effective management of decontamination processes.

RECOMMENDATIONS FOR LOCAL POLICY

RECOMMENDATION **5.2.1** The level of responsibility for decontamination of reusable medical devices within the perioperative setting should be clearly defined. A nominated lead staff member should have clear lines of responsibility and accountability for decontamination matters throughout the operating department.

RECOMMENDATION **5.2.2** The perioperative setting must have comprehensive policies and procedures in place to ensure that decontamination processes are undertaken in a controlled manner to protect the health and safety of patients and staff.

RECOMMENDATION **5.2.3** A used surgical instrument is a potential source of infection to another patient and to anyone handling the instrument. Appropriately qualified key personnel should be in place within decontamination or sterile services. These personnel should work within legislative and best practice guidance in order to minimise the risk to patients and staff.

RECOMMENDATION **5.2.4** All staff involved in decontamination processes must have access to up-to-date legislation and guidance. This is essential for the organisation to carry out the statutory duties imposed upon it by law and the mandatory duties imposed by the Department of Health.

RECOMMENDATION **5.2.5** As a minimum, staff should have access to key references found in Controls Assurance for decontamination of reusable medical devices HSC 1999/179 (NHS Executive 1999a):

- The NHS Estates (England and Wales) website contains much of this information – www.decontamination.nhsestates.gov.uk
- Department of Health guidance can be accessed on the internet on the DH COIN database – www.dh.gov.uk
- Advice and guidance documents are also listed on the Medicines and Healthcare Products Regulatory Agency MHRA website – www.mhra.gov.uk
- The Health and Safety Executive website contains up-to-date information on legislation and guidance – www.hse.gov.uk
- The Controls Assurance Support Unit website – www.casu.org.uk – also provides up-to-date guidance. Controls Assurance standards exist for decontamination processes, and organisations are legally required to undertake risk assessments and complete audit returns as part of a risk management system.
- In Scotland decontamination guidance is included and referred to in the 'Glennie' Report NHS Scotland Sterile Services Provision Review Group – 1st report NHS Scotland – www.show.scot.nhs.uk/sehd/publications/GlennieFramework.pdf

- Scottish Health Technical Memoranda (SHTM) provide healthcare facilities with a framework of best practice in the choice of purchasing, installation, validation, and monitoring and routine operation of equipment. They are compatible with existing European and British standards.
- More detailed guidance on local decontamination in Scotland is available from the Property and Environment Forum – www.show.scot.nhs.uk/pef

5.3 ACQUISITION

STANDARD There is a system in place for the safe procurement and acquisition of reusable medical devices and decontamination equipment.

Before acquiring reusable medical devices and decontamination equipment, all decontamination issues must be considered.

RECOMMENDATIONS FOR LOCAL POLICY

RECOMMENDATION **5.3.1** Organisations should have a specialist group to consider the full implications of procurement and disposal of medical devices and non-medical equipment. Key representatives may include:

- users
- medical physicists
- electro-medical engineers (EME) or electro-bio-medical engineers (EBME)
- risk managers
- infection control team
- sterile services department
- estates
- procurement/purchasers
- decontamination lead.

The purpose of the group is to ensure that the technical specifications of the equipment purchased meet the user's needs.

RECOMMENDATION **5.3.2** The specialist group should ensure that the decontamination instructions provided by the medical device manufacturer demonstrate compatibility between the medical device and the available decontamination equipment, and that appropriate policies are in place. Advice on the purchase of decontamination equipment and medical devices may be sought from the authorised person (sterilisers) or the decontamination lead.

RECOMMENDATION **5.3.3** Consideration should also be given to the following:

- Regulatory compliance information
- Device/equipment evaluation reports
- User experience and preferences
- Comparable costs and features of alternative devices
- Standardisation on a single model where possible
- Training and maintenance implications
- Organisational and departmental policy
- Safety and hazard notices issued by the Medicines and Healthcare Products Regulatory Agency (MHRA) or NHS Estates.

RECOMMENDATION **5.3.4** A procurement policy must be in place which ensures that all purchased medical devices are compatible with available decontamination processes. It is recommended that the Microbiology Advisory Committee (MAC) manual (MDA 1999a) and MDA Device Bulletin 9801 (MDA 1998a) are referenced when formulating the policy.

RECOMMENDATION **5.3.5** There should be an audit process in place for verifying the appropriateness of medical devices and equipment purchased.

RECOMMENDATION **5.3.6** To assist organisations with their purchasing decisions, the NHS Purchasing and Supply Agency (PASA) has established framework agreements for purchasing medical devices. Details are available from their website – www.pasa.nhs.uk

5.4 LOAN SURGICAL INSTRUMENTS AND EQUIPMENT

STANDARD There is a system in place for managing the decontamination of loan equipment.

RECOMMENDATIONS FOR LOCAL POLICY

RECOMMENDATION **5.4.1** All surgical instruments and equipment entering the organisation should be cleaned and sterilised before and after use in accordance with manufacturer's instructions MDA SN 2000(18) (MDA 2000a). When medical devices are loaned from the organisation the same principles apply.

RECOMMENDATION **5.4.2** Procedures should be identified to ensure that the decontamination of loan equipment is suitably controlled, validated and recorded.

RECOMMENDATION **5.4.3** There should be evidence of an audit process to verify compliance with policies and procedures related to borrowed or loaned equipment.

RECOMMENDATION **5.4.4** If new equipment is being introduced for a trial and staff are unfamiliar with it, then it is essential that adequate time for decontamination training is provided.

RECOMMENDATION **5.4.5** Items requiring disassembly should always be dismantled and processed in accordance with manufacturer's instructions.

5.5 DECONTAMINATION TRAINING

STANDARD There is a system in place for ensuring that all personnel involved in decontamination are competent to perform decontamination processes.

Personnel undertaking decontamination must be competent and supervised where necessary. Inadequately trained staff will fail to decontaminate devices effectively and will put patients at risk. They may also risk their own health and safety if they are unaware of safe practice standards.

RECOMMENDATIONS FOR LOCAL POLICY

RECOMMENDATION **5.5.1** There should be evidence of individual training records detailing decontamination training provided.

RECOMMENDATION **5.5.2** All personnel involved in decontamination should have a personal development plan, with learning objectives clearly stated and training needs identified and facilitated.

RECOMMENDATION **5.5.3** There should be evidence of an audit process to verify compliance with policies and procedures related to staff training in decontamination processes.

5.6 CLEANING

STANDARD There is a system in place for the cleaning of medical devices before disinfection to reduce the risk of transmission of infectious agents.

RECOMMENDATIONS FOR LOCAL POLICY

RECOMMENDATION **5.6.1** Surgical instruments and associated accessories should be decontaminated immediately after use, or as soon as is reasonably practicable.

RECOMMENDATION **5.6.2** The Department of Health recommends that the washing of instruments be undertaken within automated equipment and that the process is validated (DH 2001). Hand washing of instruments should only occur if the instrument is unsuitable for immersion in water.

RECOMMENDATION **5.6.3** The recommendations of the Department of Health (DH 2001) are that *'local reprocessing should be the exception rather than the norm.'* Automated mechanical cleaning provides an efficient, reproducible process whose effectiveness can be validated. This is the preferred method of cleaning as it is more consistent and easily controlled than manual methods. *'All reprocessing of surgical instruments should be undertaken outside the perioperative setting where possible and preferably within the sterile services department.'*

5.7 MANUAL CLEANING

STANDARD There is a system in place for the manual cleaning of medical devices and equipment.

Manual cleaning must only be considered where manufacturer's instructions specify that the device is not compatible with automated processes. Where manual cleaning is undertaken, it should be carried out in accordance with the protocol for the local decontamination of surgical instruments issued by NHS Estates (2001) which can be accessed at www.decontamination.nhsestates.gov.uk

RECOMMENDATIONS FOR LOCAL POLICY

RECOMMENDATION **5.7.1** Equipment consisting of more than one component must be dismantled so that each part can be adequately cleaned.

RECOMMENDATION **5.7.2** The area to be used for manual cleaning should be dedicated for the purpose with a sink (not a hand wash basin) to contain water, and detergent for cleaning instruments. There should also be a second dedicated sink (not a hand wash basin) for rinsing items.

RECOMMENDATION **5.7.3** To minimise the risk to personnel undertaking manual cleaning, splashing and the creation of aerosols must be avoided at all times.

RECOMMENDATION **5.7.4** Detergent dilution and water temperature should be used in accordance with manufacturer's instructions or local policy.

RECOMMENDATION **5.7.5** It is important to be aware that protein coagulates at 35°C so the water temperature should be monitored before immersion.

RECOMMENDATION **5.7.6** The operator should wear personal protective equipment (PPE), dismantle or open the instrument to be cleaned and fully immerse it in the solution in order to displace trapped air and to ensure penetration of the lumen if hollow instruments are being cleaned.

RECOMMENDATION **5.7.7** Consideration should be given to the use of protein enzyme-dissolving solutions when cleaning medical devices with lumens or complex parts, or those which may be identified as 'difficult to clean'.

RECOMMENDATION **5.7.8** The operator should brush, wipe, agitate, jet-wash or hand spray the item to dislodge all visible bio-burden, taking care to ensure that the item remains under the water at all times to prevent aerosols.

RECOMMENDATION **5.7.9** When removing the item from the sink any excess detergent should be drained thoroughly prior to placing in the second sink to rinse in clean water.

RECOMMENDATION **5.7.10** The item should be rinsed thoroughly with clean water or water jet gun under the surface of the water.

RECOMMENDATION **5.7.11** The item should be removed and drained before drying.

RECOMMENDATION **5.7.12** All necessary documentation should be completed, including the item being processed and the method and solutions used.

5.8 DISINFECTION

STANDARD There is a system in place for the disinfection of medical devices and equipment before sterilisation to reduce the risk of transmission of infectious agents.

Disinfection is defined as a process used to reduce the number of viable microorganisms in a load, but which may not necessarily inactivate some viruses and bacterial spores.

RECOMMENDATIONS FOR LOCAL POLICY

Disinfection may be achieved by a number of methods but the two most common are moist heat or thermal disinfection and liquid chemicals.

Moist heat

Moist heat is the method of first choice as it is easily controlled, leaves no toxic residues and is relatively safe to those involved in the process.

RECOMMENDATION **5.8.1** Disinfection can be achieved by washing or rinsing at 73–90°C. Most automated washer-disinfectors manufactured for the reprocessing of surgical instruments incorporate a disinfection stage.

Liquid chemicals

Medical devices that cannot withstand the relatively high temperatures required for disinfection by moist heat should be disinfected by using chemical solutions. But these should only be employed where no practical alternative exists.

RECOMMENDATION **5.8.2** Receptacles used for chemical disinfectant solutions must be cleaned and steam-sterilised before being used.

RECOMMENDATION **5.8.3** The user must take care to ensure that the device is clean, that the correct chemical concentration is used and that the device is properly submerged to ensure contact with all parts.

RECOMMENDATION **5.8.4** When preparing chemical disinfectants, the user must wear the appropriate PPE which may include, but is not limited to, goggles or visors, gloves and waterproof apron.

RECOMMENDATION **5.8.5** The room used for chemical disinfection must be well-ventilated or contain an appropriate Class 1 exhaust-protective cabinet.

RECOMMENDATION **5.8.6** Control of Substances Hazardous to Health (COSHH) assessments must be undertaken regarding the toxicity of substances used. This includes personal monitoring or monitoring by occupational health services when required as part of COSHH requirements (HMSO 2002).

RECOMMENDATION **5.8.7** When immersing medical devices with lumens, it may be necessary to agitate the devices in the disinfectant to dislodge any air trapped inside, as disinfectants will only be effective if the solution reaches all surfaces.

RECOMMENDATION **5.8.8** Appropriate exposure times as recommended by the manufacturer must be adhered to.

RECOMMENDATION **5.8.9** If the device is for immediate use after disinfection, staff must use an aseptic technique when removing it from the chemical solution.

RECOMMENDATION **5.8.10** The device must be rinsed in sterile water and carefully dried using a sterile, non-linting cloth.

RECOMMENDATION **5.8.11** If the device is to be stored before being used, it can be removed from the liquid, rinsed in sterile water, dried with a non-linting cloth and stored in a secure area.

RECOMMENDATION **5.8.12** Where a sterile product is required, it should be processed immediately before being used and not stored before use.

5.9 AUTOMATED WASHER-DISINFECTORS

STANDARD There is a system in place which, as far as is reasonably practicable, utilises automated washer equipment to disinfect medical devices, according to the manufacturer's instructions.

RECOMMENDATIONS FOR LOCAL POLICY

Decontamination processes are less effective on instruments that are difficult to clean or are in poor condition.

RECOMMENDATION **5.9.1** For certain complex medical devices, it may be necessary to disassemble the device prior to decontamination. The manufacturer's instructions must be followed and all the surfaces exposed to the cleaning processes.

RECOMMENDATION **5.9.2** It is also important that medical devices are correctly loaded into the automated washer-disinfectors so that the maximum cleaning efficacy can be achieved.

RECOMMENDATION **5.9.3** Consideration should be given to purchasing medical devices that can be mechanically cleaned or replaced by a single use alternative.

RECOMMENDATION **5.9.4** Mechanical washer-disinfectors used for decontamination should be purchased against the Model Engineering Specification NHS Estates C30, and specified in accordance with BS 2745 and monitored in accordance with HTM 2030, SHTM 2030 (Scotland) Washer-Disinfectors (NHS Estates 1997a, 2002).

RECOMMENDATION **5.9.5** Washer-disinfector logbooks and records should be kept by the designated user. Such records should include a description of any loads processed, cycle parameters, product release with details of routine testing and maintenance of equipment used.

RECOMMENDATION **5.9.6** Endotoxin levels in rinse water should be included in the process control and monitoring procedures.

5.10 INSPECTION AND FUNCTION TESTING

STANDARD There is a system in place for the competent inspection, maintenance and testing of all medical devices that have been decontaminated within the department.

RECOMMENDATIONS FOR LOCAL POLICY

RECOMMENDATION **5.10.1** The inspection, maintenance or testing of devices must be undertaken by competent staff trained in accordance with manufacturer's instructions and local policy.

RECOMMENDATION **5.10.2** Where practical, the inspection and function-testing of surgical instruments should not be carried out by the staff responsible for cleaning the devices. These staff members have a responsibility for ensuring the item is thoroughly cleaned and fit for reuse.

RECOMMENDATION **5.10.3** Devices that are dirty, wet or stained should be rejected and returned to the wash area for manual cleaning, followed by an automated wash process, before continuing through to packaging and sterilisation.

RECOMMENDATION **5.10.4** Instruments must be handled with care since any scratches and roughened surfaces will harbour dirt and bacteria.

RECOMMENDATION **5.10.5** Instruments that have an outer insulation coating require close inspection to ensure that the insulation is intact.

RECOMMENDATION **5.10.6** As part of the decontamination process all instruments should be subject to function testing following cleaning to ensure that they will perform the tasks for which they are designed. Staff undertaking such testing must adhere to the following basic tests:

- There is free movement of all parts and joints do not stick.
- The edges of clamping instruments meet with no overlap and teeth mesh together.
- Scissor edges meet to the tip and move freely across each other with no overlap or rough edges.

- All screws on jointed instruments are tight and have not become loose during the cleaning process.

RECOMMENDATION **5.10.7** Where hinged instruments are found to be stiff, a water soluble lubricant should be used occasionally to avoid interference with the sterilisation process.

RECOMMENDATION **5.10.8** In preparing instruments for wrapping and sterilisation it is essential that all surfaces are presented to the sterilisation process and that, where devices can be taken apart, they are sterilised in this state wherever practicable.

RECOMMENDATION **5.10.9** Instruments with ratchets should be closed on the first ratchet only to ensure steam can penetrate to all surfaces.

RECOMMENDATION **5.10.10** A procedure should be established for the reporting of any defects and the need for items to be repaired or replaced. In the case of instrument sets, the contents sheet may be used to indicate faulty instruments, but the actual item must be identified in case there are a number of similar devices on the set.

RECOMMENDATION **5.10.11** Where an instrument must be removed from a set and sent away for repair, the set must be removed from circulation until the repaired instrument is returned.

RECOMMENDATION **5.10.12** Instruments for repair should be returned to the manufacturer or a reputable repair company. They should be decontaminated in accordance with MHRA DB 2003(05) (MHRA 2003) and accompanied by a decontamination certificate.

RECOMMENDATION **5.10.13** Records should be kept of all inspection and testing work undertaken.

5.11 SINGLE USE MEDICAL DEVICES

STANDARD There is a system in place which ensures that all medical devices intended for single use are not reprocessed for reuse.

RECOMMENDATIONS FOR LOCAL POLICY

RECOMMENDATION **5.11.1** Medical devices intended for single use only must not be reprocessed for reuse. The reuse of single use medical devices can affect their safety, performance and effectiveness, exposing patients and staff to unnecessary risk. Devices designated for single use must not be reused under any circumstances, as stated in HSC 1999/179 and MDA DB 2000(004) (NHS Executive 1999a, MDA 2000b).

RECOMMENDATION **5.11.2** A policy should be in place to ensure that medical devices designated for single use are never reused.

RECOMMENDATION **5.11.3** There should be an adequate audit process to verify compliance with policies and procedures relating to single use medical devices.

RECOMMENDATION **5.11.4** There should be evidence of a training programme to ensure that staff involved in the decontamination process are aware of the European standard symbol (from EN 980) that denotes single use only.

5.12 PACKAGING

STANDARD There is a system in place for the appropriate packaging of medical devices.

RECOMMENDATIONS FOR LOCAL POLICY

RECOMMENDATION **5.12.1** Where packaging is recommended, for example in porous-load sterilisers, only materials which comply with appropriate packaging standards for sterilisation, as detailed in the BS EN 868 series, should be used. The packaging materials must be compatible with the sterilisation process and may be either rigid or flexible.

RECOMMENDATION **5.12.2** Packaging of products after sterilisation is not recommended.

RECOMMENDATION **5.12.3** Peel-apart pouches or plain paper bags are often used for single instruments or small loads. These are bags with a see-through front and paper backing. It is essential that peel-apart pouches are sealed to ensure that the product remains sterile after autoclaving.

RECOMMENDATION **5.12.4** Non-self-sealing pouches/bags require a heat sealing machine or autoclave tape to seal them.

RECOMMENDATION **5.12.5** Paper bags can have either a plain top which requires autoclave tape for sealing, or a heat seal top which requires a crimping and sealing machine.

RECOMMENDATION **5.12.6** Sterile surgical instruments should be labelled in accordance with the requirements of BS EN 980 – graphical symbols for use in the labelling of medical devices.

RECOMMENDATION **5.12.7** The following information should be available for the device being processed:

- Name of the device/pack
- Name of the manufacturer (ie: the reprocessor)
- Date of the manufacture/sterilisation
- Date of the expiry, where appropriate
- Method of sterilisation used (this may be obvious by the sterilisation indicator panel on the packaging material)
- Cycle number/machine number of the steriliser used.

5.13 STERILISATION

STANDARD There is a system in place which ensures validation of the sterilisation process for all medical devices.

RECOMMENDATIONS FOR LOCAL POLICY

RECOMMENDATION **5.13.1** Unless the item to be sterilised is known to be damaged by the application of heat or moisture, moist heat sterilisation using saturated steam under pressure should always be used in preference to other methods, since it is more reliable and can be monitored effectively.

Exposure to saturated steam at 134°C, under pressure for a period of at least three minutes, in the total absence of air, will eliminate infective microorganisms.

RECOMMENDATION **5.13.2** There are a number of sterilisers used within healthcare and particular attention should be paid to the following areas:

- Validation and management of sterilisation equipment using HTM 2010/SHTM 2010 (NHS Estates 1997b)
- Monitoring of steam supply of porous load sterilisers using HTM 2031/SHTM 2031 (NHS Estates 1997c)
- Ensuring ethylene oxide steriliser installations meet HBN 13/SHBN 13 (NHS Estates 1992).

Benchtop sterilisers

RECOMMENDATION **5.13.3** The withdrawal of benchtop sterilisers from the clinical area is recommended to prevent '*the inappropriate use of processes*' MDA DB 2002(06) (MDA 2002a). This should discourage the reprocessing of instruments in the clinical area and encourage the sterilisation of decontamination processes HSC 2000/032 (NHS Estates 2002).

RECOMMENDATION **5.13.4** MDA DB 2002(06) and HTM 2010/SHTM 2010 provide detailed guidance on the use and testing of benchtop sterilisers. MDA DB 2000(05) (MDA 2000c) provides guidance as to when porous loads can be processed in vacuum sterilisers if required. However, organisations should ensure that the following are not sterilised using a downward displacement benchtop steriliser:

- Single use devices
- Devices in any form of wrapping including pouches
- Equipment with lumens or cavities
- Porous loads.

RECOMMENDATION **5.13.5** To ensure the safety of the device the following must be adhered to:

- Each steriliser will have a reservoir chamber from which the water is delivered for steam generation. This must be filled daily using sterile water for irrigation. At the end of the day or following final use, the chamber should be drained when the water is cooled. It should be cleaned, dried, covered with a lid and left empty for future use in accordance with HTM 2031/SHTM 2031 (NHS Estates 1997c).
- A schedule for periodic testing should be planned and performed in accordance with documented procedures HTMs and SHTMs 2010, 2031 and MDA Device bulletin 2002(06) (MDA 2002a). The schedule should provide details of daily, quarterly and yearly testing.
- Each steriliser should have a logbook in which details of maintenance, validation, faults, modifications, routine tests, and each load processed are recorded.
- Some benchtop sterilisers require a warm-up cycle before instruments can be processed according to manufacturer's instructions.
- Daily tests should be performed by the operator or user. These should consist of a stem penetration test (vacuum benchtop sterilisers only) and an automatic control test. Sterilisers must not be used until the daily tests have been carried out and the results are satisfactory.
- Before carrying out the daily tests the user should clean the rubber door seal with a clean, damp, non-linting cloth, check the chamber and shelves for cleanliness and debris, fill the reservoir with sterile water for irrigation, turn the power source on, and record these tasks with the date and signature of the operator in the logbook.
- If the steriliser fails to meet any of the test requirements, it should be withdrawn from service and advice sought from the manufacturer or estates department.
- Benchtop sterilisers must be fitted with independent process monitoring or recording equipment. Their efficacy should be reviewed regularly against relevant guidance.

Planned maintenance

RECOMMENDATION **5.13.6** Equipment such as washer-disinfectors and sterilisers to be used in validated processes require planned preventative maintenance and periodic calibration and testing to ensure they remain in the same condition as when validated. Validation processes require the monitoring of the critical variables of each cycle. This should be independent of monitoring used to control the decontamination equipment.

RECOMMENDATION **5.13.7** HTM 2010/SHTM 2010, HTM 2030/SHTM 2030, MDA DB 9804, MDA2002(05) and MDA DB 2002(06) define the minimum standards required to ensure safe operation of the decontamination process (NHS Estates 1997b, c, MDA 1998b, 2002a, b).

5.14 PROCESSING OF RIGID AND FLEXIBLE ENDOSCOPES

STANDARD There is a system in place for the decontamination of rigid and flexible endoscopes.

RECOMMENDATIONS FOR LOCAL POLICY

RECOMMENDATION **5.14.1** Decontamination, storage and preparation of endoscopes should be undertaken in accordance with MDA DB 2002(05), MDA DB 2004(028) (MDA 2002b, MHRA 2004) and current legislative requirements.

RECOMMENDATION **5.14.2** In accordance with the manufacturer's instructions, rigid endoscopes should be cleaned, disinfected, inspected, packaged and sterilised using validated automated processes, in a sterile services department wherever possible. Rigid endoscopes that cannot tolerate steam sterilisation should be cleaned and subjected to a high level disinfection process using a compatible liquid chemical disinfectant, or sterilised using a suitable low temperature process.

RECOMMENDATION **5.14.3** In accordance with manufacturer's instructions, the channels of flexible endoscopes should be flushed immediately after use.

RECOMMENDATION **5.14.4** Cleaning brushes should be single use only.

RECOMMENDATION **5.14.5** In accordance with the manufacturer's instructions, flexible endoscopes which cannot be autoclaved should be cleaned and subjected to high-level disinfection using a suitable and compatible liquid chemical disinfectant in an automated endoscope reprocessor.

RECOMMENDATION **5.14.6** When practical, single use accessories should be used and should never be reused.

RECOMMENDATION **5.14.7** Reusable endoscopic accessories should be reprocessed in a sterile service department using a validated automated process in accordance with the device manufacturer's instructions.

RECOMMENDATION **5.14.8** Flexible endoscope usage should be traceable in accordance with the requirements of HSC 1999/178 (NHS Executive 1999b).

RECOMMENDATION **5.14.9** Rigid endoscopes must be stored sealed in the container or packaging in which they were sterilised.

RECOMMENDATION **5.14.10** Flexible endoscopes should be dried and stored suspended vertically in ventilated storage cabinets, to allow circulation of air. They should not be in contact with other endoscopes or flat surfaces and should be reprocessed prior to use.

RECOMMENDATION **5.14.11** It is important that the outer covering of the endoscope is tested before use by leak testing, in accordance with MDA DB 2002(05) (MDA 2002b).

Detailed guidance for the cleaning and high level disinfection of endoscopy equipment can be found in MDA DB 2003(05) (MHRA 2003).

5.15 TRANSPORT

STANDARD There is a system in place for the safe transport of reusable medical devices.

All reusable medical devices should be handled, collected and delivered in a manner that reduces the risk of contamination to the product, patients, staff and any area of the healthcare facility. The recommendations below are from the Institute of Sterile Service Management (ISSM 2002).

RECOMMENDATIONS FOR LOCAL POLICY

RECOMMENDATION **5.15.1** Personnel should be trained to handle, collect and transport medical devices/equipment. Where appropriate, personnel should wear protective clothing in accordance with local safety policies and procedures, which should include methods for dealing with spillages. Personnel collecting and transporting medical devices should be vaccinated against hepatitis B.

RECOMMENDATION **5.15.2** Persons aware of the potential infection hazards should separate reusable devices from clinical waste at the point of use.

RECOMMENDATION **5.15.3** Reusable textiles should be placed in appropriate linen bags and returned to the laundry service.

RECOMMENDATION **5.15.4** Contaminated medical devices should be confined and contained in closed leak-proof plastic bags or containers to avoid spills, the generation of aerosols, or contact with staff and environmental surfaces. They should be transported as soon as possible after use to the decontamination area. The contents of the containers should be labelled to facilitate processing.

RECOMMENDATION **5.15.5** The container used for transportation should be easy to clean, should close securely, and be clearly labelled to identify the user and the contents.

RECOMMENDATION **5.15.6** Used equipment should be safely contained and transported to the decontamination area, and records kept of vehicles and containers used.

RECOMMENDATION **5.15.7** Contaminated medical devices and equipment must be kept separate from clean medical devices and equipment during transportation. This is achieved by using separate containers to provide physical barriers between clean and dirty items.

RECOMMENDATION **5.15.8** Contaminated medical devices/equipment must only enter the department through the decontamination area.

RECOMMENDATION **5.15.9** Where contaminated medical devices are to be transported outside the healthcare premises and onto a public highway, those responsible for such transportation must refer to the requirements of the Carriage of Dangerous Goods by Road Act (HMSO 1996) and the Health and Safety at Work Act (HMSO 1974).

5.16 STORAGE

STANDARD There is a system in place for the safe storage of medical devices.

It is important to ensure that storage conditions maintain packs in the condition in which they are required for use.

RECOMMENDATIONS FOR LOCAL POLICY

RECOMMENDATION **5.16.1** A storage area should be dedicated for the purpose and not used for other activities.

RECOMMENDATION **5.16.2** The storage area should be appropriately designed to prevent damage to packs and to allow for the strict rotation of stock.

RECOMMENDATION **5.16.3** Shelving should be easily cleaned and allow free movement of air around the stored product.

RECOMMENDATION **5.16.4** Products must be stored above floor level, away from direct sunlight and water, and in a secure, dry and cool environment.

RECOMMENDATION **5.16.5** Products should not be packed tightly together on shelves, in drawers or containers, as this may damage the packaging – MDA SN 1999(32) (MDA 1999b).

RECOMMENDATION **5.16.6** Products found to be wet or damaged should be returned for reprocessing.

RECOMMENDATION **5.16.7** Before use, the sterile product should be checked to ensure that it is intact, and that the steriliser indicator confirms that the pack has been subjected to an appropriate sterilisation process. The product should also still be within the expiry date.

5.17 STERILE SERVICES DEPARTMENT FACILITIES

STANDARD There is a system in place that ensures, as far as is reasonably practicable, that all medical devices are decontaminated within a designated sterile services department.

Effective cleaning of medical devices prior to disinfection or sterilisation is of the utmost importance in reducing the risk of transmission of infectious agents.

RECOMMENDATIONS FOR LOCAL POLICY

RECOMMENDATION **5.17.1** Sterile services departments should conform to controls assurance and meet HBN13/SHBN13 (NHS Estates 1992) design and building standards, and requirements for the segregation of controlled environments.

RECOMMENDATION **5.17.2** To achieve the required standard there must be segregation of soiled returns and clean supply, as described in HBN13/SHBN13 Scotland.

RECOMMENDATION **5.17.3** There must be separate areas for the following:

- Reception, sorting and decontamination of reusable medical devices and equipment
- Inspection and function testing of decontaminated devices/equipment
- Preparation and assembly of packs
- Pre-sterilisation holding areas
- Sterilisation
- Processed goods storage
- Distribution of processed items
- Raw materials preparation and storage
- Administration and training
- Staff change and rest areas.

RECOMMENDATION **5.17.4** All personnel entering and leaving the clean room must do so through a dedicated entrance/exit and wear appropriate clothing whilst in the area.

RECOMMENDATION **5.17.5** All persons requiring entry into the clean production area should:

- enter through the dedicated gowning area
- wear head cover and dedicated footwear
- thoroughly wash and dry hands and don a clean, non-linting gown
- exit through the gowning area where clean room clothing will be removed and discarded into an appropriate facility. The use of clean room clothing outside of the clean area contributes to the risk of contamination and should be prohibited.

RECOMMENDATION **5.17.6** HBN 13 refers to the design of new SSD facilities. Standards should be compared with those in existing departments as part of the risk assessment process. Action plans to bring existing facilities up to this standard should form part of the organisation's risk management plan.

RECOMMENDATION **5.17.7** Any location in which decontamination processes take place should:

- be physically separate from all other work areas, including patient treatment areas
- be accessible from a service corridor
- be mechanically ventilated – HTM 2025/SHTM 2025 (Scotland), HTM 2040 (NHS Estates 1994a, b)
- have walls and other surfaces which are finished with flush junctions, smooth, water resistant and able to withstand frequent cleaning
- have floors sealed with a washable non-slip finish

- have adequate lighting available to permit good working practices
- have hand washing and personal protective equipment facilities located in or near to the decontamination area.

5.18 TRACKING AND TRACEABILITY

STANDARD There is a system in place for effective tracking and traceability of medical devices throughout the decontamination process.

All surgical instrument sets should be able to be tracked through the decontamination process so that they can be traced to individual patients in the event of an adverse incident, such as a sterilisation failure.

HSC 2000/032 states: *'It is important that systems are in place to allow sets of surgical instruments to be tracked through decontamination processes in order to ensure that the processes have been carried out effectively. Systems should also be implemented to enable the identification of patients on whom the instruments have been used. This is important so that the relevant patients can be identified in the event of exposure to potential risk'* (NHS Executive 2000).

The tracking system should be part of a computerised electronic system, as a manual tracking system has limited opportunities for data retrieval.

RECOMMENDATIONS FOR LOCAL POLICY

RECOMMENDATION **5.18.1** The organisation should have a policy in place for tracing sets of surgical instruments to the patients on whom they have been used.

RECOMMENDATION **5.18.2** The tracing system should allow for details of the decontamination process for each used instrument set or medical device to be traced to the patient.

RECOMMENDATION **5.18.3** It is important that patient confidentiality is maintained in whatever tracking system is used.

RECOMMENDATION **5.18.4** There should be evidence of an audit process to verify that the systems for tracking and traceability are implemented and that records are maintained including links to the patient's notes.

RECOMMENDATION **5.18.5** A chemical indicator should be clearly visible on the outside of packs to be sterilised. Chemical indicators show that items have been exposed to physical conditions during a sterilisation cycle.

Chemical indicators do not replace quality assurance measures such as time, pressure, temperature monitoring, biological monitoring, proper packaging, proper steriliser maintenance, and proper storage and handling.

RECOMMENDATION **5.18.6** The sterilising process should be monitored at regular intervals with reliable biological indicators. Commercially manufactured biological indicators prepared in accordance with minimum performance criteria should be stored and used according to the indicator manufacturer's written instructions. Measurements should be performed with a biological indicator that employs spores of established resistance in a known population.

RECOMMENDATION **5.18.7** Records should be maintained for all instrument sets cleaned, identifying:

- the cleaning and sterilisation method used
- the name of the person undertaking the decontamination
- details of the actual item being processed.

RECOMMENDATION **5.18.8** Records relating to documentation should be maintained by the organisation for a minimum of 11 years or in accordance with local data policies.

Decontamination guidance for Northern Ireland

General considerations for decontamination guidance in Northern Ireland:

- For staff working in Northern Ireland healthcare establishments, decontamination guidance is available from the Department of Health, Social Services and Public Safety (DHSSPS) – www.dhsspsni.gov.uk/ and the Northern Ireland Adverse Incident Centre – www.dhsspsni.gov.uk/niaic
- Guidance already issued by the DHSSPS, circular HSS(MD)4/01, states that centralised reprocessing of instruments in departments which meet current best practice and standards is the preferred model of care. Local reprocessing of medical devices should be the exception rather than the norm.
- When reprocessing rigid and flexible endoscopes, practitioners in Northern Ireland are recommended to adhere to Device Bulletin DB(NI)2002/05 which is available to download on the NIAIC website – www.dhsspsni.gov.uk/niaic

NORTHERN IRELAND REFERENCES

Northern Ireland Adverse Incident Centre 2002 Device Bulletin DB(NI)2002/05 *Decontamination of Endoscopes* www.dhsspsni.gov.uk/niaic

British Society of Gastroenterology 2003 *Endoscopy Guidelines* www.bsg.org.uk

Northern Ireland Department of Health and Social Services 2001 *Decontamination of Reusable Medical Devices*

HSS(MD)4/01 and addendum 3 of HSS(MD)4/01 *Protocol for Local Decontamination of Surgical Instruments* Belfast, DHSSPS

Microbiology Advisory Committee to the Department of Health 1999 *Sterilization, Disinfection and Cleaning of Medical Equipment: Guidelines on Decontamination* (MAC Manual) London, DH

REFERENCES

Department of Health 2001a *Decontamination Programme Technical Manual: a protocol for local decontamination of surgical instruments* London, DH

Health Care Standards Unit 2003 *Decontamination of Reusable Medical Devices: controls assurance standard* London, DH. www.hcsu.org.uk

HMSO 1974 *The Health and Safety at Work Act* Norwich, The Stationery Office. www.healthandsafety.co.uk

HMSO 1996 *The Carriage of Dangerous Goods by Road Regulations* Norwich, The Stationery Office. www.hmso.gov.uk

HMSO 2002 *The Control of Substances Hazardous to Health Regulations (COSHH)* Norwich, The Stationery Office. www.hmso.gov.uk

Institute of Sterile Services Management 2002 *Standards and Practice* Edinburgh, ISSM **(NB This document is currently under revision)**

Medical and Healthcare Products Regulatory Agency 2003 *Management of Medical Devices Prior to Repair, Service or Investigation* MHRA DB 2003(05) London, MHRA. http://devices.mhra.gov.uk

Medicines and Healthcare Products Regulatory Agency 2004 *Flexible and Rigid Endoscopes* MHRA DB 2004(028) London, MHRA. www.medical-devices.gov.uk

Medical Devices Agency 1998a *Medical Device and Equipment Management for Hospital and Community Based Organisations* MDA DB 1998(01) London, MDA. http://devices.mhra.gov.uk

Medical Devices Agency 1998b *The Validation and Periodic Testing of Benchtop Vacuum Steam Sterilisers* MDA DB 1998(04) London, MDA. http://devices.mhra.gov.uk

Medical Devices Agency 1999a *Sterilisation, Disinfection and Cleaning of Medical Equipment: Guidance on decontamination from the Microbiology Advisory Committee to Department of Health (MAC Manual)* London, MDA. http://devices.mhra.gov.uk

Medical Devices Agency 1999b *Storage of Medical Devices* MDA SN 1999(32) London, MDA. http://devices.mhra.gov.uk

Medical Devices Agency 2000a *Handling of Surgical Instruments on Loan from Another Organisation* MDA SN 2000(18) London, MDA. http://devices.mhra.gov.uk

Medical Devices Agency 2000b *Single Use Medical Devices: implications and consequences of reuse* MDA DB 2000(004) London, MDA. http://devices.mhra.gov.uk

Medical Devices Agency 2000c *Guidance on the Purchase, Operation and Maintenance of Vacuum Benchtop Steam Sterilisers* MDA DB 2000(05) London, MDA. http://devices.mhra.gov.uk

Medical Devices Agency 2002a *Benchtop Steam Sterilisers – guidance on purchase, operation and maintenance* MDA DB 2002(06) London, MDA. http://devices.mhra.gov.uk

Medical Devices Agency 2002b *Decontamination of Endoscopes* MDA DB 2002(05) London, MDA. http://devices.mhra.gov.uk

NHS Estates 1992 *Sterile Services Departments Health Building Note* HBN 13/SHBN 13(Scotland) Leeds, NHS Estates **(NB This document is currently under revision)** www.knowledge.nhsestates.gov.uk

NHS Estates 1994a *Ventilation in Healthcare: validation and verification* Health Technical Memorandum HTM 2025/SHTM 2025 (Scotland) Leeds, NHS Estates. www.knowledge.nhsestates.gov.uk

NHS Estates 1994b *The Control of Legionallae in Healthcare Premises* Health Technical Memorandum HTM 2040 Leeds, NHS Estates. www.knowledge.nhsestates.gov.uk

NHS Estates 1997a *Washer-Disinfectors* Health Technical Memorandum HTM 2030/SHTM 2030 Leeds, NHS Estates. www.knowledge.nhsestates.gov.uk

NHS Estates 1997b *Sterilisation* Health Technical Memorandum HTM 2010/SHTM 2010 (Scotland) Leeds, NHS Estates. www.knowledge.nhsestates.gov.uk

NHS Estates 1997c *Clean Steam for Sterilisation* Health Technical Memorandum HTM 2031/SHTM 2031 (Scotland) Leeds, NHS Estates. www.knowledge.nhsestates.gov.uk

NHS Estates 2002 *Washer/Disinfectors: a model engineering specification* C30 Leeds, NHS Estates. www.knowledge.nhsestates.gov.uk

NHS Executive 1999a *Controls Assurance in Infection Control: decontamination of medical devices* HSC 1999/179 Leeds, DH. www.dh.gov.uk

NHS Executive 1999b *Variant Creutzfeldt-Jakob Disease (vCJD): minimising the risk of transmission* HSC 1999/178 Leeds, DH. www.dh.gov.uk

NHS Executive 2000 *Decontamination of Medical Devices* HSC 2000/032 Leeds, DH. www.dh.gov.uk

FURTHER READING

British Standards Institution 2002 *Graphical Symbols for Use in the Labelling of Medical Devices* BS EN 980 London, BSI. bsonline.techindex.co.uk

Department of Health – Spongiform Encephalopathy Committee 1998 *Transmissible Spongiform Encephalopathy Agents: safe working and the prevention of infection* Advisory Committee on Dangerous Pathogens (ACDP) Spongiform Encephalopathy Advisory Committee (SEAC). www.nhsis.co.uk. Amended parts to the document June 2003 are available from: www.dh.gov.uk

Department of Health 1998 *Guidance for Clinical Health Workers: protection against infection with blood-borne viruses* HSC 1998/063 London, DH. www.dh.gov.uk

Department of Health 1999 *Variant Creutzfeldt-Jakob Disease (vCJD): minimising the risk of transmission* HSC 1999/178 London, DH. www.dh.gov.uk

Department of Health 2000 *Decontamination of Medical Devices* HSC 2000/032 London, DH. www.dh.gov.uk

Department of Health 2001 *The Epic Project Developing National Evidence-based Guidelines for Preventing Healthcare Associated Infections* London, DH. www.dh.gov.uk

Department of Health 2003 *Winning Ways: working together to reduce healthcare associated infection in healthcare.* Report by the CMO London, DH. www.dh.gov.uk

HMSO 1992 *Personal Protective Equipment Regulations* Norwich, The Stationery Office. www.hmso.gov.uk

HMSO 1999 *Management of Health and Safety at Work Regulations: approved code of practice and guidance* Norwich, The Stationery Office www.hmso.gov.uk

HMSO 1999 *Transport of Dangerous Goods (Safety Advisors' Regulations)* Norwich, The Stationery Office. www.hmso.gov.uk

HMSO 2000 *Statutory Instrument No 128. The Pressure Systems Safety Regulations (PSSR)* Norwich, The Stationery Office

Infection Control Nurses Association 2003 *Infection Control Guidance for General Practice* Bathgate, ICNA. www.icna.co.uk

McNeil B 2004 Management of a CJD Case Part 1: preoperative organisation of the case *British Journal of Perioperative Nursing* 14 (4) 164–170

McNeil B 2004 Management of a CJD case Part 2: the patient with CJD in the operating theatre *British Journal of Perioperative Nursing* 14 (5) 223–226

Medical Devices Agency 2001 *Compatibility of Medical Devices and Reprocessing Equipment with Decontamination Agents* MDA SN 2001(28) London, MDA. http://devices-mhra.gov.uk/mda/mdawebsitev2.nsf

Medical Devices Agency 2001 *Safe Use and Disposal of Sharps* MDA SN 2001(19) London, MDA. www.medical-devices.gov.uk

NHS Estates 2001 *A Review of the Decontamination of Surgical Instruments in the NHS in England* Leeds, NHS Estates

NHS Estates 2001 *Infection Control in the Built Environment* Leeds, NHS Estates. www.nhsestates.gov.uk/download/publications_guidance/infectn.pdf

NHS Estates 2003 *Decontamination Guidance* CD-ROM Leeds, NHS Estates

NHS Estates 2004 *A Protocol for the Local Decontamination of Surgical Instruments* Leeds, NHS Estates. www.decontamination.nhsestates.gov.uk/downloads

NHS Executive 1999 *For the Record – managing records in NHS Trusts and Health Authorities* HSC 1999/53 Leeds, DH. www.info.doh.gov.uk/doh/coin4.nsf

NHS Executive 1999 *Clinical Governance in the New NHS* HSC 1999/065 Leeds, DH. www.info.doh.gov.uk/doh/coin4.nsf

NHS Executive 1999 *Governance in the New NHS: controls assurance statements 1999/2000 and risk management and organisational controls* HSC 1999/123 Leeds, DH. www.info.doh.gov.uk/doh/coin4.nsf

NHS Executive 2002 *Governance in the New NHS: controls assurance statements 2000/2001 and establishment of the Controls Assurance Support Unit* HSC 2001/005 Leeds, DH. www.info.doh.gov.uk/doh/coin4.nsf

NHS Scotland Property & Environment Forum – www.show.scot.nhs.uk/pef

NHS Scotland 2001 *Sterile Services Provision Review Group First Report: the Glennie framework.* www.show.scot.nhs.uk

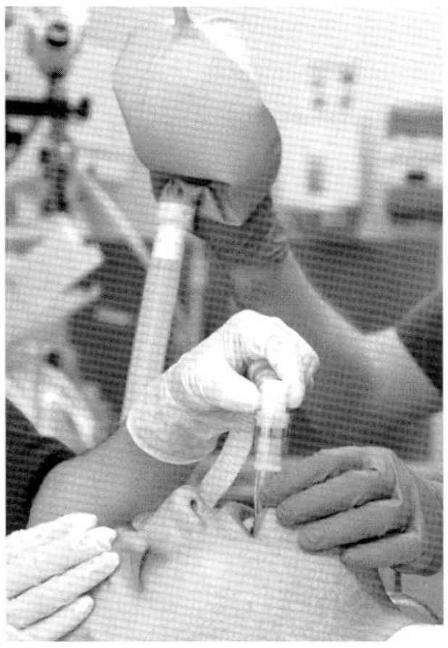

6 PRINCIPLES OF ANAESTHETICS

6.1 PREOPERATIVE ASSESSMENT

STANDARD There is a system in place that minimises any risks of surgery and anaesthesia in order to ensure the best possible outcome for the patient.

Today's healthcare is patient-centred, tailored to the convenience of patients and, through accurate information, allows the patient to have a greater say in and influence on their treatment. Preoperative assessment is fundamental to the patient's surgical pathway. It ensures that the patient is fully informed about the risks and benefits of surgery, and that the patient is in optimal health for the surgery to be undertaken. It also ensures that the limited resources such as beds and theatre time are effectively utilised.

INTRODUCTION

Preoperative assessment has been around for many years and is used very successfully in day surgery. In the inpatient elective surgery pathway developments are slower, but progress has been substantial over the past 2–3 years. Publications have included:

- *National good practice guidance on preoperative assessment for inpatient surgery* and *National good practice guidance on preoperative assessment for day surgery* by the Modernisation Agency (2003a, b)
- *Preoperative Assessment: setting a standard through learning* (which includes a CD-ROM) by Janke et al (2002)
- *Preoperative Tests: the use of routine preoperative tests for elective surgery* by the National Institute for Clinical Excellence (2003).

The degree of preoperative assessment depends on whether patients require emergency, urgent or elective surgery, but the Modernisation Agency recommend that all patients should undergo preoperative assessment. For the elective inpatient, preoperative assessment ideally should occur 6–8 weeks prior to the proposed date of surgery.

Government initiatives such as patient choice and reducing waiting lists have meant that patients now agree a date for surgery, that is they are able to choose within a reasonable range of dates. This is ideally placed to coincide with the patient's preoperative assessment.

Preoperative assessment can take place in a variety of settings either in primary or secondary care. For patients undergoing major surgery, assessment usually takes place within secondary care. Input from therapies, social services, anaesthetists, pain control nurses and other specialities is readily accessible and can be co-ordinated through the pre-assessment clinic.

The aim of preoperative assessment is to:

- assess a patient's fitness for surgery and anaesthesia
- identify if further investigations and treatment are required in order to reduce the perioperative morbidity and mortality
- identify the individual patient's specific cultural, ethnic or religious needs, and any communication or special needs requirements
- plan a patient's stay in hospital from admission to discharge
- liaise with external agencies if necessary to facilitate a safe return to the community
- provide an opportunity for the patient to discuss their treatment, gain further information and request additional explanations about the risks and benefits
- provide staff with the opportunity to explain specific preoperative instructions, provide information about expected postoperative outcomes, and other self-help matters which may improve the surgical outcome, such as smoking and diet
- minimise a patient's fears and anxieties.

Preoperative assessment can be performed as part of a primary care assessment prior to referral to the consultant, or by telephone, health questionnaire or face-to-face interview.

The benefits of preoperative assessment are that:

- the patient fully understands the proposed procedure and therefore is able to give informed consent
- there is a reduction in postponement of the patient's surgery due to the patient being unfit, as there has been adequate time for investigations to be carried out and actions taken prior to surgery
- the patient is prepared psychologically and emotionally for the surgery ahead and has knowledge of expected outcomes.

Research has shown that preoperative assessment clinics increase patient admission rates, reduce rates of those who do not attend, and reduce cancellations, all of which impact resources such as beds and theatre time.

RECOMMENDATIONS FOR LOCAL POLICY

RECOMMENDATION **6.1.1** Preoperative assessment can be nurse-led. Research studies have shown that a nurse-led service can be safe and efficient and that nurses are as effective as medical staff in pre-admission clerking.

RECOMMENDATION **6.1.2** Nurses who provide a nurse-led service must be trained and assessed to agreed protocols to undertake clerking and physical examination. Nurses can also request basic investigations (blood, x-rays, etc).

RECOMMENDATION **6.1.3** Evidence-based protocols must guide practice and individual staff must recognise and acknowledge their limitations. Training for pre-assessment staff must be comprehensive and competency-based.

RECOMMENDATION **6.1.4** The preoperative assessor must encompass all roles identified within the Modernisation Agency (2002, 2003a, b) guidance.

RECOMMENDATION **6.1.5** Preoperative assessment for all patients must be included within the hospital's surgical pathway and NHS waiting list management policies.

RECOMMENDATION **6.1.6** All patients requiring surgical intervention must undergo preoperative assessment, whether this is at outpatient clinic where they are health screened or at an established preoperative assessment clinic.

RECOMMENDATION **6.1.7** A patient's notes must be available for their preoperative assessment.

RECOMMENDATION **6.1.8** There should be communication strategies to refer patients to other professionals (eg: therapies, social services, dieticians) and follow-up such referrals.

RECOMMENDATION **6.1.9** Communication pathways should also be established with theatres, anaesthetics departments and relevant medical staff (eg: consultants, other medical areas).

RECOMMENDATION **6.1.10** Preoperative assessment staff must have the autonomy to cancel or postpone the patient, although it is the anaesthetist's responsibility to determine whether a patient is fit or not.

RECOMMENDATION **6.1.11** Investigations must be undertaken in accordance with the NICE (2003) guidance (posters and booklets are available).

RECOMMENDATION **6.1.12** Written information and patient records must be completed indicating the assessment process and any actions/referrals to be taken.

RECOMMENDATION **6.1.13** Auditing of the preoperative assessment service should be carried out, following the Modernisation Agency guidance.

6.2 PREOPERATIVE FASTING

STANDARD Clear guidance on preoperative fasting is provided before all types of anaesthesia and surgical interventions, in accordance with national and local guidelines and recommendations.

The preoperative fasting of surgical patients before the administration of a general anaesthetic is a widely established practice. It is considered essential to reduce the risk of vomiting and regurgitation and the possible aspiration of gastric contents (Seymour 2000).

There should also be agreement within the multidisciplinary team as to whether patients undergoing regional anaesthesia should also be fasted. Fasting facilitates the administration of a general anaesthetic in the event of failed regional anaesthesia.

Specific guidance relating to fasting periods for trauma patients, paediatrics and obstetric patients as well as other patients with specific needs should also be incorporated into the policy.

RECOMMENDATIONS FOR LOCAL POLICY

RECOMMENDATION **6.2.1** The patient should be given a clear explanation as to the reason and importance of preoperative fasting prior to anaesthesia.

RECOMMENDATION **6.2.2** To aid the timing of preoperative fasting and patient comfort and safety, the order of the operating list should not be changed unless it is essential to do so.

RECOMMENDATION **6.2.3** Patients should be restricted from eating solid foods, infant formula, or any other milk or milk products for six hours before their operation.

RECOMMENDATION **6.2.4** Breast milk must be withheld from infants for four hours preoperatively.

RECOMMENDATION **6.2.5** All patients may drink clear non-particulate and non-carbohydrate fluids until two hours preoperatively.

RECOMMENDATION **6.2.6** The chewing of gum is controversial, but should be considered as if it were oral fluid and prohibited for two hours preoperatively. The greatest danger from chewing gum is as a foreign body, which may partially block the airway (AAGBI 2001).

RECOMMENDATION **6.2.7** Patients who are vulnerable to dehydration such as the elderly, children, breast-feeding mothers, pregnant women, critically ill patients, and patients who have undergone bowel preparation, should not be left for long periods without hydration. Intravenous fluid therapy may be required preoperatively if a prolonged fast is encountered.

RECOMMENDATION **6.2.8** It is essential to take additional precautions with patients who have suffered trauma, as gastric emptying may be delayed. This is also the case for patients who have an increased likelihood of vomiting and regurgitation on induction such as obese patients, pregnant women, patients with hiatus hernia or gastric reflux problems, and anxious patients. For these patients the use of cricoid pressure during induction is required even though the recommended period of preoperative fasting has occurred.

6.3 PREOPERATIVE HANDOVER

STANDARD The theatre reception area operates efficiently and promotes patient comfort and safety at all times.

Patients should be received into the perioperative area by a practitioner into a safe, clean and adequately prepared environment that promotes an air of confidence and privacy. This area should be exclusively used for the reception of preoperative patients.

RECOMMENDATIONS FOR LOCAL POLICY

RECOMMENDATION **6.3.1** All patient care must be delivered in a safe and professional manner in the immediate preoperative phase.

RECOMMENDATION **6.3.2** The reception area should be free from any unnecessary noise.

RECOMMENDATION **6.3.3** The receiving theatre practitioner must have validated training and experience to undertake this role.

RECOMMENDATION **6.3.4** The receiving theatre practitioner must introduce themselves to the patients.

RECOMMENDATION **6.3.5** The escorting practitioner must hand over the relevant information to the receiving practitioner.

RECOMMENDATION **6.3.6** The receiving theatre practitioner must verify verbally with the patient (where the patient is able to speak for themselves) and/or carer or escort practitioner, the following details, as well as checking all relevant documentation in a confidential manner:

- Name and date of birth
- Time and type of premedication (if any)
- Time of fasting
- Patient allergies

- Prosthesis removed
- Presence of caps/crowns/bridges which cannot be removed
- Jewellery taped/removed including body piercing
- The site of surgery.

RECOMMENDATION **6.3.7** The receiving theatre practitioner must check to ensure that all relevant patient documentation is available. This should include the following:

- Medical notes
- Nursing notes
- X-rays
- Drug prescription chart
- Consent form
- Patient labels
- Relevant investigation results.

RECOMMENDATION **6.3.8** The receiving theatre practitioner must ensure that the consent form has been completed correctly, has been signed by the patient and that the patient is aware of the procedure to be carried out.

RECOMMENDATION **6.3.9** The receiving theatre practitioner should document that the patient has been checked into the department.

RECOMMENDATION **6.3.10** The receiving theatre practitioner must give a full explanation of the procedure to the patient prior to transfer to the anaesthetic/operating room.

RECOMMENDATION **6.3.11** Where a practitioner other than the reception practitioner is to escort the patient to the anaesthetic/operating room, the practitioner must be introduced to the patient and a full handover given.

RECOMMENDATION **6.3.12** The patient should be escorted into the anaesthetic/operating area only after the area has been adequately prepared to receive the patient.

RECOMMENDATION **6.3.13** A minimal patient waiting time in the preoperative area is recommended.

RECOMMENDATION **6.3.14** The patient should not be left unattended at any time.

Additional recommendations for patients with other needs

RECOMMENDATION **6.3.15** Provision must be made for patients wishing to retain personal effects (eg: spectacles, hearing aids, head coverings or prostheses) with minimum problems. The ward staff must document this and inform the receiving practitioner of these effects.

RECOMMENDATION **6.3.16** Provision must be made for patients who cannot speak English by ensuring that there is an interpreter/carer with the patient who can facilitate communication during transfer and until induction of anaesthesia. The reception practitioner must introduce themselves to the interpreter/carer in a professional manner and ensure that they have signed the relevant section of the consent form. An identified member of staff must be allocated to accompany the interpreter/carer throughout all perioperative stages. Provision must be made to return them to the ward and arrangements made for the postoperative phase.

RECOMMENDATION 6.3.17 Provision must be made for patients who have special requirements (eg: special needs patients, disabled patients, and patients who have hearing or visibility impairment) to ensure that there is a carer to facilitate communication and transfer of the patient until induction of anaesthesia or other appropriate stage of the patient's care. The reception practitioners must introduce themselves to the carer in a professional manner and ensure that the consent form has been signed correctly and, where necessary, that the parent/guardian/carer has signed the appropriate section. An identified member of staff must be allocated to accompany the carer throughout all perioperative stages. Provision must be made to return them to the ward and arrangements made for the postoperative phase.

RECOMMENDATION 6.3.18 Provision must be made for children, to ensure that there is a carer with the patient to facilitate communication and transfer until induction of anaesthesia or appropriate stage of the patient's care. The child must be permitted to bring a personal comfort item with them if they wish to. The child should be allowed to walk/be carried to theatre and to wear their own pyjamas that should be freshly laundered. The reception practitioners must introduce themselves to the child and carer in a professional manner and ensure that the consent form has been signed correctly and, where necessary, the parent/guardian has signed the appropriate section. The child should be escorted to an appropriate reception area. An identified member of staff must be allocated to accompany the parent/carer throughout all perioperative stages. Provision must be made to return them to the ward and arrangements made for the post-operative phase where local policy permits.

6.4 PATIENTS UNDERGOING ANAESTHETIC PROCEDURES

STANDARD Patients receive anaesthetic care in a safe environment and are monitored appropriately by competent personnel.

Safe patient care in the anaesthetic area should ideally start with preoperative care in the surgical ward or preoperative assessment clinics. These environments provide an opportunity to give information to the patient and increase the understanding of the planned anaesthesia care.

It is well documented that patients' anxiety levels are reduced when they are well informed and have met the staff involved in their care. The assessment, planning, evaluation and documentation of care is essential for the patient's well-being, however it is not always possible for anaesthetic practitioners to assess the patient preoperatively given the working demands of the operating department. If a preoperative assessment has not been carried out, good communication skills and an awareness of a patient's needs are vital.

Maintaining a safe environment and current clinical practice with regard to the checking of equipment within a framework of infection control guidelines, ensures a holistic approach to safe practice.

The patient undergoing an anaesthetic intervention requires individual support at all times. Many operative departments recognise the need for a nominated practitioner to provide this support for patients in the anaesthetic room.

RECOMMENDATIONS FOR LOCAL POLICY

Personnel issues

RECOMMENDATION **6.4.1** Staff who work in the anaesthetic room, who assist the anaesthetist and who undertake direct patient care, must hold a professionally validated qualification to a minimum requirement of a recognised and related higher education diploma.

RECOMMENDATION **6.4.2** Qualified anaesthetic practitioners must take every opportunity to keep up to date with current professional knowledge and be able to evaluate its use in patient care.

RECOMMENDATION **6.4.3** All qualified anaesthetic practitioners must accept responsibility for their own continuing personal and professional development. This can be outlined by a personal development plan.

Patient care

RECOMMENDATION **6.4.4** Qualified anaesthetic practitioners must be aware of the psychological, social and cultural factors which influence the patient's response to illness and disease. Staff must be able to develop supportive and understanding relationships with patients awaiting anaesthetic intervention by demonstrating understanding of particular needs.

RECOMMENDATION **6.4.5** There should be a dedicated trained anaesthetic assistant present for all procedures requiring the presence of an anaesthetist (AAGBI 1998).

RECOMMENDATION **6.4.6** Qualified anaesthetic practitioners must understand the importance of good interpersonal and communication skills with particular reference to:

- the use/non-use of face masks
- the effects of hearing or visual loss
- the importance of effective and instrumental touch
- facial expression and the importance of non-verbal cues
- the giving of information to patients.

RECOMMENDATION **6.4.7** Qualified anaesthetic practitioners must be able to demonstrate skills in assessment, planning, implementation and evaluation of patient care and document this information accordingly.

RECOMMENDATION **6.4.8** Parents should be allowed to escort children to the anaesthetic room and remain with them until induction.

RECOMMENDATION **6.4.9** A local protocol should be in place for thromboprophylaxis. This should include timing of anticoagulant administration to ensure safe neuraxial (spinal and epidural) analgesia.

Preparation and maintenance of anaesthetic equipment

RECOMMENDATION **6.4.10** All routine safety checks on anaesthetic equipment must be carried out in accordance with published guidelines and the manufacturer's instructions. This includes:

- the anaesthetic delivery system
- filters
- connectors and airway devices
- suction
- scavenging
- monitoring
- accessories.

A laminated sheet entitled *Checklist for Anaesthetic Equipment* has recently been published (AAGBI 2004a). A copy of this checklist should be attached to each anaesthetic machine and used as a basis for all checks.

RECOMMENDATION **6.4.11** All anaesthetic equipment must be checked, prepared and demonstrated as functional before induction of anaesthesia is commenced. A major cause of anaesthetic critical incidents has been when anaesthetic machines and breathing systems have not been adequately checked by an anaesthetist before the commencement of the operating list.

RECOMMENDATION **6.4.12** A record should be kept with the anaesthetic machine as evidence that this check has been undertaken. The record should include the name of the practitioner and anaesthetist, and the date and time when the check was undertaken. These should also be recorded in the patient's anaesthetic record.

RECOMMENDATION **6.4.13** All anaesthetic equipment must undergo regular maintenance checks by medical engineers and/or service contractors in accordance with national guidelines and local policies. Maintenance should be registered accordingly. The first user check after servicing is especially important and must be recorded.

RECOMMENDATION **6.4.14** A capnograph must be available in all settings where anaesthesia is provided.

RECOMMENDATION **6.4.15** Additional specific checks should be undertaken for each new patient during an operating session, or for any alteration or addition to the breathing system, monitoring or accessories. The anaesthetist is responsible for these checks and must be satisfied that they have been carried out correctly (AAGBI 2004a).

RECOMMENDATION **6.4.16** Any device marked as single use must be used for one patient only and not reused.

RECOMMENDATION **6.4.17** Qualified anaesthetic staff must be aware of the relative costs of anaesthetic equipment and the need for reasonable economy in its preparation, use and maintenance.

Infection control/clinical practice

RECOMMENDATION **6.4.18** In order to ensure control of infection, it is essential to maintain a high standard of asepsis in the anaesthetic room at all times. All staff must be encouraged to apply and maintain this.

RECOMMENDATION **6.4.19** Clear guidelines must be in place for the effective disinfection and decontamination of anaesthetic devices and equipment. These must be strictly observed at all times. It will be necessary to refer to the manufacturer's guidelines, the local infection control team and the

AAGBI *Infection Control in Anaesthesia* guidelines (AAGBI 2004b) when developing local policy.

RECOMMENDATION **6.4.20** A new bacterial/viral filter should be used for every patient.

RECOMMENDATION **6.4.21** Manufacturing instructions must be adhered to for the reuse of breathing circuits.

RECOMMENDATION **6.4.22** Disposable receptacles for anaesthetic equipment are recommended for each individual patient. Where non-disposable receptacles are used, it is essential that these can be autoclaved and processed accordingly for each patient.

RECOMMENDATION **6.4.23** Specific and detailed protocols should be available which relate to clinical anaesthetic procedures, for example, insertion of central venous catheters, spinal and epidural procedures.

RECOMMENDATION **6.4.24** Syringes and needles are sterile single use items. After entry or connection to a patient's vascular system or attached infusion, a syringe or needle should be considered contaminated and used only for that patient (AAGBI 2002).

A syringe should not be used for multiple patients, even if the needle is changed.

RECOMMENDATION **6.4.25** If syringes are prepared in advance of the procedure, they must be stored in a clean container and not left on work preparation surfaces.

RECOMMENDATION **6.4.26** It is recommended that anaesthetic masks are either for single patient use or are sterilised within a sterile supplies unit between patient use.

RECOMMENDATION **6.4.27** It is recommended that oral, naso-pharyngeal, tracheal tubes, bougies and catheter mounts are for single patient use. Laryngeal masks should be decontaminated according to manufacturer's instructions.

RECOMMENDATION **6.4.28** Reusable laryngoscope blades should be decontaminated by a sterile supplies unit after patient use. Provision should be made to ensure enough blades are in the system for this to be effective. Laryngoscope handles should, if suitable, be periodically decontaminated by the sterile supplies unit.

RECOMMENDATION **6.4.29** Flexible laryngoscopes should be decontaminated by an automated system in accordance with manufacturer's instructions and Medical Device Agency guidelines (MDA 1996).

RECOMMENDATION **6.4.30** The anaesthetist and assistant should wear gloves during intubation and should place used devices in a designated receptacle to prevent decontamination of pillows, drapes and linen.

Patient safeguards

RECOMMENDATION **6.4.31** Qualified anaesthetic staff must be aware of potential hazards to patients and take all necessary precautions to prevent any untoward incidents related to environmental safety. National guidelines and local policies must be adhered to at all times, in particular with regard to:

- explosions and fire
- electrical and radiation hazards
- pollution
- chemical substances.

RECOMMENDATION **6.4.32** Careful identification and checking procedures must be carried out with regard to each individual patient, the accompanying documentation and sites of operation. The checks must be conducted:

- when sending for the patient from the ward
- when the patient arrives in the operating department
- in the anaesthetic room prior to induction
- in the theatre prior to surgery.

RECOMMENDATION **6.4.33** Qualified anaesthetic staff must be competent in identifying and minimising potential hazards to unconscious and sedated patients.

RECOMMENDATION **6.4.34** Patients must be supported at all times by a nominated staff member when awaiting induction of anaesthesia.

RECOMMENDATION **6.4.35** Standard procedures for the identification, storage, security and administration of drugs, intravenous fluids and blood products must be rigorously applied at all times by qualified anaesthetic staff, in line with local policies and procedures.

RECOMMENDATION **6.4.36** All anaesthetic drugs must be drawn up by a qualified medical practitioner, or by appropriately trained anaesthetic personnel where local policy permits. Drugs should be placed in a disposable receptacle and remain with the patient throughout surgery prior to disposal at the end of the procedure.

RECOMMENDATION **6.4.37** During a critical incident, qualified anaesthetic staff may be required to administer drugs for intravenous use. This should be done only under the direct supervision of a qualified medical practitioner.

6.5 MALIGNANT HYPERTHERMIA

STANDARD There is a system in place that facilitates early diagnosis and prompt treatment of malignant hyperthermia.

Malignant hyperthermia (MH), also known as malignant hyperpyrexia, is a rare inherited autosomal dominant myopathy. It is characterised by a hypermetabolic state which is triggered by exposure to some anaesthetic agents.

Classic MH most often manifests in the operating theatre, but it can also occur within the first few hours of recovery from anaesthesia. The syndrome is thought to be due to a reduction in the reuptake of calcium by the sarcoplasmic reticulum. The reuptake of calcium is necessary for the termination of muscle contraction. Consequently, muscle contraction is sustained, resulting in signs of hypermetabolism, including acidosis, tachycardia, hypercarbic glycosis, hypoxaemia and hyperthermia.

Unsafe drugs

- Depolarising muscle relaxants
- Volatile anaesthetic agents (eg: halothane isoflurane, enflurane, desflurane, sevoflurane)

Safe drugs

- Antibiotics
- Antihistamines
- Antipyretics
- Barbiturates
- Benzodiazepines (diazepam, midazolam)
- Ketamine
- Local anaesthetics
- Nitrous oxide
- Non-depolarising muscle relaxants (eg: vecuronium, rocuronium)
- Opioids
- Propofol
- Propranolol
- Vasoactive drugs

Some patients may develop MH despite multiple prior uneventful exposures to triggering drugs. Typically MH is triggered by suxamethonium chloride or volatile anaesthetic agents. Some other drugs have been found to be safe in patients susceptible to MH.

An unexplained tachycardia is usually the first sign of MH. Other signs are an increase in end-tidal carbon dioxide and a decrease in arterial oxygen saturation, tachycardia and dysrhythmias, generalised muscular rigidity including masseter spasm, tachypnoea, hyperthermia and cyanosis.

When clinical signs suggest MH, there are several lab tests which can be performed although the halothane-caffeine contracture test remains the gold standard. This is performed on muscle obtained by biopsy of the vastus lateralis, which is bathed in a solution containing 1–3% halothane and caffeine. These agents decrease the muscle contraction and facilitate diagnosis.

RECOMMENDATIONS FOR LOCAL POLICY

Early diagnosis and prompt treatment of MH should reduce mortality. The only currently available specific treatment is sodium dantrolene which should be available wherever general anaesthesia is administered. A protocol for the management of MH should be in place. Dantrolene interferes with calcium release from the sarcoplasmic reticulum, thus reducing muscle contraction and the hypermetabolic manifestations.

RECOMMENDATION **6.5.1** If MH is suspected the practitioner should follow simple guidelines:

- Call for help
- Stop causative agents
- Hyperventilate patient with 100% oxygen
- Finish or abort the procedure
- Administer dantrolene as prescribed
- Change to a clean circuit not exposed to volatile agents
- Cool patient
- Monitor and treat acidosis
- Promote urine output
- Treat hyperkalaemia
- Monitor creatinine kinase, urine myoglobin and coagulation for 24–48 hours.

RECOMMENDATION **6.5.2** If a patient is deemed susceptible to MH, a regional anaesthetic should be considered with close monitoring of vital signs. If general anaesthetic is essential, clear guidelines should be followed:

- Clean anaesthetic machine, remove vaporisers, replace soda lime and circuit
- Flush machine with oxygen for 20 minutes at 10 litres/minute
- Patient should be first on the operating list and all necessary departments informed
- Crash trolley, dantrolene and MH management guidelines should be immediately accessible
- Anaesthetist should check creatinine kinase and do a complete blood count preoperatively
- Postoperatively, anaesthetist should check laboratory values and monitor the patient in recovery.

6.6 PATIENT HANDOVER FROM THEATRE TO RECOVERY

STANDARD There is a system in place that facilitates a comprehensive handover to ensure continuity of care and patient safety in the transfer from the intraoperative phase to the immediate postoperative phase.

It is an important aspect of patient care that all relevant information is shared with all practitioners caring for a patient in the perioperative setting. The transfer of a patient from theatre to the recovery area is a crucial element of patient care which requires effective communication in both verbal and written forms.

RECOMMENDATIONS FOR LOCAL POLICY

RECOMMENDATION **6.6.1** The anaesthetist should accompany the patient to recovery, and formally hand over the care of the patient to an appropriately validated trained member of staff. A member of the intra-operative team should escort the patient with the anaesthetist.

RECOMMENDATION **6.6.2** The following information should be available at the handover:

- Patient's name, date of birth and theatre they are being transferred from
- The ward the patient is scheduled to return to, if known
- The procedure that was carried out
- The type of anaesthetic used, or combination of anaesthesia such as general anaesthetic and regional block
- The duration of anaesthetic if appropriate
- Details of any local anaesthetic infiltration to the wound, including the local anaesthetic agent, strength and dose administered
- Patient prescription documents
- Intravenous fluid therapy records if appropriate
- Type of dressings used
- Type of wound closure used
- Type of drain, how it is secured and the position
- Presence of stoma, urinary catheter or other similar item
- Any allergies
- Whether there is a need for an interpreter, carer or parent to assist in patient care and the arrangements that are in place for contacting such individuals
- Whether the patient has any personal items such as dentures or spectacles that must accompany the patient on transfer
- Any item of clothing that may have been removed, and details of whether the patient was told in advance that this would happen
- Relevant medical history (eg: the presence of a pacemaker)
- Any communication difficulties (eg: hearing loss or partially sighted)
- Skin condition and integrity
- Position of diathermy plate, if relevant
- Any other information that is specific to the patient
- Any specific security needs, such as a patient who is serving a custodial sentence.

6.7 POST-ANAESTHETIC RECOVERY

STANDARD A designated post-anaesthetic recovery area is provided for immediate post-anaesthetic care. Post-anaesthetic care practitioners are competent to administer one to one patient care until the patient is fully conscious and able to maintain a clear airway.

The purpose of the post-anaesthesia recovery area is to provide care until the patient can be safely discharged, either to a general ward or home in an awake and stable condition, or transferred to a high dependency or intensive care unit (NHS Quality Improvement Scotland 2003).

RECOMMENDATIONS FOR LOCAL POLICY

Design

A dedicated recovery unit is required which should be located centrally in the operating theatre department. A number of acute hospitals have now increased the functional capacity of their recovery units to a 24-hour, seven-day per week basis. The implication for the built environment is that staff facilities need improving and facilities for visitors will be required (NHS Estates 2004).

RECOMMENDATION **6.7.1** The recovery area should be located near to the theatre reception area to allow free access of patients to and from wards.

RECOMMENDATION **6.7.2** An increasing number of patients are transferred on their beds from the operating theatre to the recovery unit. Each space must therefore be large enough to accommodate an adult bed, with additional space for the monitoring equipment and immediate access for staff in case of emergency. Bed space area should comply with the requirement for dealing with an emergency situation.

RECOMMENDATION **6.7.3** Postoperative theatre recovery facilities that provide short-term intensive care have been approved by the DH (HSC 2000/17) (NHS Executive 2000). To meet these requirements and those set out in *Comprehensive Critical Care* (DH 1999) and for maximum flexibility, some of the bed spaces in the recovery unit should be equipped to accommodate a critically ill patient (minimum Level 2) on a planned care, short-term basis (for further guidance see NHS Estates 2003).

- A minimum space of 3.6 x 3.8m is required in each bed area (NHS Estates 2004).
- A clinical wash hand basin with non-touch taps is required at the front of each bed space.
- Natural daylight enhances the feeling of well-being and is an essential requirement. The main overhead lighting should be dimmable.
- A central station should be positioned in order to allow observation of the whole recovery area.

RECOMMENDATION **6.7.4** Maintaining privacy and dignity is a basic human right. This must be maintained during the post-anaesthetic period. Every bed space should be separated by lead-lined solid partitions with a lead-lined curtain at the foot end of each bed space. This ensures that the radiation protection requirements have been met (NHS Estates 2004).

RECOMMENDATION **6.7.5** Facilities for storage of clean and sterile equipment should be available and subject to local operational policies (eg: storage of drugs).

RECOMMENDATION **6.7.6** Access to utility rooms and sluice facilities are required.

RECOMMENDATION **6.7.7** It is essential that the recovery room is fully equipped to deal with emergency resuscitation, whilst ensuring immediate access to emergency equipment from all parts of the recovery area.

A system of summoning aid in the event of an emergency must be available, including the provision of alarm and telephone or intercom links to operating theatres and rest areas. The system should be tested daily before the start of an operating list.

An individual anaesthetist should be identified who is available at all times during a session, should an emergency occur.

RECOMMENDATION **6.7.8** The decor should be pleasant and comply with regulations to allow cleaning to take place in accordance with a planned preventative maintenance programme.

RECOMMENDATION **6.7.9** If the recovery area is used for patients who have undergone local and general anaesthetic procedures, consideration should be given to the placement of patients who are awake and fully orientated to their surroundings.

Environment

RECOMMENDATION **6.7.10** The recovery area should be kept clean at all times.

RECOMMENDATION **6.7.11** The room temperature should be maintained at 19–22°C and should be free from draughts.

RECOMMENDATION **6.7.12** There should be a positive pressure ventilation facility in the recovery area to ensure that exhaled anaesthetic gases are removed effectively.

RECOMMENDATION **6.7.13** In order to promote a peaceful recovery for postoperative patients, noise levels should be controlled.

RECOMMENDATION **6.7.14** Lighting should allow for effective patient observation but should be conducive to patient comfort. Local lighting should be available to assist in clinical examination.

RECOMMENDATION **6.7.15** Post-anaesthetic care staff should be aware of safe practice related to storage of equipment, the handling of blood and bodily fluids and disposal of contaminated waste.

Equipment

RECOMMENDATION **6.7.16** Each bed space must be equipped with:

- pipeline outlets for suction, oxygen and air
- electric sockets

- individual lamps
- sphygmomanometer and stethoscope
- monitoring equipment for the observation of electrocardiograph, pulse oximetry, non-invasive blood pressure, arterial pressure, central venous pressure and temperature.

RECOMMENDATION **6.7.17** The recovery bed or trolley, must have an operational two way tilt facility. Trolleys should have padded sides.

RECOMMENDATION **6.7.18** Emergency equipment must be accessible and should include that required for endotracheal intubation, defibrillation, tracheotomy, malignant hyperthermia and anaphylaxis.

RECOMMENDATION **6.7.19** Equipment should be available to deal with inadvertent hypothermia.

RECOMMENDATION **6.7.20** It is essential that all equipment in recovery is in working order and that it is checked daily and checks are documented. Any faulty equipment should be replaced and sent for repair immediately.

Nursing

RECOMMENDATION **6.7.21** The anaesthetist must formally hand over care of a patient to a recovery room nurse or operating department practitioner (AAGBI 2002).

RECOMMENDATION **6.7.22** The post-anaesthetic area is a specialist clinical area – therefore practitioners working in this area must possess the competencies to provide safe and effective care without direct supervision. The practitioner must understand the implications of the surgery the patient has undergone and the complications which can be expected. When critically ill patients are managed in the recovery room because of bed shortages, the primary responsibility for the patient lies with the critical care team. The standard of nursing and medical care should be equal to that within the critical care unit (AAGBI 2002).

RECOMMENDATION **6.7.23** Post-anaesthetic practitioners must be competent in airway management and in managing a patient with a laryngeal mask in situ. The removal of endotracheal tubes is the responsibility of the anaesthetist. The anaesthetist can delegate removal of an endotracheal tube to a non-medical post-anaesthetic care practitioner who has received validated training for the task and is deemed competent to perform the duty. This must be supported by a local policy.

RECOMMENDATION **6.7.24** Post-anaesthetic practitioners must be competent in assessing the patient's condition including vital signs, basic life support, intravenous administration, assessment of homeostasis, patient controlled analgesia, epidurals, sedation and administration of pain relief.

RECOMMENDATION **6.7.25** At least one member of the recovery team should be a certified Advanced Life Support provider and, if caring for children, must hold an appropriate paediatric life support qualification.

RECOMMENDATION **6.7.26** Patients must be kept under clinical observation at all times and vital signs recorded. The introduction of automatic recording systems is encouraged. The frequency of observations will depend on the stage of recovery, nature of surgery and clinical condition of the patient. The Association of Anaesthetists of Great Britain and Ireland (2002) recommend the recording of:

- level of consciousness
- haemoglobin oxygen saturation and oxygen administration
- blood pressure
- respiratory frequency
- heart rate and rhythm
- pain intensity
- intravenous infusion
- drugs administered
- temperature, urinary output, central venous pressure, end tidal CO_2, surgical drainage – depending on circumstances.

RECOMMENDATION **6.7.27** No fewer than two staff should be present in the recovery area when there is a patient who does not fulfil the criteria for discharge to the ward (AAGBI 2002).

RECOMMENDATION **6.7.28** Validated training should be available for practitioners to administer intravenous analgesia, including opiates prescribed by anaesthetists. This must be managed within protocols agreed by the anaesthetic directorate within the hospital organisation. The Association of Anaesthetists of Great Britain and Ireland (2002) recommend that non-medical practitioners should not administer opioids unless there is the immediate availability of an anaesthetist.

RECOMMENDATION **6.7.29** Patients should not be returned to the ward until emesis and postoperative pain is managed and the patient is in a comfortable state to return to the ward. Agreed discharge criteria of patients from the recovery room to the ward should be in place in all units (AAGBI 2002).

Post-anaesthetic care of the paediatric patient

RECOMMENDATION **6.7.30** The Kennedy Report recommendations for children's services have implications for all theatre and surgical facilities (DH 2002). A segregated area for children is essential in the recovery unit, with provision for parents to stay with them. The designated recovery area for post-anaesthetic care of children should be child-orientated and decorated with artwork conducive to a child-friendly healthcare environment. Artwork can be paintings, murals, prints, photographs, sculptures, decorative tiles, ceramics, textile hangings and furniture (NHS Estates 2004). The advantages of such a therapeutic environment are that it:

- mitigates the stress of the environment
- creates a sense of safety and security
- promotes a bond between patient and caregiver
- perpetuates an image of excellence for the hospital.

RECOMMENDATION **6.7.31** Paediatric equipment should include a full range of face masks, breathing systems, airways, nasal sponges and tracheal tubes. Monitoring equipment should include a full range of non-invasive blood pressure cuffs and small pulse oximeters.

RECOMMENDATION **6.7.32** If children are to be recovered in the area, then a paediatric nurse should be a member of the team, or the area should have access to the advice of a qualified paediatric nurse (RSCN) in accordance with local policy. Children have specific care needs as they are more likely to be disorientated postoperatively and at risk of vomiting and laryngeal spasm.

RECOMMENDATION **6.7.33** Paediatric patient postoperative pain should be managed effectively using pain assessment tools. Intramuscular injections should be avoided so as not to distress children.

6.8 POSTOPERATIVE NAUSEA AND VOMITING

STANDARD Postoperative nausea and vomiting are managed effectively in the recovery area.

Nausea, retching and vomiting may exist independent of each other and therefore should be assessed individually. There are a number of factors within surgery and anaesthesia that can produce postoperative nausea and vomiting (PONV) such as preoperative starving, opioids, dehydration, noxious chemicals, gut distension and interference in the labyrinthine apparatus.

The patient who experiences nausea and vomiting should be cared for in an empathetic and professional manner within the theatre environment. The patient should be discharged from the unit in a safe and stable condition.

RECOMMENDATIONS FOR LOCAL POLICY

RECOMMENDATION **6.8.1** Patients should be managed by a preoperative fasting policy. There should not be an excessive starvation time.

RECOMMENDATION **6.8.2** Patients at risk of PONV should be identified in the preoperative period.

RECOMMENDATION **6.8.3** Patients suffering nausea and vomiting should be afforded privacy and dignity.

RECOMMENDATION **6.8.4** Tissues and face wash should be provided for patients who suffer PONV.

RECOMMENDATION **6.8.5** Drug therapy can be administered for persistent or symptomatic PONV.

RECOMMENDATION **6.8.6** A fan can be provided to agitate air for a cooling breeze around patient.

RECOMMENDATION **6.8.7** Mouthwash can be provided for hygiene and comfort.

RECOMMENDATION **6.8.8** Any vomiting must be recorded on the fluid chart.

RECOMMENDATION **6.8.9** If a nasogastric tube is in situ, any aspirate from this must be recorded. Aspiration via suction can be performed where necessary.

RECOMMENDATION **6.8.10** Reassurance must be given to the patient if required.

RECOMMENDATION **6.8.11** Distraction therapies and breathing techniques can be used to control emesis.

6.9 PAIN MANAGEMENT

STANDARD Pain is managed effectively for patients in the perioperative setting.

Pain can be defined as: *'an unpleasant sensory and emotional experience associated with actual or potential tissue damage or, described in terms of such damage'* (International Association for the Study of Pain 1979) and *'whatever the experiencing persons say it is and existing whenever they say it does'* (McCaffery & Pasero 1999).

Pain is a subjective experience, thus all patients should receive multi-disciplinary care in an empathetic and professional manner within the perioperative environment. Postoperative pain management should be multi-disciplinary, based on the best available evidence, and should reduce or eliminate pain and discomfort with the minimum of side effects. Patients should be transferred from the recovery unit in a safe and stable condition.

RECOMMENDATIONS FOR LOCAL POLICY

Pain management in recovery

RECOMMENDATION **6.9.1** There should be a simple pain assessment tool incorporating a numerical (eg: 0–10) or descriptive (mild, moderate, severe) scale.

RECOMMENDATION **6.9.2** Pain assessment and documentation should be regarded as the fifth vital sign.

RECOMMENDATION **6.9.3** Pain intensity should be assessed and recorded on the patient's care plan on admission, and on discharge from recovery. Pain intensity on discharge should be at a level acceptable to the patient.

RECOMMENDATION **6.9.4** Patients should participate in the assessment process wherever possible.

RECOMMENDATION **6.9.5** Non-verbal clues and physiological signs (blood pressure, heart rate) should also form part of the assessment.

RECOMMENDATION **6.9.6** There should be an interpreter present if the patient is a non English speaker. Pain assessment tools should be available in languages other than English. These are available online from The Pain Society – www.painsociety.org/pain_scales.html

RECOMMENDATION **6.9.7** The recovery practitioner must be aware of the cultural differences related to pain behaviours.

RECOMMENDATION **6.9.8** Facilities need to exist for a carer or relative to be present at a defined stage, if the recovery practitioner feels it to be beneficial.

RECOMMENDATION **6.9.9** The recovery practitioner must act as advocate for the patient if they feel the patient needs that support.

RECOMMENDATION **6.9.10** Staff should be proficient in undertaking therapeutic analgesic interventions by a number of routes including intravenous, rectal and subcutaneous.

RECOMMENDATION **6.9.11** Staff should be competent in initiating and monitoring advanced interventions after additional education, training and assessment where necessary.

RECOMMENDATION **6.9.12** Diversional therapy should be employed to assist in pain management where the practitioner thinks necessary (ie: change of position, tactile reassurance or other appropriate measures).

RECOMMENDATION **6.9.13** Patients experiencing pain must be afforded some privacy and dignity when receiving treatment.

RECOMMENDATION **6.9.14** There must be a referral process to the acute pain team for follow-up if appropriate.

RECOMMENDATION **6.9.15** At handover of care, pain assessment and the effectiveness of interventions must be a principal point in the process.

RECOMMENDATION **6.9.16** All documentation must be complete, with a signed handover to the receiving nurse indicating a complete transfer of care.

Patient controlled analgesia (PCA)

RECOMMENDATION **6.9.17** The checking and administration procedure should be undertaken by a registered and competent practitioner.

RECOMMENDATION **6.9.18** A record should be kept of the identity of the infusion device and patient details.

The infusion devices must be checked before each use.

The infusion devices must be cleaned after each use.

Where applicable, the infusion site should be checked for patency and assessed using a visual phlebitis score (VIP). Any reaction must be reported and acted upon.

RECOMMENDATION **6.9.19** All records should be contemporaneous and complete (PCA chart, vital signs chart, prescription sheet, fluid balance and care documentation).

Epidural administration: management of equipment and assessment of patients

RECOMMENDATION **6.9.20** A protocol should exist that describes the overall management of patients, troubleshooting guidelines, instructions for changing epidural infusion solutions and the management of patients receiving anticoagulants and thromboprophylaxis.

RECOMMENDATION **6.9.21** A record should be kept of the identity of the infusion device and patient details.

The infusion devices must be checked before each use.

The infusion devices must be cleaned after each use.

RECOMMENDATION **6.9.22** Preparation of the pump and the prescribed analgesic regime should be undertaken by a registered and competent practitioner.

RECOMMENDATION **6.9.23** All observations should be performed regularly and recorded on a specific observation chart.

RECOMMENDATION **6.9.24** The infusion rate and volume administered must be checked regularly and recorded, as well as being checked against the prescription.

RECOMMENDATION **6.9.25** Troubleshooting guidelines should be available.

RECOMMENDATION **6.9.26** Specified emergency drugs must be readily available.

RECOMMENDATION **6.9.27** Any change in the patient's condition must be recorded contemporaneously and reported where necessary.

6.10 PATIENT DISCHARGE FROM RECOVERY

STANDARD There is a system in place that facilitates a comprehensive handover of information from a recovery practitioner to a member of the ward staff, at the time of a patient's discharge from the recovery area.

It is essential that there is a comprehensive record of all care given to a patient during the perioperative phase of their treatment, and that this is reported to the practitioner who will be returning them to, and subsequently caring for them in, a ward environment. As with the transfer of a patient from theatre to recovery, the handover from recovery to the ward is a crucial element of patient care that requires effective verbal and written communication skills.

RECOMMENDATIONS FOR LOCAL POLICY

Criteria for discharge

RECOMMENDATION **6.10.1** The patient should be conscious and able to maintain their own airway.

RECOMMENDATION **6.10.2** Physiological observations should be within acceptable parameters.

RECOMMENDATION **6.10.3** Patient should be free from pain and emesis as far as is possible.

RECOMMENDATION **6.10.4** Appropriate drugs have been prescribed/administered as appropriate.

Handover information

RECOMMENDATION **6.10.5** The following information should be included in the handover from recovery practitioner to ward staff:

- Patient's name and date of birth
- The procedure carried out
- The type of anaesthetic or combination of anaesthesia such as general anaesthetic and regional block
- The duration of the anaesthetic, if appropriate
- Any local anaesthetic infiltration to the wound including the local anaesthetic agent, strength and dose administered
- Patient prescription documentation
- Care records regarding drugs given during the perioperative phase
- Records of intravenous therapy if applicable, including fluid balance chart
- Type of dressing
- Type of wound closure
- Type of drain, how it is secured and the position
- Amount of exudates in the drain and, if this is excessive, what action has been taken such as informing the surgeon
- Presence of stoma, urinary catheter or other similar item, and a report of any drainage as appropriate
- Any allergies
- Whether the patient needs to have an interpreter, carer or parent to assist in patient care and the arrangements that are in place for contacting such individuals if they are not accompanying the patient back to the ward
- Whether the patient has any personal items, such as dentures or spectacles that must accompany the patient on transfer, or if these items have been returned to him/her
- Relevant medical history such as the presence of a pacemaker
- Any communication difficulties such as hearing loss or partially sighted
- Skin condition and integrity (tissue viability assessment)
- Any changes at the site of the diathermy plate if appropriate
- Any other information that is specific to the patient
- Any specific security needs such as a patient who is serving a custodial sentence.

Transfer to the ward

RECOMMENDATION **6.10.6** During the transfer from recovery to the ward, the patient should be accompanied by a validated trained member of staff and a porter.

RECOMMENDATION **6.10.7** Suitable equipment such as oxygen and suction should also be available.

6.11 RESUSCITATION GUIDELINES

STANDARD There is a system in place that outlines resuscitation practices and equipment in accordance with the Resuscitation Council UK guidance.

The Resuscitation Council (UK) has made recommendations for the standards in resuscitation and resuscitation training in hospital settings. These standards relate to:

- Basic Life Support (BLS) for children and adults
- Advanced Life Support (ALS) for adults
- Paediatric Advanced Life Support (PALS)
- Newborn Life Support.

The provision of an effective resuscitation service has wide ranging implications with respect to training, standards of care, risk management and clinical governance. In many hospitals, specific resuscitation officers and teams have responsibility for providing and maintaining the service. They liaise closely with each department to ensure that all training needs, equipment checks and regular updates are met, and to ensure staff comply with the required standards to fulfil their duty of care. In many hospitals it is mandatory to attend resuscitation training on an annual basis.

Cardiopulmonary resuscitation in a theatre environment is likely to be a controlled situation as there will be trained staff immediately at the scene complete with all the necessary equipment. However, in situations where there are fewer trained staff, such as at the end of the day in a day surgery unit, there is a need to call a cardiac arrest team. All team members should hold a current Resuscitation Council (UK) Advanced Life Support certificate.

RECOMMENDATIONS FOR LOCAL POLICY

Staff responsibilities

RECOMMENDATION **6.11.1** All staff must receive adequate instruction on induction programmes.

RECOMMENDATION **6.11.2** All staff must receive orientation as to the type and location of resuscitation equipment in the department. This may involve daily orientation if new and/or agency staff are in the operating department.

RECOMMENDATION **6.11.3** All staff should be familiar with the equipment kept in their department, in particular the method of interchange for adult and paediatric paddles.

RECOMMENDATION **6.11.4** Staff should undertake regular checks to ensure that equipment is ready for use at all times. Staff need to be aware of their accountability when signing to say that they have completed these checks. Their signature indicates that all is well and that they are familiar with the equipment.

Equipment provision

Recommended suggested minimum equipment for management of adult cardiopulmonary arrest is listed below.

RECOMMENDATION **6.11.5** AIRWAY EQUIPMENT

- Pocket masks with oxygen port
- Self-inflating resuscitation bag with oxygen reservoir and tubing
- Clear face masks, sizes 4, 5 and 6
- Oro-pharyngeal airways, sizes 2, 3 and 4
- Yankauer suckers x 2
- Endotracheal suction catheters x 10
- Laryngeal mask airway (size 4) or Combitube (small)
- McGill forceps
- Endotracheal tubes – oral, cuffed, sizes 6, 7 and 8
- Gum elastic bougie
- Lubricating jelly
- Laryngoscopes x 2 – normal and long blades
- Spare laryngoscope bulbs and batteries
- 1″ ribbon gauze/tape
- Scissors
- Syringe, 20mls
- Clear oxygen mask with reservoir bag (eg: Hudson mask)
- Oxygen cylinders x 2 (if no wall oxygen)
- Cylinder key

RECOMMENDATION **6.11.6** **CIRCULATION EQUIPMENT**

- Intravenous cannulae, 18 gauge x 3, 14 gauge x 3
- Hypodermic needles, 21 gauge x 10
- Syringes 2mls x 6, 5mls x 6, 10mls x 6, 20mls x 6
- Cannula fixing dressings and tapes x 4
- Seldinger wire central line kits x 2
- 12G Non-Seldinger central venous cannulae x 2
- Intravenous giving sets x 3
- 0.9% sodium chloride, 1000mls x 2

DRUGS

RECOMMENDATION **6.11.7** Immediately available prefilled syringes:

- Adrenaline/epinephrine, 1mg (1:10,000) x 4
- Atropine, 3mgs x 1
- Amiodarone, 300mgs x 1

RECOMMENDATION **6.11.8** Other readily available drugs:

- Adrenaline/epinephrine, 1mg (1:10,000) x 4
- Sodium bicarbonate 8.4%, 50mls x 1
- Calcium chloride 13.24%, 10mls x 2
- Lignocaine, 100mgs x 2
- Atropine, 1mg x 2
- Normal saline, 10mls ampoules x 10
- Naloxone, 400mcqs x 2
- Adrenaline/epinephrine, 1:1,000 x 2
- Amiodarone, 150mgs x 4
- Magnesium sulphate 50% solution, 2g (4ml) x 1
- Potassium chloride, 40mmols x 1
- Adenosine, 6mg x 10
- Midazolam, 10mg x 1
- Hydrocortisone, 200mg x 1
- Glucose, 10% 500mls x 1

RECOMMENDATION **6.11.9** **ADDITIONAL ITEMS**

- ECG electrodes
- Defibrillation gel pads
- Clock
- Gloves/goggles/aprons

NB A sliding sheet or similar device should be available for safer handling.

Paediatric equipment

RECOMMENDATION **6.11.10** Consultation with paediatricians as well as the resuscitation officer is essential in compiling paediatric equipment. In many cases, it is simply a case of having similar but smaller ranges of equipment available.

RECOMMENDATION **6.11.11** A pharmacist should always have been consulted to ensure that the correct drugs have been included in the resuscitation packs, and that these are clearly identified. This is extremely important if different strengths are required according to the child's weight.

RECOMMENDATION **6.11.12** Although wall or piped oxygen and suction should be used, portable suction and oxygen devices are also necessary so that equipment is available in the event of a systems failure.

RECOMMENDATION **6.11.13** Other equipment should be available, including:

- stethoscope
- ECG machine
- blood pressure measuring device
- pulse oximeter
- blood gas syringes
- oesophageal detector device.

RECOMMENDATION **6.11.14** Defibrillators should be standardised throughout the hospital and paediatric paddles should be available in areas where children are treated.

RECOMMENDATION **6.11.15** The paediatric resuscitation team should ideally be separate from the adult team and should have at least one member who holds the Paediatric Advanced Life Support certificate. The team leader must be knowledgeable about equipment, drug doses and the aetiology of paediatric cardiac arrests.

RECOMMENDATION **6.11.16** Hospitals which admit trauma patients should develop a separate trauma team. One member of the team should be an anaesthetist who has the experience to manage the patient's airway.

RECOMMENDATION **6.11.17** Standard national and international guidelines for resuscitation must be followed and resuscitation should be regularly audited.

REFERENCES

Association of Anaesthetists of Great Britain and Ireland 1998 *Risk Management* London, AAGBI

Association of Anaesthetists of Great Britain and Ireland 2001 *Preoperative Assessment: the role of the anaesthetist* London, AAGBI

Association of Anaesthetists of Great Britain and Ireland 2002 *Immediate Post-Anaesthetic Recovery* London, AAGBI

Association of Anaesthetists of Great Britain and Ireland 2004a *Checklists for Anaesthetic Machines* London, AAGBI

Association of Anaesthetists of Great Britain and Ireland 2004b *Infection Control in Anaesthesia* London, AAGBI

Department of Health 1999 *Comprehensive Critical Care* London, DH

Department of Health 2002 *Government's Response to Kennedy Report (Children's heart surgery at the Bristol Royal Infirmary)* London, DH

International Association for the Study of Pain. Subcommittee on Taxonomy 1979 Pain Terms: a list with definitions and notes on usage *Pain* 6 249–252

Janke E, Chalk V, Kinley H 2002 *Preoperative Assessment: setting a standard through learning* University of Southampton, New Generation Project

McCaffrey M, Pasero C 1999 *Pain: clinical manual* St Louis, Mosby

Medical Device Agency 1996 *Decontamination of Endoscopes* MDA DB 9607 London, MDA

Modernisation Agency 2002 *Operating Theatre and Preoperative Assessment Programme* London, DH

Modernisation Agency 2003a *Operating Theatre and Preoperative Assessment Programme: national good practice guidance on preoperative assessment for inpatient surgery* London, DH

Modernisation Agency 2003b *Operating Theatre and Preoperative Assessment Programme: national good practice guidance on preoperative assessment for day surgery* London, DH

National Institute for Clinical Excellence 2003 *Preoperative Tests: the use of routine preoperative tests for elective surgery* London, NICE

NHS Estates 2003 *Facilities for Critical Care* Norwich, The Stationery Office

NHS Estates 2004 *Facilities for Surgical Procedures* Health Building Note HBN 26 London, The Stationary Office

NHS Executive 2000 *Modernising Critical Care Services* HSC 2000/17 Leeds, DH

NHS Quality Improvement Scotland 2003 *Clinical Standards: anaesthesia care before, during and after anaesthesia* Edinburgh, DH

Seymour S 2000 Preoperative Fluid Restrictions: hospital policy and clinical practice *British Journal of Nursing* 9 (14) 925–930

FURTHER READING

American Operating Room Nurses Association 2004 *Standards, Recommended Practices and Guidelines* Denver, AORN Inc

Arnold A 2002 Postoperative Nausea and Vomiting in the Perioperative Setting *British Journal of Perioperative Nursing* 12 (1) 24–32

Association of Anaesthetists of Great Britain and Ireland 1991 *Role of the Anaesthetist in the Emergency Services* London, AAGBI

Association of Anaesthetists of Great Britain and Ireland 1994 *Recommendations for Standards of Monitoring during Anaesthesia and Recovery* London, AAGBI

Association of Anaesthetists of Great Britain and Ireland 1998 *Risk Management* London, AAGBI

Association of Anaesthetists of Great Britain and Ireland 1998 *The Anaesthesia Team* London, AAGBI

Association of Anaesthetists of Great Britain and Ireland 1998 *Guidelines for Obstetric Anaesthesia Services* London, AAGBI and Obstetric Anaesthetists Association

Association of Anaesthetists of Great Britain and Ireland 1998 *Anaesthesia and Anaesthetists: information for patients and relatives* London, AAGBI

Association of Anaesthetists of Great Britain and Ireland 2001 *Preoperative Assessment: the role of the anaesthetist* London, AAGBI

Association of Anaesthetists of Great Britain and Ireland 2001 *Anaesthesia and Perioperative Care of the Elderly* London, AAGBI

Association of Anaesthetists of Great Britain and Ireland 2002 *Immediate Post Anaesthetic Recovery* London, AAGBI

Association of Anaesthetists of Great Britain and Ireland 2003 *Theatre Efficiency: safety, quality of care and optimal use of resources* London, AAGBI

Australian Colleges of Operating Room Nurses 2004 *Standards for Perioperative Nursing* Sydney, ACORN

Bird C 2000 No Need to Starve *Nursing Times* 14 (41) 20

Bramhall J 2002 The Role of the Nurses in Preoperative Assessment *Nursing Times* 98 (40) 34–35

British Medical Association Resuscitation Council (UK) and Royal College of Nursing 2001 *Decisions Relating to Cardiopulmonary Resuscitation: a joint statement* London, BMA

Burden N 2000 *Ambulatory Surgical Nursing* 2nd ed, USA, WB Saunders Company

Casey D, Ormrod G 2003 The Effectiveness of Nurse-led Surgical Pre-Assessment Clinics *Professional Nurse* 18 (12) 685–687

Clarke P, Jones J 1998 *Brigden's Operating Department Practice* Edinburgh, Churchill Livingstone

Craft TM, Upton PM 2001 *Key Topics in Anaesthesia Clinical Aspects BIOS* Oxford, Scientific Publishers Ltd

Dean A, Fawcett T 2002 Nurses' Use of Evidence in Preoperative Fasting *Nursing Standard* 17 (12) 33–37

Department of Health 1997 *The Caldicott Committee: report on the review of patient identification information* London, DOH

Eltringham R, Durkin M, Andrews S, Casey W 1998 *Post-Anaesthetic Recovery – a practical approach* London, Springer-Verlag

Forunto N 2001 *Berry and Khon's Operating Room Technique* Missouri, Mosby

Hung P 1992 Preoperative Fasting *Nursing Times* 88 (48) 57–60

Jackson A 1998 Infection Control: a battle in vein infusion phlebitis *Nursing Times* 94 (4) 68–71

Jester R, Williams S 1999 Preoperative Fasting: putting research into practice *Nursing Standard* 13 (39) 33–35

Jevon P 2002 Resuscitation in Hospital: Resuscitation Council (UK) recommendations *Nursing Standard* 16 (33) 41–44

Jolley S 2001 Managing Postoperative Nausea and Vomiting *Nursing Standard* 15 (40) 47–54

Justins D 2004 Good Practice in Continuous Epidural Analgesia for Acute Pain Management *Royal College of Anaesthetists Bulletin* 26 1309–1312

Kumar B 1990 *Working in the Operating Theatre* Edinburgh, Churchill Livingstone

National Association of Theatre Nurses 2002 *Risk and Quality Management System* Harrogate, NATN

National Association of Theatre Nurses 2003 *Staffing for Patients in the Perioperative Setting* Harrogate, NATN

Neacsu A 2002 Prediction of Difficult Intubation *British Journal of Perioperative Nursing* 12 (7) 249–253

NHS Executive 1996 *Clinical Guidelines: using clinical guidelines to improve patient care within the NHS* London, DH

NHS Quality Improvement Scotland 2003 *Clinical Standards: anaesthesia care before, during and after anaesthesia* Edinburgh, NHS QIS

O'Callaghan N 2002 Preoperative Fasting *Nursing Standard* 16 (36) 33–37

Pain Society 2002 *Recommendations for Nursing Practice in Pain Management* London, The Pain Society. www.painsociety.org

Pain Society 2003 *Pain Management Services Good Practice* London, The Pain Society. www.painsociety.org

Radford M 2003 Recovery Nursing Services – an evolution *British Journal of Perioperative Nursing* 13 (4) 155–161

Rai M, Pandit J 2003 Forum-day of Surgery Cancellations After Nurse-led pre-assessment in an Elective Surgical Centre *Anaesthesia* 58 684–711

Resuscitation Council 2000 *CPR Guidance for Clinical Practice and Training in Hospitals* London, Resuscitation Council

Rowe J 2000 Preoperative Fasting: is it time for a change? *Nursing Times Plus* 96 (17) 14–15

Royal College of Anaesthetists 1999 *Guidelines for the Provision of Anaesthetic Services: anaesthetic practice in respect of resuscitation* London, RCA

Royal College of Anaesthetists 2002 *Implementing and Ensuring Safe Sedation* London, RCA

Royal College of Anaesthetists 2002 *Anaesthesia Explained* London, RCA

Royal College of Anaesthetists 2003 *Your Child's General Anaesthetic: information for parents and guardians of children* London, RCA

Royal College of Nursing 2003 *Standards for Infusion Therapy* London, RCN

Royston D, Cox F 2003 Anaesthesia: the patient's point of view *The Lancet* 262 1648–1658

Shields L, Werder H 2002 *Perioperative Nursing* Oxford, Blackwell Science

Smith AF, Vallance H, Slater RM 1997 Shorter Preoperative Fluid Fasts Reduce Postoperative Emesis *British Medical Journal* 314 1486

Starritt T 1999 Recovery. In *Back to Basics* Harrogate, NATN

Walsgrove H 2004 Piloting a Nurse-Led Gynaecology Preoperative Assessment Clinic *Nursing Times* 100 (3) 38–41

Watson K, Rinomhota S 2002 Preoperative Fasting: we need a new consensus *Nursing Times* 98 (15) 36–37

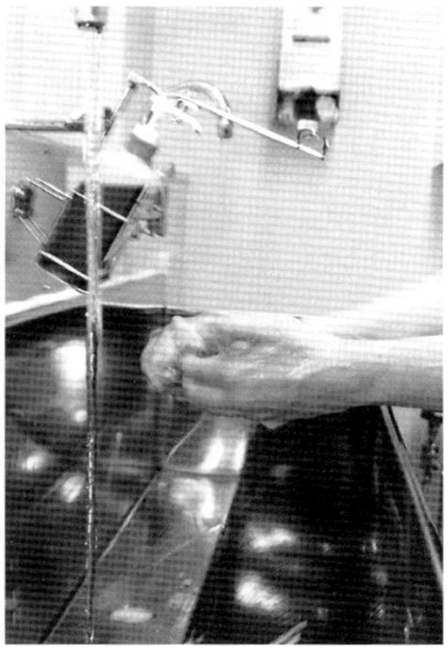

7 CLINICAL EFFECTIVENESS

7.1 CARE OF THE PATIENT IN THE DAY CARE SETTING

STANDARD There are established criteria for selecting patients for day surgery. Patients receive treatment in a day surgery setting that is suited to their needs and in an environment which is conducive to high quality care. Patients are fully informed about their operation and fit for surgery on the agreed date resulting in an improved experience of surgery.

Day surgery is defined by the Audit Commission (2001) as the admission of carefully selected patients to hospital for a planned surgical procedure, with the patients returning home on the same day.

The need for more day surgery is widely recognised by patients, clinicians, NHS managers and the Department of Health. An increase in day surgery to 75% of all elective surgery is a central feature of the *NHS Plan* (DH 2002). The *NHS Plan* places the patient at the centre of a framework for a modern NHS, with the aim of reducing waiting times, implementing efficient booking systems and introducing patient choice. Initiatives such as the treatment centre programme will increase the overall capacity for day surgery. By the end of 2005 there will be at least 60 treatment centres operating in England, which will boost capacity by at least 250,000 operations. Day surgery can assist the NHS in achieving its target of treating more patients faster.

Day surgical care should not be regarded as a sub-speciality of surgery. It is an appropriate surgery performed on a day basis from within a dedicated day surgery unit. It therefore requires the same facilities as those available for inpatient surgery.

Day surgical nursing care should be of the same high standard as inpatient care. It is essential to provide adequate information to patients who are required to arrive prepared for same-day surgery, and who are expected to care for themselves with minimal, non-expert assistance within hours of surgical intervention and the administration of general, local, regional anaesthesia or sedation (Mitchell 2002).

Day surgical treatment should not be regarded as a cheap option. Surgery, anaesthesia and nursing care must only be carried out by senior personnel to ensure a swift, safe and sympathetic progress through an area dedicated solely to the care of day surgical patients. Patients must not be treated as secondary to patients who require major or emergency treatment in an acute situation.

Day surgery provides benefits to patients as they receive treatment that is suited to their needs and which allows them to recover in their own homes. The risk of hospital acquired infection is also reduced.

Patients treated in day surgery units can be divided into four main categories (Audit Commission 2001):

True day surgery patients

Day case patients who require full operating theatre facilities and/or a general anaesthetic.

Minor day cases

Day case patients who generally do not require full operating theatre facilities or general anaesthetic. Procedures include endoscopy, pain relief procedures and minor surgery.

Inpatients

Although inpatients should not be mixed with day cases because their needs are different, some day surgery units do treat inpatients, so they need to be included in any assessment of activity. Inpatients are treated in day surgery units for two main reasons:

- A patient admitted as an emergency needs a bed but no beds are available elsewhere in the hospital.
- Operations on inpatients (elective or emergency) are sometimes carried out in the day unit operating theatre.

Patients having preoperative assessment

It is important to ensure that only the appropriate patients are offered day surgery. Patients with complex medical conditions require medical assessment and may not be suitable for day surgery. Preoperative assessment is the key to ensure that only suitable patients are offered treatment in the day unit setting.

RECOMMENDATIONS FOR LOCAL POLICY

Patient selection

RECOMMENDATION **7.1.1** Quality care and safe nursing practice can only be effective when patients are rigorously and suitably selected for day surgical care. Suitable selection is the responsibility of the referring general practitioner and the consultant surgeon at the outpatient consultation. Advice should also be sought from consultant anaesthetists practising in day surgery. The following are basic guidelines:

- All patients must be escorted home accompanied by a responsible and informed adult.
- All patients must be adequately supervised during their recovery at home for a minimum period of 24 hours. The 24-hour period of restriction will need to be extended to 48 hours when benzodiazepines, sedatives or opioids have been administered in conjunction with general, regional or local anaesthesia.
- Patients must have suitable home conditions with adequate toilet facilities.
- Anxious or phobic patients may benefit from a night in hospital if pre-medication is considered desirable.
- Over-anxious parents may prefer professional support in hospital to assist in the care of their child in the immediate postoperative period.
- Physiological fitness should be considered, rather than a strictly chronological age limit. It is necessary to screen all patients for physiological suitability regardless of age.
- No operative procedure should be performed if it carries a risk of excessive postoperative pain, haemorrhage or prolonged immobility. Community assistance may be sought for follow-up arrangements and wound dressing. It is the responsibility of the day surgery nurse to liaise with community services to arrange follow-up care.
- Patients with cardiovascular or respiratory disease, diabetes or gross obesity are not suitable to be treated as day cases. Borderline cases may be referred to the relevant anaesthetist.
- The patient should have access to a telephone for advice and in an emergency.
- Distances to be travelled postoperatively should not exceed one hour.

Pre-admission assessment and preparation

RECOMMENDATION **7.1.2** Preoperative assessment ensures that the patient is fit for surgery and anaesthetic. It should also ensure that the patient fully understands the proposed operation.

RECOMMENDATION **7.1.3** Preoperative assessment in day surgery should:

- confirm that the patient wishes to have the operation recommended by the surgeon
- assess the patient's suitability for day surgery
- assess the patient's fitness for surgery and anaesthesia, including the risks of the combined effects of surgery and anaesthesia
- ensure that the patient fully understands the proposed procedure by providing further oral and written explanation of the information provided by the surgeon
- provide the opportunity for explanation and discussion and minimise any fears or anxiety the patient may experience
- provide information about the preoperative process and any specific preoperative instructions (eg: who to contact if they want to cancel the operation, fasting instructions)
- identify any special requirements for the surgical procedure
- provide an opportunity to discuss with patients any self-help matters which may improve the outcome of their surgery (eg: stopping smoking or losing weight)
- identify any cultural requirements and any communication or other special needs
- assess the home support available to the patient post-discharge and identify any special requirements to facilitate prompt discharge. (DH 2003)

RECOMMENDATION **7.1.4** All patients receiving appointments for day surgical treatment must be reassessed before admission by suitably experienced nursing staff to ensure that borderline cases are referred to the relevant anaesthetist.

RECOMMENDATION **7.1.5** Detailed verbal information about operative procedure, mode of anaesthetic, and possible postoperative restrictions and symptoms, must be explained before the admission date. The day surgery practitioner should be assured that informed consent for the operation has been obtained by clinicians.

RECOMMENDATION **7.1.6** All patients should receive written preoperative instructions with regard to social arrangements, preparation for surgery (ie: fasting) and the nature of their anaesthetic and surgical treatment. Written information about attendance time, anticipated waiting time and the expected sequence of events, including a description of the procedure, discharge time and car parking arrangements should be provided at initial assessment interview.

RECOMMENDATION **7.1.7** Assessment and future plan of care should be initiated. Documentation of health status prior to the day of surgery, preferably following outpatient visit, will ensure that preoperative investigations (ie: Hb, x-ray) can be completed before the admission date.

Admission

RECOMMENDATION **7.1.8** Initial establishment of patient/nurse rapport is essential immediately on admission. Any undue anxiety or adverse psychological state detrimental to favourable outcome will need to be resolved prior to administration of the chosen anaesthetic and before surgical intervention. Pre-medication is not normally indicated for day surgical procedures, thus nursing care will involve the strategic use of highly refined communication skills, sensory information, verbal and non-verbal support to reduce anxiety.

RECOMMENDATION **7.1.9** Any alteration in current health status, social arrangements or discharge plan must be documented and communicated to the relevant clinicians prior to treatment. All day surgery patients undergo the same careful preparations for surgery as do their inpatient counterparts.

RECOMMENDATION **7.1.10** Allergic reactions, baseline monitoring, physiological abnormalities, patient identity, suitable skin preparation and electrosurgery precautions need to be carefully documented and communicated to the perioperative environment personnel.

Perioperative care

RECOMMENDATION **7.1.11** The day surgery practitioner must possess a sound knowledge of all forms of anaesthesia, their adverse reactions, potential physiological effects and the potential minor sequelae which patients may experience regardless of the type of anaesthetic used. All patients are monitored for reaction to anaesthetic drugs throughout and immediately after completion of procedure. Basic observations should include blood pressure, heart rate and rhythm, respiratory rate, oxygen saturation, skin condition and psychological state.

RECOMMENDATION **7.1.12** The rigorous adherence to standard and safe nursing practice that is recommended for all operating theatres is also applicable in the day surgery operating theatre. Infection control, manipulation of the environment, surgical preparation of the patient, safe positioning, skin preparation, aseptic technique, swab, instrument and needle counts must be of uniform standard and carried out in accordance with local policy.

RECOMMENDATION **7.1.13** Privacy, dignity and confidentiality of all day surgery patients must be preserved at all times. No information must be disclosed to relatives, escorts or friends without prior permission from the patient. Examination of patients under the effect of general anaesthesia by medical students must be regulated and prior written consent obtained from the patient.

RECOMMENDATION **7.1.14** Day care surgery may potentially be conducted under general, regional or local anaesthetic. Practitioners caring for these patients in the recovery phase should be competent in the following skills:

- Total support of the unconscious patient
- Management of the airway and extubation
- Monitoring levels of consciousness and minimising disorientation
- Assessing and treating postoperative pain
- Treating nausea and vomiting
- Managing a respiratory or cardiac emergency
- Performing cardiopulmonary resuscitation.

RECOMMENDATION **7.1.15** Discharge criteria should be set in consultation with medical practitioners. If the day surgery nurse discharges the patient it will be necessary to ensure that patients are adequately informed, in writing and verbally, about the nature of the operative procedure, anticipated postoperative progress and future follow-up arrangements. The nurse should also ensure that:

- vital signs have returned to baseline parameters
- fluids can be tolerated and patient has voided
- pain is controlled and analgesics supplied
- haemorrhage or wound haematoma is absent
- mobility aids are provided as necessary
- follow-up and community care arrangements are made
- a responsible and informed escort is available
- social support and close supervision is available for 24 hours following general anaesthesia.

Guidelines should be incorporated into local policy for patients who may be requiring to be admitted for inpatient care.

Pain management

RECOMMENDATION **7.1.16** Uncontrolled pain followed by nausea and vomiting are the main causes of readmission to an inpatient bed following day surgery and are a leading cause of patient dissatisfaction with it (Mitchell 2004). Poor pain management is also one of the most common reasons for unanticipated contact with GP services following discharge from the day surgery unit. Therefore a pain management protocol should be in place. Pain should be assessed and documented before discharge and patients should be informed of the necessity to take analgesia as prescribed for the first 24 hours following discharge.

Evaluation and audit

RECOMMENDATION **7.1.17** The quality of surgical treatment, anaesthetic agent, nursing care, postoperative self-management and pain control can be assessed by the use of questionnaires, postoperative phone calls, by analysis of readmission rates, incidence of infection or complications at follow-up consultation, and by canvassing community personnel. Patient and carer satisfaction can be ascertained in a similar fashion. A patient satisfaction survey is recommended at least every two years.

RECOMMENDATION **7.1.18** The continual review of written and verbal information, and consultation with other health professionals, will be required in order to improve the information offered and to ensure that a day surgical patient has full understanding of the procedure.

RECOMMENDATION **7.1.19** Collection of relevant statistics, budgetary control and costings are important aspects of day surgical audit.

Management

RECOMMENDATION **7.1.20** It is important that the rate of patients that did not attend (DNA) for surgery without giving notice is monitored and audited.

RECOMMENDATION **7.1.21** Patients should be reminded of their appointments just before their operations to minimise the likelihood of a patient forgetting to attend and therefore wasting a theatre slot.

RECOMMENDATION **7.1.22** Patients should be allotted individual appointment times close to the time of their procedures rather than expecting them to all arrive at the same time.

RECOMMENDATION **7.1.23** Patients should receive specific appointment times at the time of the decision to admit.

RECOMMENDATION **7.1.24** Written information should be provided at discharge including advice on how to deal with common postoperative problems such as control of pain, nausea and vomiting.

RECOMMENDATION **7.1.25** Discharged patients should be informed who to contact for further advice and help.
A telephone number at the hospital for advice and emergencies should be provided before discharge.

RECOMMENDATION **7.1.26** Discharged patients should be telephoned at home to check that they are progressing without any complications.

RECOMMENDATION **7.1.27** The numbers of day case patients that have to be transferred to inpatient facilities rather than go home should be monitored and audited.

7.2 ELECTROSURGICAL EQUIPMENT

STANDARD There is a system in place that facilitates the safe use of all electrosurgical equipment within the perioperative setting. Hazards of these products are identified and minimised to reduce the risks to patients and staff. All members of the perioperative team have sufficient knowledge of the principles and processes of electro-surgery.

INTRODUCTION

Electrosurgery or diathermy is defined as *'the cutting and coagulation of body tissue with a high frequency (ie: radio frequency) current'* (AORN 2004).

Monopolar diathermy

Monopolar diathermy is the passage of a high frequency current through the patient from the live or active electrode (diathermy forceps or pencil) to the return or indifferent electrode (patient plate). Where the flow of the current is resisted in body tissue, there is a localised rise in temperature which will create a high enough temperature to produce the relevant effect of coagulation or cut.

Bipolar diathermy

In bipolar diathermy, the active and return electrodes are combined within the diathermy forceps, one point is the active electrode and the other is the return electrode. The current passes between the two points which, with the exception of the tips, are separated with insulating material. Bipolar diathermy is perceived to be safer as the current pathway is much shorter than in monopolar diathermy. Bipolar diathermy is generally used when:

- coagulation only is required.
- coagulation is required in peripheral areas of the body such as hands or feet or other areas where 'channelling' may occur.
- pinpoint or microcoagulation is required.
- patient has a pacemaker in situ.

Ultrasound

In addition to electrosurgery and diathermy, ultrasound equipment can also cut or coagulate tissue using high frequency sound waves. For example, the UltraCision instrument or Harmonic Scalpel from Ethicon Endo Surgery, Ligasure from Tyco Healthcare, or the Radiofrequency Vapouriser from Mitek facilitate the transformation of electrical energy into mechanical energy. These instruments, developed for use in both open and laparoscopic procedures, have a range of attachments which are designed for use with a hand-piece. This in turn is activated by a foot switch controlled by the user to generate power from the main unit. The transformation of power generally occurs within the handset. Although ultrasound instruments are not normally associated with electrosurgery products, many of the principles relating to electrosurgery are also applicable to ultrasound instruments.

ELECTROSURGERY EXPLAINED

Electrosurgery requires an electrosurgical generator which produces the radio frequency current, a cable, active electrode, and return plate or indifferent electrode for monopolar diathermy. Bipolar diathermy uses the same items except that the return or indifferent electrode is not required. The electrosurgical generator or unit can produce three distinct surgical effects, known as fulguration, desiccation and cutting. The electrosurgical generator creates different wave forms which are determined by the setting on the machine, universally known as COAG, CUT and BLEND. The settings and desired effects are linked as follows:

Desiccation and COAG

The COAG waveform consists of bursts of radio frequency which, when used on low power, create the effect known as desiccation. Desiccation is defined as a relatively slow drying out of tissues by current. Desiccation does not produce sparks which in turn lead to coagulation.

Fulguration and COAG

When the COAG waveform is used at a high power setting it will create the effect known as fulguration. The high power generates sparks which create intermittent heating of tissue causing cells to dry out quickly rather than explode into steam.

Cutting

The CUT waveform is a continuous waveform at a lower voltage but higher current than COAG. It creates a high density of current in a specific tissue area in a short period of time. This results in cell explosion due to the localised but intense heat.

Blend

Blend is a combination of CUT and COAG and is used where haemostasis is required as tissue is cut.

HAZARDS OF ELECTROSURGERY

There are a number of hazards that can be identified in relation to the use of electrosurgery in the perioperative environment, and it is important to be aware of these in order to minimise the risk of adverse incidents.

Accidental burns

The source of an accidental burn is often linked to the return electrode. Some burns are found directly below the return electrode and are associated with a failure of the electrode. This problem has largely been eliminated due to the development of contact quality monitors (CQMs) and return electrode monitor plates (REM plates). These systems are designed to monitor the patient to pad interface. Many return electrodes are now single use and consist of a dual pad which is adhesive. In the event of a patient's electrode pad being ineffective, the monitoring unit will sound an alarm and cut the current, thus reducing the chances of a burn. The cause of the ineffectiveness may be due to the pad being positioned badly or not being fully in contact with the patient. There is also the possibility of the pad being defective.

There are also concerns about the site of the return electrode in relation to surgical implants or prostheses. In some situations, there is a need to place a return electrode close to the site of a metallic implant. This is safe to do, as an established metallic implant such as a bone screw or larger implant will safely conduct the current. The current will be diffused over a relatively large surface area of metal that is in contact with the patient's tissue, resulting in a subsequent loss of heat that cannot cauterise tissue.

Another source of accidental burns occurs when an alternative pathway has been found. Alternative pathways occur when the current is diverted from the return electrode and finds an alternative path from the patient to the 'ground'. In an isolated generator, ground represents the negative phase of the isolation transformer within the electrosurgical generator. In an 'earthed' generator, ground represents the common earth of the mains electricity system. If the point of contact between the patient and the grounded object is small, sufficient current density can be generated to cause a burn. The most likely alternative pathway is created by the patient coming into contact with a metal part of the operating table, a table accessory or an ECG electrode. This problem is reduced but not eliminated by the use of isolated electrosurgical units which have little or no reference to earth, although it is pertinent to be aware that earthed referenced currents can still be produced from isolated units in certain circumstances. Another source of an alternative site burn is one that is due to 'leakage current'. However, it is pertinent to be aware that earthed generators are still available from some companies for use in specialised applications.

Surgical plume

This is the name given to the vapour containing particles that is released when an electrosurgery, laser or ultrasonic device is used on body tissue. There is evidence to suggest that the content of this plume could contain toxic chemicals, carbonised tissue, blood particles, viral DNA particles, bacteria and carbon dioxide, to name but a few. As a result of this it is recommended that specific smoke evacuators with ultra low penetrating air filter(s) are used to remove this plume from the perioperative environment. NATN recommendations are as follows (NATN 2001):

- All thermal instruments used in surgery produce smoke which potentially contains infective agents that may be hazardous to staff.
- Dedicated smoke evacuators must be used and the filters checked and changed as per the manufacturer's recommendations.
- Piped or free standing suction units must not be used for smoke evacuation as they do not have particulate filters.
- High filtration face masks should be worn in all procedures that produce surgical plume to minimise the inhalation of carbonaceous particles.

Minimal access surgery

Minimal access surgery (MAS) has increased dramatically in recent years and has specific hazards in relation to electrosurgery. These are primarily related to the number of instruments and cannulae that are contained within the operative field. The principle hazards associated with these procedures are:

- direct coupling, which occurs when an active instrument touches an inactive one
- capacitive coupling, which occurs when current is conducted from one instrument to another with no direct contact
- insulation failure, where breaks in insulation materials are not noticed prior to use.

All of the above may lead to accidental burns to patients undergoing minimal access surgery.

Endoscopic surgery

Endoscopic surgery uses metal instruments in confined spaces, increasing the risk that an active electrode will come into contact with a metal endoscope, resulting in a burn for either the patient or the surgeon. Endoscopic electrosurgery may be deemed to be of a lower power than other electrosurgery and thus less harmful. Clinical evidence may suggest otherwise, particularly in view of Medicines and Healthcare Products Regulatory Agency alerts to these types of products (MDA 2002, MHRA 2003).

Other types of hazard

Interactions of electrosurgery equipment can occur with skin preparations and other alcohol-based or aerosol products. The pooling of alcoholic prep solutions must be avoided and these solutions should be allowed to dry or be dried with a surgical swab prior to the start of any surgical procedure (MDA 2000).

Interference can also occur with other medical devices such as pacemakers, ECG machines and video equipment used in minimal access surgery. Wherever possible, patients with pacemakers in situ should only be subject to bipolar diathermy and every effort should be made to ensure that the current flows away from the pacemaker. Under no circumstances should the path of the current pass through the pacemaker. The use of electrosurgical equipment should be stopped immediately if an arrhythmia occurs.

RECOMMENDATIONS FOR LOCAL POLICY

Safeguards for staff

RECOMMENDATION **7.2.1** It should be ensured that:

- all members of the perioperative team have been trained in the principles of electrosurgery and ultrasound
- all staff are aware of the potential hazards of electrosurgery products and that procedures and techniques are in place to minimise these hazards
- all members of the team have received instruction on the use of the electrosurgical equipment within the perioperative setting
- regular audits of practice are undertaken, which highlight areas of best practice and identify areas where improvement in relation to technique and/or education is required
- there are adequate supplies of high filter face masks for staff
- adequate smoke evacuation is undertaken to minimise the risks of plume to all in the perioperative setting.

Preparation and use of electrosurgical equipment

RECOMMENDATION **7.2.2** Equipment must be prepared and used in accordance with the manufacturer's instructions, including the instructions relating to checking the alarm systems prior to use.

RECOMMENDATION **7.2.3** All cables and electrodes must be checked prior to use to ensure there are no insulation or other defects.

RECOMMENDATION **7.2.4** Cables must not become looped (for example around a towel clip holding the insulated container) as this may cause an inductive impedance in the circuit and thus reduce the effectiveness of the electrosurgical electrode.

RECOMMENDATION **7.2.5** There must be a robust maintenance programme to prevent defects as far as possible, in accordance with manufacturer's instructions. All types of maintenance undertaken on electrosurgical products must be recorded.

Safe practice

RECOMMENDATION **7.2.6** All connections must be secure prior to the commencement of surgery.

RECOMMENDATION **7.2.7** The active electrode should be housed in an insulated container and kept well away from the operative field except when in use.

RECOMMENDATION **7.2.8** Pre-gelled, self adhesive patient plates are recommended, but in the event that electrode gel is required, it should be used in accordance with the manufacturer's instructions.

RECOMMENDATION **7.2.9** Single use return electrodes should **not** be reused.

RECOMMENDATION **7.2.10** The electrosurgical generator or unit should be switched off or set to standby before touching the live electrode terminal.

RECOMMENDATION **7.2.11** It is the responsibility of the user to ensure that the equipment is suitable to the task.

RECOMMENDATION **7.2.12** The activation of the active electrode is the responsibility of the surgeon and/or a trained non-medical surgical assistant.

Safeguards for patients

RECOMMENDATION **7.2.13** The return electrode should be sited as close as possible to the operative site.

RECOMMENDATION **7.2.14** It is essential that the return electrode site is free from hair, skin blemishes, lesions or scars, prior to the application of the electrode.

RECOMMENDATION **7.2.15** The return electrode should be sited over a vascular, muscular area.

RECOMMENDATION **7.2.16** The return electrode must remain in direct and complete contact with the patient's skin. This is to ensure that the CQM or REM system is fully operational. If the CQM or REM alarm sounds or the patient is moved during surgery, it is necessary to recheck the return electrode site.

RECOMMENDATION **7.2.17** The return electrode should remain dry during surgery, and precautions should be taken to prevent pooling of inflammable liquids in any cavity under the patient's body or under the return electrode itself.

RECOMMENDATION **7.2.18** The patient should not come into contact with 'grounded' metal objects.

RECOMMENDATION **7.2.19** Skin condition should be checked immediately before and after surgery as well as prior to leaving the perioperative setting.

RECOMMENDATION **7.2.20** The site of the return electrode should be documented in the patient's perioperative record and any other comments should also be documented.

RECOMMENDATION **7.2.21** All necessary precautions should be taken for patients with medical devices such as pacemakers.

7.3 SPECIMEN MANAGEMENT

STANDARD There is a system in place which reduces the risk of error when tissue and other product samples are obtained in the perioperative setting. This system will address the necessary precautions for patients and staff when sample collection occurs.

Specimens are regularly taken during interventional procedures. It is essential that every specimen reaches the pathology, microbiology, histology or cytology department without undue delay and in optimum condition.

The laboratory examination of specimens is important for determining subsequent treatment of the patient. The care and handling of specimens is therefore a crucial step in the investigations. Perioperative staff should be aware of the procedures involved in the care of specimens, including correct documentation, safe handling and appropriate despatch. Further information is available from the local hospital pathology services handbook.

RECOMMENDATIONS FOR LOCAL POLICY

RECOMMENDATION **7.3.1** It is strongly advised that the policy is developed in conjunction with the laboratory services that specimens will be sent to, to ensure that all requirements are met.

Collection of sample

RECOMMENDATION **7.3.2** The scrub practitioner must determine the nature and site of the specimen that is being taken. This information will then guide staff as to the actions that are required for the specific type of specimen being collected.

RECOMMENDATION **7.3.3** It is imperative that the scrub practitioner checks whether the sample should be placed in a container containing preservative or other transport medium, or whether it should be a dry specimen. This decision will be guided by the type of specimen. For example, a majority of histopathology specimens will be placed in formalin or other specific fixative.

RECOMMENDATION **7.3.4** The scrub practitioner should relay all this information to the circulating practitioner who will assist in the specimen collection process.

RECOMMENDATION **7.3.5** It is recommended that care is taken in selecting an appropriate specimen container, in relation to its size and purpose. For histopathology specimens, the container should be large enough to ensure that the specimen floats freely, is completely covered by appropriate fixative and is sealed for transportation.

RECOMMENDATION **7.3.6** The circulating person must follow standard blood and body substance isolation precautions when placing the specimen in the container. Precautions also need to be taken to prevent any contamination of the outside of the specimen container.

RECOMMENDATION **7.3.7** All staff should adhere to COSHH regulations (HMSO 2002) and local policies for treatment in respect of splash injuries from specimen fixative or body fluids.

RECOMMENDATION **7.3.8** All specimens for microbiology should be placed in a specified biohazard bag which is sealed before dispatch. Similarly any other specific requirements for the transport of specimens should be actioned in accordance with local requirements.

RECOMMENDATION **7.3.9** Standard blood and body substance isolation precautions should always be used when handling specimens, as all specimens are considered a potential source of infection.

RECOMMENDATION **7.3.10** If specimens cannot be taken to the laboratory within the specified time limits (eg: specimens taken at night when there is no collection service) they should be stored in accordance with local instructions from the labs concerned. Some specimens without fixatives may need to be stored in a dedicated specimen fridge at a temperature of 4°C, thus minimising the potential for bacterial growth. However, storage at 4°C is inappropriate for specimens in formalin as this will delay fixation of the specimen. Similarly, in the event of blood cultures being collected arrangements should be made for immediate transfer to microbiology in accordance with local policy.

Documentation requirements

RECOMMENDATION **7.3.11** After checking with the patient's notes, the following details should be recorded on the specimen pot label:

- Patient's full name, identification number and date of birth
- Ward, hospital, theatre
- Nature of the specimen
- Date/time specimen was taken
- Nature of fixative
- Consultant's name.

These details should be recorded on an adhesive label that is attached to the body of the specimen container.

RECOMMENDATION **7.3.12** The same details should also be recorded on the request form, along with the following:

- Medical practitioner's name, clearly and legibly written
- Medical practitioner's signature
- Contact details (eg: bleep number of the medical practitioner for use in the event that the laboratory may need a contact for further clarification or results)
- Details of who the report should be submitted to.

RECOMMENDATION **7.3.13** Prior to the specimen being placed into the container it is essential that a member of the perioperative team labels the specimen container. This must be done after the details have been provided but before the specimen is placed in the container. The label must **not** be placed on the lid of the container, as this could cause confusion over the specimens.

RECOMMENDATION **7.3.14** The labelled container must be shown to the scrub practitioner in conjunction with the details as they are recorded in the patient's notes. This may be achieved by showing the scrub practitioner the notes, consent form or operating list. The documentation used must previously have been checked for accuracy of the details.

RECOMMENDATION **7.3.15** The information on the investigation request form must correspond with the details on the specimen container and the patient's notes. It must also contain relevant clinical information to assist the laboratory staff.

RECOMMENDATION **7.3.16** It is the responsibility of the medical practitioner to sign the request form and state what particular investigations are required. This should generally be the surgeon, but on occasions may be another medical practitioner such as the anaesthetist. Whoever provides the details should supply all the information, including clear identification of who they are and their contact details.

RECOMMENDATION **7.3.17** It is extremely important that all information is checked and accurate before the specimen leaves the operating theatre. The specimen must be accompanied by the documentation.

RECOMMENDATION **7.3.18** The urgency of the specimen should be determined and in the event of it being urgent, a clear protocol should be developed to ensure that the specimen is delivered to the labs and dealt with, with minimum delay.

RECOMMENDATION **7.3.19** In the event of urgent specimens laboratory staff should be notified. Those responsible for transport of the specimen to the laboratory should be aware of their responsibilities, particularly the delivery point in each lab.

RECOMMENDATION **7.3.20** It is recommended that a signed record is kept of all specimens dispatched from the perioperative setting. Names must be printed as well as signed.

Specimens requiring special consideration

FROZEN SECTIONS

RECOMMENDATION **7.3.21** It is the responsibility of the medical staff to notify the histology department of specimens requiring frozen section and to complete the investigation request form prior to starting the operation.

RECOMMENDATION **7.3.22** Specimens for frozen section are placed in dry containers, labelled as stated and must be despatched immediately to the appropriate department.

FOREIGN BODIES

RECOMMENDATION **7.3.23** Foreign bodies must be clearly labelled and retained for inspection.

RECOMMENDATION **7.3.24** Forensic specimens must be saved in accordance with local policies, ensuring that there is total traceability of the specimen at all times until it reaches its destination.

RECOMMENDATION **7.3.25** Some forensic samples will not necessarily be body tissue (eg: a bullet removed during surgery from gunshot wounds).

RECOMMENDATION **7.3.26** Policy must be clear on the type of forensic samples that may be required. The method of collection, storage and destination should be determined. It is advisable that advice is sought from the forensic services for this section of the policy.

ORTHOPAEDIC IMPLANTS

RECOMMENDATION **7.3.27** When orthopaedic implants are to be removed, care should be taken to ascertain:

- whether the implant is to be sent for bacterial, pathological, metallurgical or mechanical examination
- the legal ownership of the implant before any destructive testing is carried out.

RETAINED PRODUCTS OF CONCEPTION

RECOMMENDATION **7.3.28** It is imperative that personal wishes are respected in relation to a foetus or foetal tissue.

RECOMMENDATION **7.3.29** Laboratory staff need to be informed of any personal wishes expressed if a foetus or foetal tissue needs to be sent for pathological examination.

RECOMMENDATION **7.3.30** Foetal tissue must be treated in accordance with Health Service Guidelines HSG 1991/19 (NHS Management Executive 1991).

7.4 SWAB, INSTRUMENT AND NEEDLE COUNT

STANDARD All swabs, needles and instruments used in clinical invasive procedures are accounted for at all times to prevent foreign body retention and subsequent injury to the patient.

A count must be undertaken for all procedures in which swabs, instruments and/or sharps could be retained.

Although it is the responsibility of the user to return all items, it is recognised as 'custom and practice' that the scrub practitioner implements the checking procedure in order to be able to state categorically that all items have been returned.

The count must be audible to those counting and must be conducted by two members of staff, one of whom **must** be an appropriately qualified member of the perioperative team (ie: a qualified nurse or a qualified ODP Diploma/NVQ Level 3). As a minimum, one count must be done before the procedure commences and a final count must be undertaken as the procedure finishes.

Countable items

Countable items may include, but are not limited to:

- blades
- bulldogs
- cotton wool balls
- gauze strips
- instruments including screws or detachable parts
- lahey swabs (peanuts, pledgets)
- liga-reels
- local infiltration needles
- needles
- opthalmic micro sponges
- packs
- patties
- red swab/packs ties
- shods
- slings/sloops
- sponges
- tapes
- x-ray-detectable gauze swabs.

RECOMMENDATIONS FOR LOCAL POLICY

Education/training

RECOMMENDATION **7.4.1** Where a hospital runs a perioperative course, the post-basic nursing student or student ODP should have supernumerary status until they have been deemed competent for this skill by an appropriately qualified member of the perioperative team.

RECOMMENDATION **7.4.2** An introduction to the local policy must be included in the new staff orientation programme.

RECOMMENDATION **7.4.3** Healthcare assistants/support workers should not be involved with the count until they have been assessed as competent to do so.

Packaging

RECOMMENDATION **7.4.4** All swabs, including lahey swabs (peanuts, pledgets), neuro patties and packs that are used during invasive procedures must have an x-ray-detectable marker fixed securely across the width of the swab.

RECOMMENDATION **7.4.5** All swabs and packs must be packed in bundles of five and be of a uniform size and weight. Any package containing fewer or more than five should be removed from the procedure area immediately. Checks should be made based on multiples of five and recorded on the count board in multiples of five.

Responsibility for counts

RECOMMENDATION **7.4.6** Each count must be performed by two members of staff, one of whom must be a qualified perioperative practitioner. The staff involved in the counting procedure must be able to recognise and identify the instruments and medical devices in use.

RECOMMENDATION **7.4.7** The same two perioperative personnel should perform all the counts that are done during a surgical procedure.

RECOMMENDATION **7.4.8** Should it be necessary to replace the scrub practitioner during the procedure, a complete count should be performed including a full instrument check, recorded and signed by the incoming and outgoing practitioners.

RECOMMENDATION **7.4.9** Should it be necessary to replace either person temporarily, the relieving practitioner should follow the standard procedure and note and sign any additions on the intraoperative record.

RECOMMENDATION **7.4.10** The name of the replacement or relieving practitioner must be recorded on the intra-operative record.

RECOMMENDATION **7.4.11** Items which are to remain in the patient by intention (eg: packing gauze, drain tubes, catheters) must be recorded in the intraoperative record/theatre register/patient's notes. When a countable item is deliberately left in a patient, this must be recorded on the intraoperative form/theatre register/patient's notes. Its removal must also be recorded.

RECOMMENDATION **7.4.12** All items must remain in the operating theatre until the procedure has been completed and all counts have been performed. This includes laundry and clinical waste containers/bags.

RECOMMENDATION **7.4.13** Swabs that are used as surface dressing must not be x-ray-detectable. The packaging for these swabs should only be opened at skin closure. It is recommended that surface dressings are a different colour from white raytec gauze (eg: blue) so that they are easily distinguishable. This is in accordance with the same risk principle which determines that anaesthetic gauze utilised during pre-anaesthesia must be green.

Checking procedure

RECOMMENDATION **7.4.14** A swab, instrument and needle count should be performed for all clinically invasive procedures and recorded immediately. This record should be retained in the patient's notes.

RECOMMENDATION **7.4.15** Provision should be made in the theatre for a dry wipe count board, which is pre-printed and states all relevant items used. This board should be permanently fixed to the theatre wall and be at a height and in a position that facilitates access and visibility during the procedure.

RECOMMENDATION **7.4.16** The initial full swab, instrument and sharps count must be performed immediately prior to the commencement of surgery. A second count should occur before closure of a cavity within a cavity, before wound closure begins and finally at skin closure or at the end of the procedure.

RECOMMENDATION **7.4.17** When additional items are added to the field, they should be counted and recorded as part of the count documentation.

RECOMMENDATION **7.4.18** In the event of a NCEPOD 1 immediate life-threatening emergency it is recognised that it is not always feasible to perform an initial swab and instrument count. In these circumstances all packaging must be retained to facilitate a count being undertaken at the earliest and most appropriate opportunity. This must be documented in the patient's and department records.

RECOMMENDATION **7.4.19** Items added during the procedure must be counted and recorded. There should be a local traceability system of accounting for instruments that are used during the procedure.

RECOMMENDATION **7.4.20** At all times during a surgical procedure the scrub practitioner must be aware of the location of all swabs, instruments and medical devices. Neatness in approach should be encouraged to ensure that only necessary equipment is in use at any given time.

RECOMMENDATION **7.4.21** If a blade, needle or instrument breaks during use, the scrub practitioner should ensure that all pieces have been returned to them and are accounted for. Any instrument found to be damaged will compromise patient safety and therefore must be immediately taken out of use and labelled for repair. It may be necessary to inform the sterile supplies department, the manufacturers and/or the Medical and Healthcare Products Regulatory Agency (MHRA) if an obvious fault is found with equipment. If appropriate, MHRA or the National Patient Safety Agency will issue a hazard warning or safety bulletin.

RECOMMENDATION **7.4.22** A full swab, instrument and sharp count should be performed at the commencement of the closure of any cavity and the final count at the commencement of skin closure. When checking swabs the scrub practitioner should ensure the item is fully opened to check its integrity. Instruments and items with screws and/or removable parts should also be included in the count at the commencement and end of the procedure. The surgical team must allow time for these counts to be undertaken without pressure.

RECOMMENDATION **7.4.23** On completion of the final count a verbal statement should be made by the scrub practitioner to the effect that all swabs, instruments and sharps are accounted for. Verbal acknowledgement should be received from the operating surgeon in order to prevent any misunderstanding.

RECOMMENDATION **7.4.24** At the end of the surgical procedure the circulating and scrub persons must record that satisfactory checks have been completed in the relevant documentation. This should include the nursing documentation, theatre records, computerised systems and the patient's notes.

CHECKING TECHNIQUES

RECOMMENDATION **7.4.25** Both practitioners must count aloud and in unison. Items should be completely separated during the checking procedure.

RECOMMENDATION **7.4.26** The integrity of the x-ray detectable markers in swabs, packs, peanuts etc, as well as the integrity of tapes on abdominal swabs/packs, must be checked during the count.

RECOMMENDATION **7.4.27** At the initial count, and when added during the procedure, swabs and packs should be counted into groups of five. These should not be added to those already counted until the number in the packet has been verified. The additions should be in multiples of five.

In the event of an incorrect number of swabs or packs (ie: not five) the entire packet must be removed from the procedure area. The batch and lot numbers must be identified, the pack removed from stock and the appropriate bodies/agencies notified.

RECOMMENDATION **7.4.28** Hypodermic and suture needles should be recorded as a total amount at the commencement of the procedure and additional items should be added individually on the dry wipe board according to the number marked on the outer package. Suture packs may be retained and used for a check-back procedure if required.

RECOMMENDATION **7.4.29** Opening all packages during the initial needle count is not recommended. Used needles on the sterile field should be retained in a disposable, puncture-resistant needle container.

RECOMMENDATION **7.4.30** Swabs should be in full view of the operating surgeon and anaesthetist where applicable throughout a clinically invasive procedure.

RECOMMENDATION **7.4.31** Swabs and packs should be counted off the sterile field. The technique used should be safe and should incorporate infection control measures in conjunction with standard precautions.

RECOMMENDATION **7.4.32** All items should be fully opened by the circulating practitioner and placed into an appropriate contained disposal system.

RECOMMENDATION **7.4.33** As part of an effective risk management strategy it is recommended that a suitable contained disposal system is in place.

If appropriate, the system used should be sealed and the number of contents recorded on the outside of the disposal system. If there is a discrepancy in the closure counts, all bags or containers should be opened and their contents recounted.

RECOMMENDATION **7.4.34** Swab racks must not be used as a system for displaying utilised swabs due to risks of sharp injury and hygiene.

RECOMMENDATION **7.4.35** If a counted item is inadvertently dropped off the sterile field, the circulating staff member should retrieve it, show it to the scrub practitioner and place it in the appropriate contained disposal system to be included in the final count.

RECOMMENDATION **7.4.36** Items should not be cut or altered unless specifically intended for the purpose. If alteration of any item is requested by the person performing the procedure this must be documented in the patient's records, highlighted on the dry wipe board and included in the count.

RECOMMENDATION **7.4.37** Instruments should be counted audibly and viewed by the scrub practitioner and another individual. Pre-printed count sheets that are identical to standardised sets should be used for documenting instrument counts.

RECOMMENDATION **7.4.38** If any interruption occurs during the counting procedure, the count should be recommenced.

COUNT DISCREPANCY

RECOMMENDATION **7.4.39** If any discrepancy in the count is identified, the operating surgeon must be informed immediately and a thorough search implemented at once.

RECOMMENDATION **7.4.40** If a thorough search does not locate the item, an x-ray should be taken before the patient leaves the operating theatre or, if this is not feasible, before the patient leaves the operating department.

RECOMMENDATION **7.4.41** Missing microitems (eg: needles which cannot be detected on x-ray) should be recorded on the intraoperative record and theatre register. X-rays should be performed at the discretion of the surgeon.

RECOMMENDATION **7.4.42** All missing items must be documented. Formal incident procedures must be followed in accordance with local policy. The discrepancy and subsequent action must be reported to the appropriate personnel and a record must be made.

DOCUMENTATION

RECOMMENDATION **7.4.43** It is the responsibility of the scrub practitioner to ensure that documentation for completion of the count is recorded accurately.

RECOMMENDATION **7.4.44** A copy of the count sheet should be retained in the patient's notes indicating the names of the scrub and circulating staff responsible for the final count.

7.5 TOURNIQUETS FOR LIMB SURGERY

STANDARD There is a system in place that facilitates the safe use of tourniquets used in specified procedures for limb surgery. The system incorporates the requirements of routine checks and maintenance.

Modern pneumatic tourniquets consist of three basic components: a cuff wrapped around a patient's limb, a compressed gas source, and a mechanism with a pressure gauge to maintain the desired cuff pressure (Kam 2002). Applying a pressurised pneumatic cuff to a limb can be used to prevent the spread of local anaesthetic during intravenous regional anaesthesia, or it can be used to reduce bleeding and therefore improve the surgical field for the operating surgeon when operating on an exsanguinated limb.

It is essential that staff receive specific instruction prior to using a tourniquet, and are made aware of the potential dangers to the patient.

It is also necessary to consider that policies and procedures devised in relation to this apparatus are in conjunction with the *Risk and Quality Management System* (NATN 2002a).

RECOMMENDATIONS FOR LOCAL POLICY

Tourniquet usage

INDICATIONS FOR USE OF A TOURNIQUET

RECOMMENDATION **7.5.1** The following constitute indications for the use of a tourniquet:

- Peripheral joint surgery (eg: athroplasty of the knee/elbow, athroscopy of the knee)
- Hand surgery (eg: tendon or nerve repair, carpal tunnel decompression)
- Foot surgery (eg: correction of hallus valgus)
- Osteotomies
- Internal fixation of fractures of the lower arm/leg
- Previous deep vein thrombosis (DVT) or pulmonary embolism (PE)
- To prevent systemic toxicity of drugs such as during intravenous regional anaesthesia.

CONTRAINDICATIONS FOR USE

RECOMMENDATION **7.5.2** The following constitute contraindications for the use of a tourniquet:

- Blood disease (eg: sickle cell)
- Localised infection of the limb
- Regional infections (eg: cellulites)
- Peripheral vascular disease
- Severe bone trauma.

Types of tourniquet

There are two types of tourniquet commonly used:

- **Leak compensating** Such tourniquets will compensate automatically for any loss of pressure.
- **Non-leak compensating** Such tourniquets require continuous observation and may require recalibration intraoperatively by an appropriately trained member of staff.

RECOMMENDATION **7.5.3** The manufacturer's instructions should always be followed on all types of tourniquet.

LEAK COMPENSATING TOURNIQUETS

RECOMMENDATION **7.5.4** The pressures usually recommended for leak compensating tourniquets for safe practice are:

- **Thigh** Double the patient's systolic blood pressure on admission
- **Arm** 50mm Hg above the patient's systolic blood pressure on admission.

The pressure may be maintained for up to two hours.

RECOMMENDATION **7.5.5** The cuffs are inflated from a compressed air supply, cylinder or pump. The equipment usually consists of a control box, which includes a pressure gauge with an air hose attachment and various sizes of cuffs for upper and lower limbs.

RECOMMENDATION **7.5.6** Tourniquets may be applied to two limbs simultaneously. Prior to use, a tourniquet should be tested and calibrated for accuracy. A pressure of 200mm Hg is used for this test.

RECOMMENDATION **7.5.7** It is recommended that the interoperative maintenance pressures of tourniquets should be recorded in the patient's perioperative record/notes.

NON-LEAK COMPENSATING TOURNIQUETS

RECOMMENDATION **7.5.8** This tourniquet is similar in principle to the former, but is not leak proof, therefore the pressure gauge must be continually observed. The pressure may be maintained for up to two hours.

RECOMMENDATION **7.5.9** The cuffs are inflated from a pressurised cylinder of liquid gas or from a hand pump.

RECOMMENDATION **7.5.10** The average pressure for this type of tourniquet is 250mm Hg for the arm and 500mm Hg for the leg. These measurements are standard for all patients irrespective of the individual patient's systolic blood pressure. Inflation pressure is set before inflating the cuff and there will be an initial fall in pressure. Adequate time should be allowed for this to happen. There is no available test apparatus to check the accuracy of this tourniquet.

RECOMMENDATION **7.5.11** It is recommended that interoperative maintenance pressures of tourniquets should be recorded in the patient's perioperative record/notes.

Care and maintenance

RECOMMENDATION **7.5.12** Routine checking of the tourniquet system should be carried out before use and on a planned maintenance programme basis. This should include observations for leaking cuff, worn tubing, loose connections and faulty gauge.

General safeguards

RECOMMENDATION **7.5.13** When applying a tourniquet cuff care should be taken to ensure that the cuff is wider than half the limb diameter and is applied over smooth padding to protect the skin.

The edges of the cuff must overlap to ensure it exerts even pressure all around the limb.

The limb can then be exsanguinated either by elevation for one minute or by the application of a Esmarch bandage or a Rhys-Davies exsanguinator.

RECOMMENDATION **7.5.14** It is the responsibility of the operating surgeon to verify and approve the operating pressure to the tourniquet cuff.

RECOMMENDATION **7.5.15** Because the function of the tourniquet is to provide a bloodless field it is essential that all connections on the system are secure at all times when in use.

RECOMMENDATION **7.5.16** In the unlikely event of the tourniquet cuff being still inflated some time after surgery (eg: when a patient is being recovered in theatre or in a recovery area) the pressure must not be released until the surgeon has been informed. He/she must decide the correct action to take. A record of the incident should be made.

RECOMMENDATION **7.5.17** The duration of the tourniquet times must be recorded in the patient's notes/records.

RECOMMENDATION **7.5.18** To maintain adequate support of the patient's limb and ensure satisfactory exsanguination, it is recommended that two people should always be available when applying the tourniquet.

RECOMMENDATION **7.5.19** Prescribed prophylactic antibiotics should be administered intravenously five minutes before tourniquet inflation to ensure adequate tissue penetration.

RECOMMENDATION **7.5.20** The tourniquet control panel should be visible throughout the procedure.

RECOMMENDATION **7.5.21** Care should be taken not to have the cuff sited over bony prominences, in order to avoid nerve compression and damage whilst inflated.

RECOMMENDATION **7.5.22** In order for the limb to be exsanguinated the following methods may be used:

- Raising the limb to allow the blood to drain
- Active exsanguination via a roll cylinder or an Esmarch's bandage.

RECOMMENDATION **7.5.23** A roll cylinder is considered safer for the patient, providing a regular pressure and a faster process at the commencement of surgery.

RECOMMENDATION **7.5.24** The use of an Esmarch bandage tourniquet to exsanguinate a limb is not recommended. This is because it can generate pressure greater than 1,000mm Hg (133.3kPa) resulting in a higher incidence of nerve injury.

RECOMMENDATION **7.5.25** Maximal exsanguinations can be achieved without mechanical compression by elevation of the arm and leg for five minutes at 90 degrees and 45 degrees respectively.

RECOMMENDATION **7.5.26** When applying an Esmarch's bandage the following guidelines apply:

- Each turn of the bandage must overlap by approximately one inch and the bandage must be held firmly and under continuous tension in order to squeeze as much blood out of the limb as possible.

- When the limb has been completely wrapped up to the cuff, the cuff is inflated to the required pressure by activating the control box.
- When the surgical procedure involves the leg, the limb should be flexed whilst applying the Esmarch's bandage, and then held in flexion until the cuff has been inflated.

RECOMMENDATION **7.5.27** A record of the time that the tourniquet cuff was inflated must be kept. This should be recorded on the wall board in bold figures. The theatre minute clock should be activated. An audible timing device may be used. It is important that the surgeon is informed when the tourniquet reaches one hour and then every 15 minutes until the operation has been completed. Such communications should be recorded in the intraoperative notes.

RECOMMENDATION **7.5.28** The responsibility for the application and release of the tourniquet is that of the operating surgeon.

RECOMMENDATION **7.5.29** Following deflation of the tourniquet the patient's central venous pressure and blood pressure may decrease to below baseline values for 15 minutes and therefore vital signs should be closely monitored. This is caused by a shift of blood back into the limb where hyperaemia causes vasodilatation in the limb.

RECOMMENDATION **7.5.30** In male patients, care must be taken not to catch genitalia under a cuff placed around the upper thigh.

RECOMMENDATION **7.5.31** A waterproof shutoff drape should be placed around the limb, distal to the cuff to prevent skin preparation fluids from seeping under the cuff into the padding. This will minimise the risk of skin burns under the tourniquet.

RECOMMENDATION **7.5.32** The roll cylinder must be cleaned according to manufacturer's instructions between patients to prevent the spread of infections such as scabies, MRSA etc.

7.6 USE AND HANDLING OF INSTRUMENTS

STANDARD There is a system in place that ensures the safe use and handling of surgical instruments. All staff are familiar with the instrumentation used in the department and also with the need to comply with decontamination and storage requirements. Actions to be taken in relation to training requirements of new products and/or loan equipment are addressed.

Most operating departments use trays of instruments which are provided by sterile services units (SSUs), which may also supply supplementary instruments as extras. Information about the decontamination of instruments, including tracking and traceability, is available in the decontamination section of this document (Section 5).

Perioperative staff should not handle instruments unless they are competent to do so and unless they understand their use in general and specific specialities.

New products should not be introduced into the operating department until staff have received training in their use. This training must be undertaken in controlled settings and not when the instruments are in use during a procedure. The need for training must also be addressed when loan instruments that are not familiar to staff are brought into the operating department.

These training needs must be addressed to ensure that both nursing and ODP staff comply with their codes of conduct.

RECOMMENDATIONS FOR LOCAL POLICY

General safeguards

RECOMMENDATION **7.6.1** In order to prevent damage, instruments must only be used for the purpose for which they are designed (eg: osteotomes are not levers). Proper selection requires a general understanding of surgical procedures and a knowledge of anatomy.

RECOMMENDATION **7.6.2** To prevent damage, delicate instruments should be handled with care and separated from other instruments.

RECOMMENDATION **7.6.3** Specialised instruments should be regularly checked by an appropriately trained person. Specialist equipment should be made available to check the integrity of diathermy cables and instruments.

RECOMMENDATION **7.6.4** In order to maintain asepsis, instruments found to be contaminated with dried blood or body tissue prior to surgery must be discarded. If found on a tray of instruments, the whole tray must be discarded and the incident reported to the appropriate person.

RECOMMENDATION **7.6.5** Each tray of instruments should contain an instrument checklist, which incorporates the information necessary for a recorded programme of use.

RECOMMENDATION **7.6.6** Instruments must be accounted for at all times during a surgical procedure.

RECOMMENDATION **7.6.7** The scrub person should ensure that instruments are handled in such a manner as to avoid personal injury, injury to the patient or to other members of the surgical team.

RECOMMENDATION **7.6.8** Special care should be taken with sharp instruments (eg: scalpels and loaded needle holders). It is strongly recommended that all sharp instruments are transferred between staff in a receiver.

RECOMMENDATION **7.6.9** Instruments must not be allowed to rest directly on the patient, which could cause injury to the patient or damage to the drapes. Consideration should be given to the use of appropriate additional sterile surfaces (eg: Mayo tables, magnetic pads).

RECOMMENDATION **7.6.10** Instruments which have been taken directly from an autoclave into the operating theatre or lay-up room must be allowed to cool naturally before use.

Storage of instruments

RECOMMENDATION **7.6.11** The storage area should be clean, dry and free of dust.

RECOMMENDATION **7.6.12** All storage surfaces should be smooth, non-porous and capable of being easily cleaned.

RECOMMENDATION **7.6.13** Sterile items should be protected from direct sunlight.

RECOMMENDATION **7.6.14** The temperature of the storage area should range between 22°C and 24°C with a relative humidity of 35–68%.

RECOMMENDATION **7.6.15** Perioperative personnel should have the knowledge and skills related to the handling of sterile items.

RECOMMENDATION **7.6.16** Sterilised items should be transferred to and from storage areas on clean, specifically designated trolleys.

RECOMMENDATION **7.6.17** All sterile items should have an event-related shelf life. The length of time an item can be considered sterile is referred to as the shelf life. The event-related outdating theory is based on the assumption that if items are properly cleaned, wrapped, sterilised, stored and handled they can remain sterile indefinitely unless the integrity of the packaging is compromised. Therefore, the shelf life of an item is dependent on storage, handling and type of packaging material.

Education and training

RECOMMENDATION **7.6.18** Full product training should be achieved before new instrumentation is introduced to the operating department.

RECOMMENDATION **7.6.19** All new staff to the department should receive training on the use, handling and storage of instruments as part of their induction training.

RECOMMENDATION **7.6.20** Loan instrumentation that is not familiar to staff should not be used until staff have had full product training.

REFERENCES

AORN 2004 Recommended Practices for Electrosurgery. In *Standards, Recommended Practices, and Guidelines* Denver, AORN Inc

Audit Commission 2001 *Day Surgery, Acute Hospital Portfolio, Review of National Findings No 4* Norwich, The Stationery Office. www.audit-commission.gov.uk

Department of Health 2002 *Day Surgery: operational guide* London, DH. www.dh.gov.uk/daysurgery

HMSO 2002 *Control of Substances Hazardous to Health Regulations* Norwich, The Stationery Office

Kam P 2002 Tourniquet: uses and precautions *Anaesthesia and Intensive Care Medicine* 3 (7) 219–221

Medical Devices Agency 2000 *Use of Spirit-Based Solutions During Surgical Procedures Requiring the Use of Electrosurgical Equipment* SN 2000(17) London, MDA

Medical Devices Agency 2002 *The Electrosurgery Team* London, MDA

Medicines and Healthcare Products Regulation Agency 2003 *Medical Device Alert MDA 2003/037* London, MHRA

Mitchell M 2002 Guidance for the Psychological Care of Day Case Surgery Patients *Nursing Standard* 16 (40) 41–43

Mitchell M 2004 Pain Management in Day Case Surgery *Nursing Standard* 18 (25) 33–38

National Association of Theatre Nurses 2001 *Laser and Electrosurgical Plume* Harrogate, NATN

National Association of Theatre Nurses 2002 *Risk and Quality Management System* Harrogate, NATN

NHS Management Executive 1991 *Disposal of Foetal Tissue* Health Service Guidelines HSG 1991/19 London, DH

FURTHER READING

American Operating Room Nurses Association 2004 *Standards, Recommended Practices and Guidelines* Denver, AORN Inc

Anthony P, MacSweer R 1997 *Recent Advances in Histopathology* London, Churchill Livingstone

Association of Anaesthetists of Great Britain and Ireland 1994 *Day Case Surgery* London, AAGBI

Audit Commission 1990 *A Short Cut to Better Services: day surgery in England and Wales* London, HMSO

Audit Commission 1998 *Day Surgery Follow Up: progress against indicators from 'a short cut to better services'* London, HMSO

Australian College of Operating Room Nurses 2004 *Electrosurgical Equipment Standards for Perioperative Nursing* Standard S6 Adelaide, ACORN

Australian College of Operating Room Nurses 2004 *Standards, Guidelines and Policy Statements* Adelaide, ACORN

Beaumont S 1997 Preoperative Assessment for Day Case Surgery: a patient-centred service *British Journal of Theatre Nursing* 7 (9) 9–13

Beesley J 2003 Answers Supplied *British Journal of Perioperative Nursing* 13 (11) 450–451

Bell S 1998 Multiple Patient Use Versus Single Patient Use Products *British Journal of Theatre Nursing* 8 (1) 1–24

Bollens S, Arciero RA 1996 The Effect of Tourniquet Use in Anterior Ligament Reconstruction *American Journal of Sports Medicine* 24 (6) 758–764

Brown A, Duxby J 1997 Day Surgery – communication and interviewing skills *British Journal of Theatre Nursing* 7 (3) 10–15

Bynom S 1998 Reflection – a lost swab *British Journal of Theatre Nursing* 8 (5) 15–18

Campbell C, Taylor M 1999 The Multi-disciplinary Team. In *Back to Basics* Harrogate, NATN

Clarke P, Jones J 1998 *Brigden's Operating Department Practice* Edinburgh, Churchill Livingstone

Cuschieri A, Steele RJ, Moosa AR 2000 *Essential Surgical Practice* London, Arnold

DesCoteaux JG, Poulis EC, Julien M, Guiduin M 1995 Residual Organic Debris on Processed Surgical Instruments *AORN Journal* 62 (1) 23–30

Dougherty L, Lister S 2000 *The Royal Marsden Hospital Manual of Clinical Nursing Procedures* Oxford, Blackwell Science

Eyers P, Ashley S, Scott DJ 2000 Tourniquets in Arterial Bypass Surgery *European Journal of Endovascular Surgery* 20 113–117

Fulbrook S 1995 Duty of Care *British Journal of Theatre Nursing* 5 (5) 18–19

Fulbrook S 1998 Medico-legal Insights: legal aspects of the reuse of single use items *British Journal of Theatre Nursing* 8 (3) 37–39

Health and Safety Executive 1999 *Five Steps to Risk Assessment* London, HSE Books

Health and Safety Executive 2003 *Health and Safety Regulation: a short guide* London, HSE Books

Hind M, Wicker P 2000 *Principles of Perioperative Practice* Edinburgh, Churchill Livingstone

HMSO 1979 *Sales of Goods Act* Norwich, The Stationery Office

HMSO 1987 *Consumer Protection Act Part 1: product liability* Norwich, The Stationery Office

HMSO 1998 *Supply of Goods and Services Act* Norwich, The Stationery Office

Hughes A, Hughes J 2001 Electrosurgical Smoke Plume *British Journal of Perioperative Nursing* 11 (6) 252–255

Klinken C 1955 The effects of tourniquet time in knee arthroscopy patients receiving intra-articular morphine combined with bupivacaine *The Clinical Forum for Nurse Anaesthetists* 6 (1) 37–42

Knowles J 1997 Pre-assessment of the Day Surgery Patient *British Journal of Theatre Nursing* 7 (3) 16–18

Medical Devices Agency 1998 *Reporting Adverse Incidents Relating to Medical Devices* SN 1998/01 London, MDA

Medical Devices Agency 2000 *Use of Spirit-based Solutions During Surgical Procedures Requiring the Use of Electrosurgical Equipment* SN 2000/17 London, MDA

Medical Devices Agency 2002 *The Electrosurgery Team* London, MDA

Medicines and Healthcare Products Regulation Agency 2003 *Medical Device Alert MDA/2003/037* London, MHRA

National Association of Theatre Nurses 1998 *Safeguards for Invasive Procedures: the management of risk* Harrogate, NATN

National Association of Theatre Nurses 2000 *Back to Basics* Harrogate, NATN

National Association of Theatre Nurses 2002 *Risk and Quality Management System* Harrogate, NATN

National Association of Theatre Nurses 2004 *Electrosurgery: Managing the Risk* Harrogate, NATN

National Institute for Clinical Excellence 2003 *Preoperative Tests: the use of routine preoperative tests for elective surgery* Clinical Guideline 3 London, NICE

NHS Modernisation Agency 2002 *National Good Practice Guidance on Preoperative Assessment for Day Surgery* London, DH. www.modern.nhs.uk/theatreprogramme/preop

Nursing Midwifery Council 2002 *Code of Professional Conduct* London, NMC

Olsen CC 1995 Sutures, Needles and Instruments. In Meeker MH, Rothrock JC *Alexander's Care of the Patient in Surgery* 10th ed, St Louis, Mosby

Pierson MA 1995 Patient and Environmental Safety. In Meeker MH, Rothrock JC *Alexander's Care of the Patient in Surgery* 10th ed, St Louis, Mosby

Phippen M, Wells MP 2000 *Patient Care During Operative and Invasive Procedures* USA, WB Saunders

Radford M, County B, Oakley M 2004 *Advancing Perioperative Practice* London, Nelson Thornes

Raltz SL, Kozarek RA, Pethigal PA, Moorhouse MA, Merrian LD 1995 Reusable Biopsy Forceps: a cost-effective measure for the endoscopy suite *Gastroenterology Nursing* 18 (5) 167–170

Ramos-Galvez J, McCrirrick A 2003 Procedures Under Tourniquet Anaesthesia *Intensive Care Medicine* 4 (3) 77–79

Reid JH 1997 Meeting the Informational Needs of Patients in a Day Surgery Setting – an exploratory study *British Journal of Theatre Nursing* 7 (3) 19–24

Royal College of Surgeons of England 1992 *Guidelines for Day Surgery* London, RCS

Shields L, Werder H 2002 *Perioperative Nursing* London, Greenwich Medical Media

Smith B, Williams T 2004 *Operating Department Practice A–Z* London, Greenwich Medical Media

Smith CD 1994 Event-related Sterility – clinical issues *AORN Journal* 59 (6) 1313–1314

Taylor M, Campbell C 1998 Surgical Preparation. In Clarke P, Jones J (eds) *Brigden's Operating Department Practice* Edinburgh, Churchill Livingstone

Tingle J 1997 Legal Problems in the Operating Theatre: learning from mistakes *British Journal of Nursing* 6 (15) 889–891

Wakai A, Winter DC, Street JT, Redmond PH 2001 Pneumatic Tourniquets in Extremity Surgery *Journal of American Academy of Orthopaedic Surgery* 9 345–351

Wicker P 1990 Electrosurgery in Perioperative Practice, parts 1–4 *British Journal of Perioperative Nursing* Vol 27, Issues 8–11

Index